Preanesthetic Assessment 1

Preanesthetic Assessment 1

Edited by
Elizabeth A.M. Frost

B

Birkhäuser
Boston • Basel

Elizabeth A.M. Frost, M.D.
Department of Anesthesiology
Albert Einstein College of Medicine
   of Yeshiva University
Bronx, NY 10461
U.S.A.

ISSN 0896-2103

CIP-Kurztitelaufnahme der Deutschen Bibliothek
Preanesthetic assessment/ed. by Elizabeth Frost.
—Boston; Basel: Birkhäuser
NE: Frost, Elizabeth [Hrsg.]
1 (1988)
   ISBN-13: 978-1-4612-9174-9   e-ISBN-13: 978-1-4612-4818-7
   DOI: 10.1007/ 978-1-4612-4818-7

The chapters in this volume are revised and updated articles that originally appeared in consecutive issues of *Anesthesiology News* from 1985 to 1987. They appear here as a service to the
medical-anesthesiology community with the cooperation and kind permission of McMahon
Publishing Company, New York.

Typeset by Asco Trade Typesetting Ltd., Hong Kong.
Printed and bound by Arcata Graphics/Halliday, West Hanover, Massachusetts.

9 8 7 6 5 4 3 2 1

Dedicated to all the residents, reviewers and to my secretary, Ms. Carolyn Burke, who worked so hard to produce each lesson on time

Foreword

The primary mission of the medical school is to create new doctors. Once the medical student has received his or her doctorate, the medical school's interest in, and acceptance of, responsibility for the continued professional development of the physician ceases almost entirely.

Yet, with scientific advances in medicine increasing exponentially and the inevitable erosion of memory with time, teachings from our schools of medicine become increasingly irrelevant, forgotten, or both. To maintain competence, the physician must continuously re-educate him- or herself. CME—Continuing Medical Education—will probably never attain the status of the medical school's degree-granting undergraduate program, but medical schools and their faculties must recognize their responsibility, not only for *creating* competent physicians but also for *maintaining* that competence.

This volume is the product of a Continuing Medical Education program initiated by the Department of Anesthesiology at the Albert Einstein College of Medicine/Montefiore Medical Center. Our Department of Anesthesiology has historically been, and continues to be, unusually active in post-doctoral education through regional and national conferences and symposia. We recognized, however, that programs that bring physicians together in one location for a limited menu of lectures, questions, and discussion reach only a fraction of the potential audience of anesthesiologists. Such programs, as valuable as they are, by their very structure exclude more anesthesiologists than they include.

By initiating the PREANESTHETIC ASSESSMENT program, in the format of monthly articles published in *Anesthesiology News*, we hoped to make state-of-the-art analyses available to all anesthesiologists. To "give credit where credit is due," a pre- and post-test were included.

Since the inception of this program in 1985, the Albert Einstein College of Medicine Office of Continuing Medical Education has received almost 2,000 completed post-tests and requests for CME credit. From the volume of telephone calls and letters and formal evaluations undertaken by the Office of Continuing Medical Education, it was clear that many other anesthesiologists were reading and profiting from the monthly articles without requesting credit.

Although it is vital to verify and record the continuing educational endeavours of each practitioner, the highest form of education is pursued for its own sake—because of its own intrinsic value to the physician apart from credentialing and licensing requirements. The PREANESTHETIC ASSESSMENT program has proven its value to anesthesiologists. In this book the lessons published in the first two years of the program have been assembled and updated to provide a convenient reference not only for anesthesiologists preparing for Oral Board examinations but for clinicians confronted daily by routine and sometimes not-so-routine cases in the operating room.

VICTOR B. MARROW, M.A.

Assistant Professor, Department of Epidemiology and Social Medicine
Division of Law and Ethics and Director, Continuing Medical Education
Albert Einstein College of Medicine

Contents

Contributors

LYDIA ALCANTARA, M.D.
Attending Anesthesiologist, Maimonides Medical Center, Brooklyn, New York.

DAVID AMAR, M.D.
Instructor in Anesthesiology, Montefiore Medical Center, Bronx, New York.

ZANAIDA AURELLANO-HOH, M.D.
Attending Anesthesiologist, Francis Scott Key Medical Center, Baltimore, Maryland.

NIRMALA BALAN, M.D.
Assistant Professor of Anesthesiology, Albert Einstein College of Medicine of Yeshiva University, Bronx, New York.

JEFFREY BERMAN, M.D.
Assistant Professor of Anesthesiology, Albert Einstein College of Medicine of Yeshiva University, Bronx, New York.

MICHAEL DOMURAT, M.D.
Assistant Professor of Anesthesiology, University of Oklahoma, Norman, Oklahoma.

ELIZABETH A.M. FROST, M.D.
Professor of Anesthesiology, Albert Einstein College of Medicine of Yeshiva University, Bronx, New York.

CLIFFORD GEWIRTZ, M.D.
Assistant Professor of Anesthesiology, Albert Einstein College of Medicine of Yeshiva University, Bronx, New York.

CATHERINE GULATI, M.D.
Resident in Anesthesiology, Albert Einstein College of Medicine of Yeshiva University, Bronx, New York.

JONATHAN HALEVY, M.D.
Resident in Anesthesiology, Montefiore Medical Center, Bronx, New York.

GARY HARTSTEIN, M.D.
Resident in Anesthesiology, Albert Einstein College of Medicine of Yeshiva University, Bronx, New York.

ROBERT HIRSH, M.D.
Resident in Anesthesiology, Memorial Sloan-Kettering Hospital, New York, New York.

INGRID HOLLINGER, M.D.
Associate Professor of Anesthesiology, Albert Einstein College of Medicine of Yeshiva University, Bronx, New York.

ASHOK KUMAR, M.D.
Acting Chief, Anesthesia Department, National University Hospital, Singapore.

RHODA LEVINE, M.D.
Associate Professor of Anesthesiology, Albert Einstein College of Medicine of Yeshiva University, Bronx, New York.

JAMES B. MUELLER, M.D.
Fellow in Neuroanesthesia, Medical College of Virginia, Richmond, Virginia.

IRENE OSBORN, M.D.
Assistant Professor, Beth Israel Hospital, New York, New York.

RICHARD B. PATT, M.D.
Assistant Professor, University of Rochester Medical Center, School of Medicine, Rochester, New York.

WERNER PFISTERER, M.D.
Assistant Professor, Albert Einstein College of Medicine of Yeshiva University, Bronx, New York.

JOHN PRINSCOTT, M.D.
Attending Anesthesiologist, Anesthesia Associates of Flushing, Flushing, New York.

GERALD M. SCHEINMAN, M.D.
Chief Resident in Anesthesiology, Albert Einstein College of Medicine of Yeshiva University, Bronx, New York.

ANNA STANEC, M.D.
Professor of Anesthesiology, New Jersey Medical Center, Patterson, New Jersey.

Introduction

About three years ago, Mr. Ward Byrne, the editor of *Anesthesiology News* asked me if I would be interested in developing an education series for clinical anesthesiologists. He suggested that while each article should be complete in itself, there should be some common theme. Thus was the Preanesthetic Assessment series born. Of course, at first I doubted that I would be able to furnish appropriate material on a monthly basis. Although many of my colleagues promised to write, articles are rarely submitted on time. Moreover, I had no idea as to the interest such a series might generate. On both counts, my fears have been dispelled. We have met every editorial deadline for the past 2½ years (sometimes with more panic than calm) and practitioners across the United States have continued to express their interest by writing letters and by registering with our office of Continuing Medical Education to receive credit for completing the lessons.

It quickly became apparent that the series was benefiting not only those that read the articles. Whenever possible, I invited residents to present and discuss their own cases. For many of them, it was the first article that they had written. For others, it represented more work than they had done since their college days. For most of them, it was far from easy. But I share their pride in their achievements and I am happy at the increased awareness and bonds that have grown up between our residents and their attending physicians and faculty from other departments who became reviewers and discussants for each case.

As the series grew, many anesthesiologists suggested that by collecting the articles together in book form we could offer a convenient, practical reference source for clinicians and those studying for the Board examinations. The first 26 lessons are gathered here. Attempts have been made to update each chapter, although the material is essentially the same as that originally published in *Anesthesiology News*. The questions have been included at the end as a self-assessment test.

I am most grateful to the staff of *Anesthesiology News* for their cooperation and to the staff of Birkhäuser for their assistance in producing what we hope will be the first of many volumes.

ELIZABETH A.M. FROST, M.D.

CHAPTER 1

The Patient with Cerebrovascular Disease*

Michael Domurat

Case History. *A 67-year-old man who sustained three transient ischemic attacks (TIA) in the prior year was scheduled for a right carotid endarterectomy. During his last TIA, which occurred one month prior to admission, he experienced left-sided weakness lasting four hours. There was no residual neurologic deficit.*

Twenty years previously, the patient was found to be hypertensive, and he has taken medication intermittently since then. Sporadic physical examinations over the years revealed poorly controlled blood pressure. Routine blood sugar analysis 12 years ago indicated adult-onset diabetes, which was treated with chlorpropamide 250mg daily. Prior to the development of neurologic symptoms, the patient had smoked 40–50 cigarettes daily for 40 years, which he had decreased recently to 5–10 cigarettes per day. He has a morning cough, shortness of breath on exertion and is subject to frequent respiratory infections.

Since suffering an inferior wall myocardial infarction three years ago for which he was hospitalized for two weeks, he experiences angina pectoris on moderate exertion. The chest pain is readily relieved with sublingual nitroglycerin.

Current medications include: hydrochlorothiazide 50mg o.d.; propranolol 40mg q.i.d.; nitroglycerin 1/150grain sublingual as necessary for chest pain; beclomethasone dipropionate inhaler, two inhalations t.i.d. He has been taking acetylsalicylic acid 300mg daily since his last TIA.

Physical exam reveals a well-nourished, well-developed man in no acute distress. His neurologic exam is within normal limits. His heart is in normal rhythm without murmur, rub or gallop. The chest is clear with distant breath sounds. Positive findings include a right carotid artery bruit and digital clubbing.

Vital Signs: blood pressure 150/96; pulse 62/min; respiratory rate 18/min; weight 75kg; height 69 inches.

---

*Reviewed by Dr. Elizabeth A.M. Frost, Professor of Anesthesiology, Albert Einstein College of Medicine of Yeshiva University, Bronx, New York.

Laboratory Findings: serum chemistries were within normal limits; Hct 48%, PT, PTT and platelet count were all within normal limits.

The chest x-ray demonstrated increased anterior-posterior diameter with flattened hemidiaphragms. The heart was also enlarged. Arterial blood gas analyses on room air revealed pH 7.36, $PaCO_2$ 60mmHg, PaO_2 70mmHg, and HCO_3^- 36mEq/L. Forced expiratory volume in one second was 75% of vital capacity. The 12-lead electrocardiogram showed normal sinus rhythm (rate 62/ min), evidence of left ventricular hypertrophy and Q-waves in leads II, III and a VF. Cerebral angiogram demonstrated 90% stenosis of the right carotid artery at its bifurcation.

Pathophysiology of Cerebrovascular Disease

Thromboembolic syndromes are classified according to the duration and severity of the clinical deficit. Transient ischemic attacks (TIA) are characterized by episodes that last less than 24 hours with complete resolution. The reversible ischemic neurologic deficit (RIND) persists greater than 24 hours and resolves within one week. A progressive stroke is characterized by a worsening deficit with serial observations. The complete stroke is a persistent deficit which at times may be only minimally disabling.

The associated lesions may be ulcerative or stenotic and can be found anywhere in the cerebral circulation. The most common sites, however, are at bifurcations. Gradual occlusion by atherosclerotic plaque does not cause symptoms until the diameter of the lumen is reduced by at least 80%. The disease is bilateral in 50% of cases. Ulcerative lesions produce their pathology secondary to intermittent embolization, usually of platelet aggregates, at more distal points in the cerebral circulation.

Cerebrovascular procedures are designed to reduce the risk of complete stroke in patients at risk, or to enhance recovery of neurologic function in patients who have progressive cerebrovascular insufficiency. This may be accomplished in the extracranial vessels by removal of the ulcerative or stenotic lesion, or by bypassing the intracranial lesion by means of an extracranial to intracranial anastomosis. Such procedures, including anastomoses of the superficial temporal artery to a cortical branch of the middle cerebral artery or occipital arteries to posterior fossa vessels are performed less frequently. A multiinstitutional study indicated questionable benefit.[1] However, the procedure may still be indicated in specific situations such as giant aneurysm clipping when the carotid vessels may have been clamped. Controversy still exists over the efficacy of the procedure.

Preoperative Evaluation

Evaluation of patients undergoing neurovascular surgery should include careful evaluation of cardiovascular status as well as a detailed history of cardiovascular function. Most patients with cerebrovascular disease have systemic arterial hypertension, 25% have a history of previous myocardial infarction and 20% have undergone previous major vascular surgery.[2]

Hypertension

Hypertensive patients pose several problems in the perianesthetic period. Unstable systemic blood pressure fluctuations predispose to myocardial and cerebral ischemia during hypotensive episodes; postoperative hypertension puts atheromatous cerebral vessels at risk of rupture. Inadequately treated hypertension with a period of intraoperative hypotension also increases the risk of postoperative myocardial infarction.[3] Chronic hypertension shifts the cerebral autoregulatory curve to the right. The brain is thus protected against increased cerebral blood flow (CBF) at higher than normal systemic blood pressure, but it is vulnerable to ischemia if CBF decreases during hypotensive episodes.

Foëx and Prys-Roberts[4] advocate control of arterial hypertension prior to induction of anesthesia. Results of their studies have demonstrated a greater risk of intraoperative hypotension and associated cerebral and myocardial ischemia in patients with inadequately controlled or uncontrolled hypertension.

Goldman and colleagues[5] determined that preoperative control of diastolic blood pressures below 110mmHg does not pose any added risk provided close monitoring and prompt therapy eliminate any hypertensive or hypotensive episodes during the perioperative period.

Antihypertensive medication should be continued up until the day of surgery. Abrupt withdrawal of beta blockers can result in myocardial ischemia.[6] Withdrawal hypersensitivity reflects an increase in beta-adrenergic receptor sites and may become apparent within 24 hours of discontinuation of the drug and persist for as long as two weeks. Profound hypertension may also accompany sudden withdrawal of the centrally acting alpha-2 agonist, clonidine.[7,8] A parenteral form of this drug is not yet available in the U.S. In anticipation of elective surgery, it is recommended that clonidine therapy be replaced with a parenteral antihypertensive agent such as hydralazine or propranolol. Naloxone has been shown to reverse the antihypertensive effect of clonidine in the experimental animal; thus, a theoretical concern exists for naloxone use in patients treated with clonidine.[9]

Pulmonary Function

The correlation between heavy smoking and atheromatous disease has been noted by Frost et al.[10] They found that 40% of patients presenting for cerebral revascularization had a greater than 80 pack-year smoking history. A similar association between smoking and subarachnoid hemorrhage was found by Bell and Symon.[11]

Chronic pulmonary pathology and chronic bronchitis are common in these patients. Decreases in arterial oxygen saturation and carbon dioxide retention are demonstrated by arterial blood gas analysis and respiratory function testing. Chest x-ray, spirometry, and arterial blood gas analyses should be included in the preoperative evaluation. Pulmonary physiotherapy and bronchodilators may be necessary in the preoperative period to mobilize excess secretions. Following stroke or TIA, patients managed with bed rest and sedation are especially prone to pulmonary infection. These patients should be followed with serial chest x-rays, arterial blood gas analyses and a white cell count immediately prior to surgery.

Vigorous pulmonary function testing is to be avoided, and testing should be limited to bedside evaluation. Any sign of infection should be treated with appropriate antibiotic therapy. Patients should be encouraged to stop smoking immediately. Cessation of smoking, even the day prior to surgery, allows carbon monoxide levels in the blood to decrease and thereby increases the oxygen carrying capacity of hemoglobin.[12] It is essential to instruct the patient in the use of an incentive spirometer in the preoperative period. Postoperative use of such a device has been shown to decrease the incidence of pulmonary complications.

Medications

Patients with a history of TIA or at risk of developing stroke are frequently treated with low-dose aspirin.[10] Acetylsalicyclic acid (ASA) has been shown to alter platelet function via irreversible inhibition of platelet cyclooxygenase and subsequent reduction of thromboxane A_2 formation. Platelets do not undergo secondary aggregation, and bleeding time is therefore prolonged. Three hundred miligrams of ASA has been shown to prolong bleeding time within two hours of ingestion; the dysfunction persists for the life of the cell. Although many recommend postponing elective surgery until the bleeding time has returned to normal, Amrein and colleagues[13] have shown that perioperative blood loss was not increased in patients undergoing total hip replacement who received 1.2–3.6 grams of ASA daily. In spite of this, we recommend waiting for return of the bleeding time to normal before attempting intracranial surgery. Hematologic evaluation should include hemoglobin, hematocrit, platelet count, PT, PTT and bleeding time in these patients.

Nearly 85% of patients with cerebrovascular disease receive several drugs on a chronic basis. These most commonly include diuretics, antihypertensives, digitalis preparations, antiarrhythmics, anticoagulants, hypoglycemic agents, steroids and antacids.[14] The anesthesiologist must be aware that the risk of complications from drug interactions increases proportionate to the number of medications administered until 10 medications are involved. When more than 10 drugs are administered concomitantly, the complication rate rises sharply; 45% of patients experience side effects when between 10 and 20 medications are being administered concurrently.[15] Side effects can include prolonged neuromuscular blockade, delayed return to consciousness and altered renal and cardiac function.[16]

Electrolytes

As in all patients, serum electrolytes must be evaluated preoperatively. Hypokalemia is a common finding with chronic diuretic therapy. When caused by acute intracellular shifts, it may manifest as impaired myocardial contractility, electrical conduction abnormalities and, ultimately, ventricular fibrillation. The potassium-depleted heart is especially sensitive to the effects of digitalis. In one-third of patients, cardiac dysrhythmias are the first evidence of digitalis toxicity. When administering potassium supplements, at least 24–48 hours are required for equilibration throughout the tissues.

Individuals with central nervous system lesions manifesting as skeletal muscle paralysis are at risk for development of exaggerated rises in serum potassium following succinylcholine administration. This phenomenon may occur as early as four days following denervation.[17] The response peaks at 14 days. The magnitude of the response is not reliably attenuated by pretreatment with a nondepolarizing relaxant.[18] It is therefore best to avoid succinylcholine in these patients. The newer, short-acting relaxants, vecuronium and atracurium, are well suited to facilitate tracheal intubation.

Diabetes

A close association between diabetes and cerebrovascular disease has been noted.[13] Oral hypoglycemics may be continued until the evening before surgery, keeping in mind that their hypoglycemic effects may last as long as 24–36 hours. Several management regimens have been suggested to prepare the insulin-dependent diabetic for surgery. One recommends that one-fourth to one-half the normal daily insulin dose be given the morning of surgery. An intravenous infusion containing 5% dextrose is started at the time of insulin administration and infused at a rate of 2ml/kg/hr in an adult. Alternatively, insulin may be withheld and administered intraoperatively guided by frequent blood glucose analyses.[19]

Coronary Artery Disease

The patient with cerebrovascular atherosclerosis is prone to concomitant involvement of the coronary arteries. This association must be carefully considered as patients undergoing coronary artery bypass grafting (CABG) with symptomatic coronary artery disease (angina pectoris, congestive heart failure or positive stress test) have a ten-fold increased operative mortality compared to their nonsymptomatic counterparts.[20] Operative mortality in patients with coexisting carotid and coronary artery disease (CAD) approaches 14%.[21,22] Berhard et al[23] showed that simultaneous carotid endarterectomy (CE) and CABG procedures can significantly reduce operative mortality when compared to CE alone. Emery et al[24] reported a 5% mortality in a series of 42 patients undergoing simultaneous procedures. In contrast, the incidence of neurologic sequelae from CABG and cardiopulmonary bypass (CPBP) in patients with coexisting carotid disease is about 6%.[25] Turnipseed[26] found a 4.7% incidence of stroke in a similar series.

It is generally recommended to perform CE prior to initiation of CPBP. This sequence avoids alterations in cerebral perfusion caused by pump-associated hypotension, fluctuations in perfusion pressure and nonpulsatile blood flow. Debate still exists concerning the timing of CE in relation to the CABG procedure: starting CE prior to sternotomy versus sternotomy prior to CE. Emery et al recommend the sequence of sternotomy, exposure of the heart and cannulation for CPBP, and initiation of CPBP when CE is completed.[24]

The benefits of simultaneous CABG and CE are a decreased risk to the organ system not being operated on and enhanced cerebral protection against ischemia caused by alterations in cerebral perfusion pressure. The performance of CE prior to CABG in these patients exposes them to only one anesthetic procedure and· enhances the cost efficiency of laboratory and operating room facilities.

Neck Movement

The preanesthetic visit must include assessment of neck movement. If any extension of the neck causes alterations in consciousness or peripheral neurologic ability, plans must be made for an awake intubation after stabilization of the neck in a neutral position. Allen's test of adequate arterial circulation to the hands should also be documented.

Radiographic Evaluation

Cerebral arteriography remains the most accurate and reliable diagnostic procedure for localization of lesions in patients with cerebrovascular insufficiency. Access to the cerebral circulation may be achieved via retrograde catheterization of the femoral, brachial, subclavian or carotid arteries. The test is invasive, however, and not without disadvantages. Hematomas and peripheral neuropathies may develop at puncture sites. Cerebral complications are related to dislodgement of a thrombus or atherosclerotic plaque, air embolus, and luminal compression of a branching artery due to subintimal injection of contrast medium.

A relatively new method of angiography is digital subtraction angiography (DSA). The technique requires a smaller quantity of contrast material, less selective catheterization is needed compared to arteriography, and an image is obtained rapidly. Contrast agent is injected into the venous or arterial system and visualized by an image-intensifying fluoroscopy unit which then processes the images by means of a digital computer. Electronic subtraction by the computer results in a video image that is highly sensitive to structures of low contrast. Film costs are reduced and long-term storage on magnetic tapes is less expensive. Venous digital angiography offers the added advantage of being less invasive and more suited for out-patient screening. However, neither arterial nor venous DSA offers the high degree of resolution obtained with standard arteriography.

A number of newly developed noninvasive techniques are also available for evaluation of the cerebral circulation. They provide dynamic evaluation of blood flow through the internal carotid artery, and are useful screening procedures to determine whether the more invasive arteriography should be performed. Such noninvasive procedures include: cerebrovascular carotid Doppler examination (CDE), oculoplethysmography (OPG), supraorbital photoplethysmography (SOPPG) and phonoangiography.

CDE and OPG evaluate two different physiologic results of carotid occlusive disease. CDE reflects changes in extracranial carotid circulation resulting from significant carotid obstruction. OPG reflects decreases in internal carotid pressure distal to an obstructive lesion. OPG entails the use of two transparent corneal cups and warm saline as a medium for transmission of the retinal artery pulse waves. The waves are then subjected to electronic amplification and recording. CDE utilizes a directional Doppler flowmeter that is placed over the supraorbital and frontal arteries. Change in flow is then noted in response to compression of the common carotid artery. Flow normally decreases with ipsilateral common carotid artery compression; it is considered abnormal if flow does not decrease with ipsilateral compression or if it decreases with contralateral compression.

Phonoangiography utilizes a specially adapted microphone which is placed over the carotid arteries at different positions to obtain audio recordings. The wave-forms are recorded on either photographic film or magnetic tape, and are then analyzed for the degree of underlying carotid stenosis. SOPPG, like CDE, evaluates extracranial circulation. Two small transducers, each containing an infrared light-emitting diode and an adjacent photosensor, are placed over the orbit. The response to common carotid and external carotid compression are detected and stored in an analogue recorder. Abnormal flow patterns are present when: 1) there is no decrease in pulse amplitude with ipsilateral common carotid compression; 2) there is a 15% or greater reduction in amplitude with compression of either the facial or infraorbital arteries; or 3) a 33% or greater reduction in pulse amplitude occurs with compression of the ipsilateral or contralateral temporal artery.

Indications for noninvasive carotid evaluation include:[27] 1) patients with typical TIAs but with relative contraindications to arteriography (e.g., allergy to contrast medium; coagulopathies); 2) patients with an evolving stroke who have minor deficits; 3) patients with a previous stroke with a good recovery; 4) patients with symptomatic bruits; 5) patients with central retinal artery occlusion, in whom the incidence of carotid disease is approximately 20%.

Premedication

Although premedication is determined on an individual basis, certain principles apply to all patients about to undergo neurovascular surgery. Attention should be directed toward management of any coexisting medical problems. Oversedation should be avoided as it may lead to arterial hypotension and/or hypercarbia in susceptible patients. Premedication should be effective in preventing any increases in heart rate and blood pressure in the anxious patient, since these responses may lead to increased myocardial oxygen demand. Adequate sedation may be attained with the use of oral diazepam (10mg) or lorazepam (2mg). Atropine should be avoided in these patients because the unpleasant dryness of the mouth may increase apprehension. However, no medication can replace a careful preanesthetic visit with direct patient contact and thoughtful, adequate explanation of the anesthetic process.

Anesthetic Management

The anesthetic management of patients with cerebrovascular disease must be directed at protecting against ischemic infarction, maintaining normal intracranial hemodynamics, and optimizing those factors favoring resolution of ischemia. Increasing cerebral metabolic demand or decreasing substrate supply tend to increase the risk of infarction.

Also, any factor that augments blood flow or decreases metabolism minimizes the chance of infarction. In addition to these principles, planning an anesthetic technique must also consider the physiologic alterations unique to the neurovascular lesion.

References

1. The EC/IC Bypass Study Group. Failure of extracranial-intracranial arterial bypass to reduce the risk of ischemic stroke. Results of an international randomized trial. *N Engl J Med* 313(19):1191–1200, 1985.
2. Frost E.A.M.: *Clinical Anesthesia in Neurosurgery*, Boston, Butterworth, 1984, pp 118–119.
3. Steen P.A., Tinker J. H., Tarban S.: Myocardial reinfarction after anesthesia and surgery. An Update incidence, mortality and predisposing factors. *JAMA* 239:2566–2270, 1978.
4. Foëx P., Prys-Roberts C.: Anesthesia and the hypertensive patient. *Br J Anesth* 46:475, 1974.
5. Goldman L., Caldera D.L., Nussbaum S.R. et al: Multifactorial index of cardiac risk in noncardiac surgical procedures. *N Engl J Med* 297:845, 1977.
6. Nattel S., Rango R.E., VanLoon G.: Mechanism of propranolol withdrawal phenomena. *Circulation* 59:1158–1164, 1979.
7. Bruce D.L., Croley T.F., Lee JS: Preoperative clonidine withdrawal syndrome. *Anesthesiology* 51:90–92, 1979.

8. Brodsky J.B., Bravo J.J.: Acute postoperative clonidine withdrawal syndrome. *Anesthesiology* 44:519–520, 1976.
9. Farsang C., Kunos G.: Naloxone reverses the antihypertensive effect of clonidine. *Br J Pharmacol* 67:161–164, 1979.
10. Frost E.A.M.: Anesthesia for elective intracranial procedures. *Anesth Rev* 7:13, 1980.
11. Bell B.A., Symon L.: Smoking and subarachnoid hemorrhage. *Br Med J* 1:577, 1979.
12. Larson C.P.: Anesthesia for cerebrovascular surgical procedures. ASA 1983 Annual Refresher Course Lectures, Lecture No. 216.
13. Amrein P.C., Ellman L., Harris W.H.: Aspirin-induced prolongation of bleeding time and perioperative blood loss. *JAMA* 245:1825–1828, 1981.
14. Frost E.A.M.: Anesthetic management of cerebrovascular disease, *Br J Anaesth* 53:750, 1981.
15. Cullen B.F., Miller M.G.: Drug interactions and anesthesia, a review. *Anesth Analg* 58:5413–5423, 1979.
16. Frost E.A.M.: *Differential Diagnosis of Postoperative Coma in Recovery Room Care*, in Frost E.A.M., Andrews I.C. (ed). *International Anesthesiology Clinics*, Boston, Little Brown & Co., 1982, pp 13–30.
17. John D.A., Tobey R.E., Homer L.D., Rice C.L.: Onset of succinylcholine induced hyperkalemia following denervation. *Anesthesiology* 45:294–299, 1976.
18. Tobey R.E.: Paraplegia, succinylcholine and cardiac arrest. *Anesthesiology* 32:359–364, 1970.
19. Walts L.F., Miller J., Davidson M.B., Brown J.: Perioperative management of diabetes mellitus. *Anesthesiology* 43:89–99, 1981.
20. Thompson J.E., Craver J.M., Murphy D.A., Jones, et al: Concomitant carotid and coronary artery reconstruction. *Ann Surg* 195:712–720, 1982.
21. Ennix C.L., Lawrie G.M., Morris G.C. et al: Improved results of carotid endarterectomy in patients with symptomatic coronary disease: An analysis of 11,546 consecutive carotid operations. *Stroke* 10:122–125, 1979.
22. Lawrie G.M., Morris G.C.: Combined coronary and carotid revascularization, in Cohn L.H. (ed). *Modern Technics in Surgery-Cardiothoracic Surgery*, New York, Futura Publishing Co, Inc, 1980, vol 1, pp 1–21.
23. Bernhard V.M., Johnson W.D., Peterson J.J.: Carotid artery stenosis: Association with surgery for coronary artery disease. *Arch Surg* 105:837–840, 1972.
24. Emery R.W., Cohn L.H., Whittemore A.D. et al: Coexistent carotid and coronary artery disease. *Arch Surg* 118:1035–1038, 1983.
25. Urschel H.C., Razzuk M.A., Gardner M.A.: Management of concomitant occlusive disease of the carotid and coronary arteries. *J Thorac Cardiovasc Surg* 72:829–834, 1976.
26. Turnipseed W.D., Berkoff M.D., Belzer F.O.: Postoperative stroke in cardiac and peripheral vascular disease. *Ann Surg* 192:365–368, 1980.
27. Ackerman R.H.: Noninvasive carotid evaluation. *Stroke* 11:675–678, 1980.

CHAPTER 2

The Trauma Victim*

Jeffrey Berman

Case History. *A 26-year-old white male was found by the highway patrol after the car he was driving struck a telephone pole. He was admitted to the emergency room within 15 minutes of the accident.*

Initial vital signs were noted to be: blood pressure 100/82; pulse 116; respiration 36 and shallow; Glasgow coma scale 13.

The patient was conscious but confused. Physical examination showed contusions to the head and chest, and the left thigh was markedly swollen. The smell of alcohol was apparent on his breath.

Introduction

Trauma is the third leading cause of death in the United States. Sixty-eight million injuries occur yearly, of which over 100,000 are lethal. It crosses all socioeconomic and age groupings. Trauma is the leading cause of death in the first four decades of life. The prognosis for trauma victims, however, has improved markedly in recent years. More efficient medical evacuation (emergency medical services) has resulted in delivery of trauma victims to emergency centers soon after occurrence of the injuries. The first hour after a traumatic injury is referred to as the "Golden Hour" because it affords a unique opportunity to intervene and improve outcome.

The anesthesiologist, as part of the trauma team, is involved early in the patient's care. The full extent of injuries to the multiply injured patient are not always immediately apparent. Although a facial laceration attracts attention immediately, it is imperative that a systematic evaluation be performed to rule out life-threatening conditions. Early stabilization can then be started.

For the anesthesiologist, the initial review serves as both preanesthetic assessment and an opportunity to initiate therapy. It allows organization of

---

*Reviewed by Dr. Steven A. Blau, Assistant Professor of Surgery, Albert Einstein College of Medicine of Yeshiva University, Bronx, New York.

the anesthetic team and development of a comprehensive care plan. Unlike the care given nonlife-threatening illness, preoperative assessment of the trauma patient cannot be separated easily from therapeutic interventions which must usually be initiated immediately.

The preoperative management of the trauma victim falls into four categories: airway evaluation and management, fluid resuscitation, neurologic assessment, and preoperative diagnosis and organization. This lesson will cover three of these; neurologic assessment will be the subject of Chapter 14.

Airway Evaluation and Management

Securing the Airway

Establishment and maintenance of a patent airway is the first priority in a trauma patient. Obstruction of the upper airway is generally due to either the tongue, foreign bodies (blood, vomitus, dentures) or edema of the glottic area including vocal cord trauma.

In the unconscious patient, there is loss of tone in pharyngeal muscles which allows the tongue to fall against the posterior pharyngeal wall. This is treated by either a chin lift or jaw thrust, both of which move the mandible and tongue anteriorly. Repositioning of the tongue can then be maintained by placement of an oropharyngeal or nasopharyngeal airway. Unless cervical spine injury has been ruled out, these maneuvers must be carried out without flexion or extension of the neck. Placement of a nasopharyngeal tube is contraindicated when facial fractures or fractures of the base of the skull are suspected. Endotracheal intubation or cricothyroidotomy is required in the trauma patient when other attempts to open the airway have failed

A properly placed and secured, cuffed endotracheal tube provides several advantages in patient management:

- protection against aspiration,
- ability to hyperventilate,
- a means of providing continuous positive pressure ventilation,
- protection against development of upper airway obstruction,
- a route for drug administration.

Evaluation of the airway and selection of the intubation technique should be performed by the anesthesiologist. Unskilled attempts at laryngoscopy and tube placement result in further trauma, edema and bleeding in the upper airway. In a combative patient or following head trauma, the presence of hypoxia or raised intracranial pressure must be suspected. The use of adjunct drugs such as sodium thiopental or muscle relaxants to facilitate endotracheal intubation must be assessed.

If cervical spine trauma has not yet been ruled out, oral intubation should be attempted only after axial traction has been established. Fiberoptic oral intubation in skilled hands is the technique of choice. Nasotracheal intubation, usually a "blind technique," requires a cooperative or somnolent, breathing patient and is rarely the route of choice for airway establishment. Prior administration of vasoconstrictors (cocaine or phenylephrine) to the nasal mucosa will minimize the risk of bleeding.

Injury to the upper airway, facial injuries, vocal cord trauma or glottic edema may preclude endotracheal intubation. In such cases, cricothyroidotomy may be a life-saving procedure. However, it is not recommended for children because injury to the cricoid cartilage may cause subsequent subglottic stenosis.

Cricothyroidotomy is performed surgically by a vertical incision over and through the cricothyroid membrane. A scalpel handle can then be rotated 90° to dilate the opening through which a small (6mm) endotracheal tube can be inserted. Alternatively, a 14-gauge plastic intravenous catheter can be inserted. The time required to perform tracheostomy is too long for this procedure to be undertaken when the airway is closed or marginally patent.

Ventilation and Respiration

As soon as the airway has been secured, adequacy of respiration and ventilation must be assessed. The chest wall is observed for extent and symmetry of motion. Decreased rate or volume suggests narcotic overdose. Naloxone 0.4mg should be given intravenously. If tachypnea is present, and especially if a history of insulin-dependent diabetes is obtained, 50ml dextrose 50% is indicated. Palpation of the chest is useful in determining the presence of flail chest or rib fractures. Having secured an adequate airway, failure to ventilate the lungs suggests one of the following life-threatening conditions.

Tension pneumothorax develops when a "ball valve" air leak occurs, and air is forced into the thoracic cavity with no means of exit. The ipsilateral lung collapses, and pleural air displaces the mediastinum to the opposite side impairing venous return. Clinically, there is tracheal deviation, respiratory distress, unilateral absence of breath sounds, distended neck veins and hyperresonance over the affected side. A large-bore needle should be inserted immediately in the second intercostal space at the midclavicular line of the affected side. Definitive treatment with a chest tube is performed under sterile conditions as soon as possible.

Flail chest results when a segment of the chest wall loses bony continuity with the rest of the thoracic cage. Paradoxical chest wall motion results in inefficient gas exchange. Diagnosis is made by observation and palpation of crepitus and rib fractures. Flail chest is best treated by splinting and ventilatory exercises. However, if hypotension develops, arterial oxygen is less than 60mmHg, or arterial carbon dioxide is greater than 50mmHg on room air, endotracheal intubation and positive pressure ventilation are indicated for internal stabilization.

Cardiac tamponade usually results from penetrating injuries. If it is associated with blunt trauma, mortality approaches 100%. The clinical triad of elevated venous pressure, hypotension and muffled heart sounds is known as Beck's triad. A high index of suspicion should be present regarding the hypotensive trauma patient with no obvious source of bleeding and a precordial penetrating injury. The differential diagnosis is often confused with that of left tension pneumothorax. However, in the case of tamponade, there is no hyperresonance. Initial management must be prompt to restore effective heart action. Subxyphoid pericardiocentesis is carried out with a plastic-sheathed needle in the stable patient. Definitive care is thoracotomy.

Massive hemothorax is suggested by hypotension and dullness to percussion over one or both sides of the chest. The patient's neck veins may be distended or flat depending on whether venous outflow is occluded by intrathoracic blood. A chest tube should not be placed first; rather, hypovolemia should be treated and only then trial drainage attempted. If hypotension worsens, intrathoracic blood may be entering the pericardium, and the drainage should be stopped. Preparation for immediate thoracotomy should be made.

Open pneumothorax (sucking chest wound) results from a penetrating injury of the thorax that is the same size or larger than the glottic aperture. Equilibration occurs between intrathoracic and atmospheric pressure. Flow of air follows the course of least resistance, and therefore large areas of the pulmonary tree are not ventilated. The open pneumothorax is treated with a sterile occlusive dressing, taped on three sides, and a tube thoracostomy (chest tube).

These injuries require immediate therapy. Further alveolar pathology may develop minutes or hours after injury and increases mortality.

Pulmonary contusion may coincide with or be secondary to blunt trauma. Adult respiratory distress syndrome is the most common potentially lethal chest pathology in the U.S. In addition to trauma, it is associated with sepsis, left ventricular failure and neurologic injury.[1,2] The syndrome is insidious in onset, and the anesthesiologist must have a high index of suspicion for its development in the multiple trauma victim. Frequent arterial blood gas measurements should be instituted as soon as the patient's airway is secured and circulation restored. Optimal oxygenation of affected patients will require varying concentrations of oxygen supplementation and mechanical support using positive end expiratory pressure (PEEP) or some form of high-frequency ventilation.[3,4]

Fluid Resuscitation

Circulatory Status

Although the multiply injured patient may present with one or more types of shock (e.g., cardiac, septic) the syndrome most commonly seen is hypovolemic shock. Tachycardia and narrowed pulse pressure are the primary presenting signs. The anesthesiologist must assess the degree of blood loss and begin to restore effective circulating volume. Activation of the sympathetic nervous system, part of the body's compensatory response, results in increased levels of circulating catecholamines. This activity causes a preferential redistribution of cardiac output to the heart and brain, with reduction in splanchnic and renal blood flow. Adequacy of renal blood flow can be followed by monitoring urine output.

Frequently, the trauma victim will arrive at the emergency room or operating room with a pneumatic antishock garment in place. Use of this device increases total peripheral resistance, but it does not effect significant translocation of blood. It is also useful for splinting and hemorrhage control in cases of pelvic and multiple leg fractures.

The anesthesiologist should be familiar with the mechanics of this device and its safe operation. Deflation of the device begins with the abdominal section. The blood pressure is monitored while a small amount of air is allowed to escape. If the pressure drops more than 5mmHg, deflation is stopped and fluid resuscitation resumed. After successful deflation of the abdominal segment, leg sections are released one at a time. Blood pressure must be continuously monitored.

Before an assessment of circulatory status is completed, two large-bore peripheral intravenous catheters must be inserted (preferably 16 gauge). At that time, blood samples for typing and crossmatching, complete blood count (CBC), serum electrolytes (SMA-6), coagulation profile (PT/PTT) and amylase should be drawn. Balanced salt solution should be infused until the need for specific component therapy has been established. A blood pressure cuff of appropriate width (⅔ length of upper extremity) should be applied. Electrocardiographic monitoring should be instituted. Attempts to start an intraarterial line should not take precedence over prompt restoration of circulating volume.

The patient in shock will present with some or all of the following clinical signs: hypotension, tachycardia, oliguria, pallor, coolness of the extremities, cyanosis, and low central venous pressure. In more severe cases (loss of 35% or more of circulating blood volume), the patient may be confused, restless and show signs of air hunger. Although signs of hypovolemia generally correlate with the degree of blood loss, geriatric patients, anemic patients and those taking various medications (diuretics, narcotics, phenothiazines) may exhibit signs out of proportion to the degree of blood loss. Patients receiving beta adrenergic blocking agents and calcium entry antagonists may not develop tachycardia.

TABLE 1. American College of Surgeons classes of acute hemorrhage

	Class I	Class II	Class III	Class IV
Blood loss (ml)	≤750	1000–1250	1500–1800	2000–2500
Blood loss (%)*	≤15	20–25	30–35	40–50
Pulse rate†	72–84	>100	>120	≥140
Blood pressure (mmHg)‡‡	118/82	110/80	70–90/ 50–60	<50–60 systolic
Pulse pressure (mmHg)	36	30	20–30	10–20
Respiratory rate	14–20	20–30	30–40	>35
Urine output (ml/hr)§	30–35	25–30	5–15	neglible
CNS-Mental status	slightly anxious	mildly anxious	anxious and confused	confused and lethargic
Fluid replacement (use 3:1 rule for fluid resuscitation)	crystalloid	crystalloid	crystalloid + blood	crystalloid + blood

* percent of blood volume in a 70kg adult, † assume normal of 72/min, ‡ assume normal of 120/80, § assume normal of 40–50ml/hr

The American College of Surgeons has developed a scheme to quantify and classify hemorrhagic shock.[5] See Table 1. Since no one sign is reliable in making a diagnosis, several of the parameters indicated should be used. Classification is intended as a guide to the type and volume of replacement required.

Class I hemorrhage is defined as acute loss of up to 15% of total circulating volume. Clinically, the diagnosis is potentially difficult to make, especially in the young and previously healthy adult. Pulse rate, blood pressure, respiration and even pulse pressure may appear to be within normal limits. Volume replacement may be with crystalloid or balanced salt solution (lactated Ringer's, Normosol®). Three milliliters crystalloid is used to replace each milliliter of blood loss (3:1 rule).

Class II hemorrhage is loss of 20–25% of circulating blood volume (1000–1250ml in the 70kg patient) and will cause tachycardia of 100 beats/minute or more, tachypnea and a narrowed pulse pressure. Urinary output begins to decline to less than 0.5ml/kg/hr. Fluid therapy in these patients should be started with balanced salt solutions. The 3:1 rule for replacement should be used here, and the need for component therapy evaluated on an individual basis. Restoration of effective intravascular volume should not be delayed pending availability of blood or colloid.

Class III hemorrhage is the acute loss of 30–35% of intravascular volume (1500–1750ml/70kg). It produces the classical signs associated with hypovolemia in virtually all patients. In addition to a tachycardia usually greater than 120 beats/minute, tachypnea of 30–40 per minute and a significantly narrowed pulse pressure, patients have altered mental status (confusion) and significant decreases in urine output due to inadequate cerebral and renal perfusion. Restoration of circulating volume requires blood therapy. Effective circulating volume and oxygen carrying capacity must be restored.

Class IV hemorrhage represents the extreme case of hemorrhagic blood loss (>40%). Heart rate reaches 140 beats/minute or more, and the pulse pressure tracing is narrowed to 10–20mmHg. All signs seen with lesser degrees of shock are manifest to a greater degree. As in Class III, blood therapy must be started immediately.

Fluids for Resuscitation

Crystalloid and Nonprotein Expanders. In cases of mild to moderate blood loss (10–25%), replacement with blood products is usually unnecessary. The rationale for using crystalloid or colloid solutions in these cases is based on avoiding the multiple risks associated with blood therapy such as transmission of hepatitis and the autoimmune deficiency syndrome (AIDS), and antibody reactions (leukocyte, Rh) and citrate toxicity.

Considerable debate lingers over the use of crystalloids versus colloids as plasma expanders. Acute blood losses of up to 50% intravascular volume have been adequately managed with balanced salt solutions. In an animal study, a 73% depletion of circulatory blood volume was replaced by salt solution only.[6] Although dilutional anemia and hypoprotenemia developed, resuscitation was successful, and spontaneous recovery of total serum protein was completed within 24 hours.

Crystalloids may leave the circulation and cause pulmonary edema.[7] Other studies suggest that colloidal solutions, although remaining in the circulation for more hours, also leak from damaged pulmonary capillaries, thus negating their advantage.[8]

The use of dextran and other nonprotein plasma expanders is currently under investigation. Half-life in the circulation is between that of crystalloid and colloid, but their use is not without complications.[9] When nonprotein expanders are administered in volumes exceeding 1000ml, increased bleeding due to platelet dysfunction occurs. Difficulty in crossmatching after administration has also been noted. Thus, the large volumes that are required for resuscitation limit the usefulness of nonprotein expanders. The routine practice of the hospital should be followed when instituting nonblood fluid therapy in the emergency room.

Blood and Blood Component Therapy. In cases of Class III and Class IV hemorrhage (>25%) the need for blood administration is immediate. When exsanguination cannot be controlled or irreversible shock is imminent, uncrossmatched type-specific blood can be used. Approximately 1 in 1000 patients with no prior transfusion history and 1 in 100 with prior transfusion history will have an unexpected antibody detected during crossmatch.[10] If time permits an additional 5 minutes, a partial crossmatch of patient's serum with donor cells should be carried out to reduce this risk by detecting Rh and Kell antibodies. The use of type O, Rh negative blood may be used in circumstances where type-specific blood is not available. Its use is limited, however, by availability and because after administration of several units, it is then difficult to type and crossmatch the patient for subsequent blood therapy.

The use of specific blood components must be evaluated on an individual basis, taking into consideration both the total amount of red cells replaced and the results of a current CBC (including platelet count) and tests of clotting function (PT/PTT). The use of component therapy and possible complications has been dealt with extensively elsewhere.[11,12] (See Chapter 24.) Several points, however, should be made. Both fresh frozen plasma (FFP) and platelet concentrate require 30–45 minutes to prepare; therefore, the need for them must be anticipated.

As a general rule, any abnormality in coagulation studies that deviates from normal by 50% or more should be treated with whole blood or fresh frozen plasma. Special attention should be paid to head trauma victims in whom release of thromboplastin from the injured brain significantly increases the risk of bleeding.

The coagulopathy most often encountered in trauma patients is dilutional thrombocytopenia. Platelet exhaustion is rare until 10 units of blood have been administered. At this point, 0.1 unit platelet pack/kg will raise the platelet count approximately $50,000/mm^3$ (6–10 packs/70kg).

Preoperative Diagnosis and Organization

Following stabilization and assessment of the patient, a systematic "head to toe" examination must begin. This process starts by completely undressing the patient to expose hidden injuries. Although attention may become focused on a particular injury, there must be a constant reappraisal of the patient's respiratory, circulatory and neurological status. Additional diagnostic and therapeutic measures may include:

Urinary Catheterization. Low output of urine with a high specific gravity indicates the need for additional fluids. Anuria in the presence of normal blood pressure may signal renal obstruction or injury. Hemoglobinuria indicates pelvic injury. Myoglobinuria accompanies severe muscle destruction (crush injury or burn).

Central Venous Catheterization. The central venous pressure serves as an indicator of the adequacy of volume replacement.

Nasogastric tube placement relieves and prevents gastric distention. In the patient with facial trauma, the possibility of cribriform fracture exists, and the oral route should be used.

Peritoneal lavage is useful in the diagnosis of occult intraabdominal bleeding, especially in the patient with head injury, alcohol or drug overdose, or spinal cord trauma in whom appreciation of abdominal pain is reduced. Contraindications include a history of multiple intraabdominal operations and a gravid uterus. This procedure can be facilitated by 3–5ml lidocaine 1% injected locally.

X-Ray Examinations. Cervical spine films should be obtained of any injury above the clavicles. All seven cervical vertebrae must be visualized. If possible, an upright chest x-ray or left lateral decubitus view should be obtained to detect free air, fractures, loss of psoas shadow and foreign bodies. Computerized tomography of the head and neck or other regions should be performed as indicated by physical exam. Although it may strain resources, an anesthesiologist should monitor any patient with cardiovascular instability or altered consciousness during radiologic testing. Appropriate sedation may then be given while ensuring adequate ventilatory exchange.

A concise and pertinent medical history should be obtained if possible. The key elements to be addressed are remembered by the mnemonic *AMPLE*:[5]

*A*llergies;
*M*edications, including drugs and alcohol, and medical problems for which the patient has been treated;
*P*ast surgical and medical history;
*L*ast food intake (NPO status);
*E*vents preceding the trauma: How did it happen (deceleration injury, closed space explosion, etc)?

As the resuscitation and diagnosis of the multiple trauma patient proceeds, operative intervention may be recommended. The anesthesiologist should ascertain that:

• The operating room staff has been notified.
• Anesthesiology staff is prepared to receive the patient.
• The blood bank has received a properly labeled specimen and has been informed of anticipated blood requirements.
• Adequate personnel to transfer the patient are available.
• The patient has been adequately resuscitated prior to transfer.
• Preoperative medications have been administered as ordered.
• Appropriate monitoring is available during transit.
• All fluid and drugs administered have been accurately recorded.

Anesthetic Management

The use of premedicant sedative and narcotic drugs must be individualized. Often because of time constraints and physical deterioration, premedication is not indicated. Any sedative or narcotic medications must be given judiciously, especially to patients with head trauma. Careful monitoring of respiration and intracranial status is essential.

General anesthesia is usually indicated because it affords complete control of the airway and ventilation. Regional block is rarely used because of the risk of hypotension and the widespread nature of injuries which often make it impractical.

It should be assumed that all trauma patients have a full stomach. Pain, anxiety and shock are all factors that delay gastric emptying. Various regimens to reduce the gastric volume of patients for emergency surgery have been advocated. These include nasogastric suction, the use of antacids,[13] H_2 receptor antagonists,[14] anticholinergics, and metoclopramide. None has proved totally effective. Furthermore, they are unnecessary in cases where the airway has been protected by a cuffed endotracheal tube. The same principles for intubation that apply in the ER apply in the OR.

The choice of specific induction agents and muscle relaxants depends on the cardiovascular status of the patient. All agents should be used in small incremental doses. The presence of alcohol and other drugs significantly reduces anesthetic requirements.

In hypovolemic/hypotensive patients, diazepam, fentanyl, midazolam or ketamine may induce less cardiovascular depression than thiopental. Nevertheless, cardiovascular instability and the possible presence of other drugs and alcohol necessitate caution. Although ketamine may offer the advantages of bronchodilation and lack of cardiac depression, it is contraindicated in cases of head trauma because it increases intracranial pressure.

The use of nitrous oxide for maintenance of anesthesia may be limited by its interference with the ability to adequately oxygenate the patient. The potent inhalation agents afford the major advantages of rapid change of anesthetic depth and amnesia at light planes. Of the short-acting narcotic agents, sufentanil ($0.4-0.6\mu g/kg/hr$) after a loading dose of $1-2\mu g/kg$) offers the best cardiovascular stability.

References

1. Rinaldo J.E., Rogers R.M.: Adult respiratory distress syndrome—changing concepts of lung injury and repair. *N Engl J Med* 306:900–909, 1982.
2. Murray J.F.: Conference report: mechanisms of acute respiratory failure. National Heart, Lung and Blood Institute. *Am Rev Respir Dis* 115:1071–1078, 1977.
3. Pontoppidan H., Wilson R.S., Rie M.A. et al: Respiratory intensive care. *Anesthesiology* 47:96–116, 1977.
4. Cotev S., Perel A., Katznelson R. et al: The effects of PEEP on oxygenating capacity in acute respiratory failure with sepsis. *Crit Care Med* 4:186, 1976.
5. Advanced Trauma Life Support Course. American College of Surgeons, 1981.
6. Cervera A.L., Moss G.: Crystalloid distribution following hemorrhage and hemodilution. *J Trauma* 14:506–520, 1974.

7. Kallos J., Smith T.C.: Replacement of intraoperative blood loss. *Anesthesiology* 41:293–295, 1974.
8. Lowe R.T., Moss G.S., Jilek J. et al: Crystalloid versus colloid in the etiology of pulmonary failure after trauma: A randomized trial in man. *Crit Care Med* 7:107–112, 1979.
9. Isbiter J.P., Fisher M.: Adverse effects of plasma volume expanders. *Anaesth Intensive Care* 8:145–51, 1980.
10. Blumberg N., Bove J.R.: Uncrossmatched blood for emergency transfusion. *JAMA* 240:2057, 1978.
11. Isbiter J.P., Scurr R.D.: Blood transfusion therapy: Components indications, complications and controversies. *Anaesth Intensive Care* 6:297–309, 1978.
12. Miller R.D.: Complications of massive blood transfusions. *Anesthesiology* 39:82–93, 1973.
13. Wrobel J., Koh T.C., Saunders J.M.: Sodium citrate: An alternative antacid for prophylaxis against aspiration pneumonitis. *Anaesth Intensive Care* 10:116–119, 1982.
14. Morison D.H., Dunn G.L., Fargas-Babjak A.M. et al: A double blind comparison of cimetidine and ranitidine as prophylaxis against gastric aspiration syndrome. *Anesth Analg 6* 1:988–992, 1982.

CHAPTER 3

The Intravenous Drug Abuse Patient*

Clifford Gewirtz

Case History. *A 37-year-old Hispanic male presented to the ER with several stab wounds to the right arm and hand. The injuries had occurred 30 minutes prior to admission during an altercation while speedballing in a shooting gallery. Prior medical history included multiple previous admissions for pneumonia, jaundice, and mitral valve replacement.*

Physical examination revealed an undernourished patient with five puncture wounds of the right upper extremity with muscle and tendons visible in the wounds. There were several crusted ulcers on both upper and lower extremities. No obvious veins were visible. The remainder of the physical exam was remarkable for râles concentrated over the right lung base and a well-healed median sternotomy scar. Cardiac examination revealed a III/VI high-pitched pansystolic murmur with maximum intensity at the apex. Examination of the abdomen was normal except for a liver span of 15cm in the right midclavicular line.

Laboratory examinations revealed the following: Hgb 14g/dl, SMA-6 within normal limits. The EKG showed a prolonged Q-T interval and prominent Q-waves in leads II, III, and aVF. The chest x-ray showed diffuse granulomatous disease, increased pulmonary vascular markings, sternotomy wires and a mitral valve annular ring. Urinalysis was positive for trace protein but otherwise negative. Microscopic examination was unremarkable. An SMA-12 analyses and HBsAg were requested as emergencies.

Abused Drugs

While there is a plethora of drugs that are abused, the two that are most commonly abused by the intravenous route are heroin and cocaine. Other than alcohol in combination, heroin and cocaine were the two drugs most frequently cited by medical examiners reporting to the Drug Abuse Warn-

---

*Reviewed by Dr. Steven Blau, Assistant Professor of Surgery, Albert Einstein College of Medicine of Yeshiva University, Bronx, New York.

TABLE 1. Street names for heroin and cocaine in English and Spanish

Heroin/Heroina	Cocaine/Cocaina
bomb, boy, brother, brown sugar, cat, chick, Chinese red, crap, dogie, doojee, dope, duji, H, Hary, horse, junk, Mexican mud, scag, scat, smack, stuff, thing	Bernice, bernies, blow, C, Carry Nation, Cecil, coconut, coke, Corrine, dream, flake, frisky powder, girl, gold dust, heaven dust, incentive, jam, love drug, moon dust, nose candy, paradise, rock, sniff, snow, star dust, toot, uptown, white snuff
blanco, caballo, carga, chiva, la cosa, la duna gato, golpe, H, manteca, stufa	coca, nieve, perico, polvito

Data from the master file, National Institute on Drug Abuse.

ing Network (DAWN) of the National Institute on Drug Abuse.[1] (See Table 1.) Similarly, heroin and cocaine were the most frequently mentioned intravenous drugs in connection with a visit to a DAWN emergency room. Other drugs abused intravenously with a much lesser frequency included pentazocine, the barbiturates and other opioids.

Heroin

Heroin, or diacetylmorphine, when injected in a bolus, produces a warm flushing of the skin and sensations in the lower abdomen that have been described by addicts as similar in intensity and quality to sexual orgasm. This *rush* or *kick* lasts about 45 seconds. Heroin may also be injected subcutaneously (*skin popping*) which delays its onset of action.

Compared to morphine, heroin has been described as a more potent analgesic causing less nausea, vomiting and constipation. Milligram for milligram, it is approximately 2.5 times as potent as morphine, and 25 to 30 times as potent as meperidine. One milligram of heroin is equal in analgesic activity to about $100\mu g$ fentanyl. (The duration of action is approximately 2–4 hours).

The typical *bag* of heroin contains approximately 5–10mg heroin, which is *cut* with about 90mg of quinine, talc or starch.

Butorphenol tartrate, pentazocine and nalorpine are narcotic antagonists, which if administered to a heroin addict, precipitate a withdrawal crisis. Naloxone has no place in the anesthetic management of the intravenous drug abuser, again because of precipitation of withdrawal crisis. Intubation and assisted ventilation are preferable.

Cocaine

Cocaine has a powerful sympathomimetic effect when administered intravenously.[2] It is sold as a powder, often diluted with procaine, and varies greatly in purity. The powder is usually arranged on glass in thin *lines*, 3–5cm long, each containing approximately 25mg. Recently, a purified form of cocaine "crack" has become popular. Inhaling the smoke from the burning substance allows immediate absorption of the free base through the lungs into the circulation.

Cocaine, which may be injected or *snorted* intranasally, potentiates the actions of catecholamines in the central nervous system by blocking re-uptake at nerve terminals, especially of dopamine. The underlying mechanism of the associated euphoria is not well understood. Dopaminergic antagonists or depletors, such as reserpine, methyldopa, the phenothiazines, haloperidol, droperidol, and metoclopramide, can block most of the euphoric effects. Use of these drugs during anesthesia in an addicted patient may cause delayed awakening, general fatigue, lassitude, hyperphagia, and depression postoperatively. The use of phenothiazines as premedication is probably ill advised, and neuroleptic anesthesia is also a poor choice.

Heroin–Cocaine Combination

A *speedball* is a line of cocaine mixed with a bag or two of heroin. The mixture is placed in a teaspoon where it is heated to form a slurry which is then injected. A euphoric state is induced which lasts approximately 30 minutes; this is followed by a period of stupor lasting 2 to 4 hours. The time course of the combination of these two drugs may be differentiated by the presence of sweaty hands in the cocaine-predominant phase. As the veracity of patients under the influence of these drugs is questionable, much reliance must be placed on the physical examination.

To plan an anesthetic induction, it is imperative to ascertain as best as possible the time of injection. Induction during the stimulation (cocaine-predominant) phase may require high doses of anesthetic, while low doses will suffice during the heroin-predominant stage.[3,4]

Medical Evaluation

When obtaining a history from an intravenous drug abuser, the anesthetist must assume a very firm attitude. Accurate and complete information is essential for safe anesthetic management. Treatment based on evasion or misinformation can have disastrous results. Patients often fear insufficient medication in the hospital, and they may inflate the amount of their daily habit to provide a margin of safety. Polypharmacy is the rule among addicts, and it is not uncommon for patients to indulge in simultaneous abuse of legal and illegal drugs. A very detailed drug intake history must be obtained.

At the time of the initial examination of the patient, record must be made of the timing and route of injection of all drugs taken in the last 24 hours and the length of addiction. The anesthetist should try to correlate signs of recent injection with physical findings. Pinpoint pupils usually indicate recent narcotic administration, while widely dilated pupils indicate use of sympathomimetic drugs (amphetamine or cocaine).

Respiratory System

Cocaine that is inhaled acts as a vaso-constrictor of the nasal mucosa. Chronic use can cause necrosis of the nasal septum as well as part of the turbinates. The nose should be thoroughly examined prior to passage of a nasogastric or nasotracheal tube as these may dislodge necrotic tissue. The pressure exerted by these tubes may also cause necrosis in areas already ischemic.

The use of cutting agents in drug mixtures that are injected may result in pulmonic foreign body granulomatosis.[5] Chronic use of street drugs will result in a loss of diffusing capacity and decreased compliance.[6]

The use of opioids decreases cough reflexes and mucociliary clearance, which decrease peak expiratory flow. As most addicts also smoke cigarettes, the effect is similar to chronic bronchitis, ie, increased $PaCo_2$, decreased PaO_2, and pulmonary hypertension. Induction via an inhalation technique is prolonged in these patients.

Pulmonary function tests should be performed routinely in addicts before any elective surgery. If intubation in the awake state was deemed necessary in the emergent situation, an estimation of forced expiratory volume can be obtained by attaching a Wright spirometer to the end of the tube and measuring vital capacity. Chest x-ray is indicated in all patients, and arterial blood gas analyses provides useful baseline information. During a *trip* the patient is often stuporous, a condition commonly accompanied by hypoventilation and predisposition to aspiration.

Cardiovascular System

Most intravenous drug addicts have signs and symptoms of cardiovascular disease. Endocarditis is very common. The tricuspid valve is the most frequently involved, followed by the mitral valve and the aortic valve.

Prophylactic antibiotics should be administered routinely prior to induction of anesthesia.[7] As intravenous infusion of antibiotics during anesthesia may cause hypotension (current recommendations for prophylaxis include a penicillin and an aminoglycoside eg, gentamycin, tobramycin, prior to induction), consultation with an infectious disease specialist is appropriate since the sensitivities of *Staphylococcus*, the most commonly involved organism, can change dramatically. Bacteria may not be community acquired as addicts often obtain their syringes and needles from hospital sources (which underscores the need to destroy all used needles and syringes). Drug resistant bacteria frequently predominate.

Addicts frequently exhibit EKG abnormalities[8] which range from a prolonged QTc interval to electrocardiographic evidence of myocardial infarction. It is therefore important that a routine EKG be available and interpreted for all addicts, regardless of their age.

Low diastolic blood pressure is common among addicts and is thought to be due to decreased sympathetic tone, which also causes a decrease in systemic vascular resistance.[9]

Liver Disease

Most heroin addicts have significant liver abnormalities manifest by elevations in SGOT, SGPT and alkaline phosphatase.[10] Pathologic studies have found changes ranging from mild lymphocytic infiltration of the portal triads to severe fibrous tissue "bridging" between the triads. The causes of the changes are controversial. Explanations such as malnutrition and chronic toxic reaction have been postulated.[11,12]

A past history of hepatitis can be elicited from 50% of addicts, with one-third having repeat epidoses. Hepatitis B surface antigen (HBsAg), the serologic marker of the virus, is an indicator of infectivity. HBsAg is reported positive in 2.2% of addicts, four times the incidence in the general U.S. population.

Cirrhosis of the liver is also prevalent among addicts, especially in young abusers.[10] The onset of cirrhosis is earlier for addicts compared to alcoholics, and the reason for this is unclear. Talc and other contaminants which pass through the pulmonary system via arterial venous shunts are often found in the liver parenchyma and may cause granulomatous disease.

The anesthesiologist must be aware of the possibility of decreased hepatic reserve in intravenous drug abuse patients. The biochemical manifestations (increased PT or decreased serum albumin) may not be present until much of the reserve has been exhausted.

Anesthetic agents and neuromuscular blocking agents that are metabolized by the liver (eg, opioids, pancuronium, halothane) should be avoided.[13] Isoflurane appears to be the agent of choice since less than 1% is metabolized by the liver, even in the presence of hepatic enzyme induction. Similarly, atracurium, which depends on Hoffman elimination, is particularly useful.

Musculoskeletal Disorders

The stuporous heroin addict exerts much pressure over bony prominances. The normal shifting response is suppressed, and this can result in ischemic necrosis of muscles and skin and edema formation (the crush syndrome).[14] The fluid shift to the injured area can be sufficient to cause hypovolemia; and with muscle tissue necrosis, myoglobinemia may result in obstruction of the renal tubules and subsequent renal failure. Rhabdomyolysis has also been described and is thought to be due to some component in adulterated heroin.[15] The diagnosis should be suspected if the urine is dark. Laboratory determinations of myoglobin and free hemoglobin are necessary. The urine should be alkalinized with sodium bicarbonate (approximately 1mg/kg). To prevent precipitation in renal tubules, a loop diuretic such as furosemide (20mg) should be given. Appropriate consultations are indicated.

Osteomyelitis is also common in these patients. The lumbar vertebrae seem to be particularly at risk.[16] The reason for this predisposition is not well understood. If a regional anesthetic is to be considered in the addicted patient, a film of the vertebral column should be obtained to rule out involvement.

Neurologic Disease

Embolic phenomena may occur following injection of contaminated drugs. This can result in central and peripheral neurologic lesions, such as individual cranial nerve palsies or isolated peripheral neuropathies. A thorough neurologic examination is indicated. If any lesions are discovered, they must be documented to prevent confusion of new onset lesions postoperatively and to forestall medicolegal problems.

Tetanus has been reported in heroin addicts who use the skin popping technique.[11, 12] The predisposition is thought to be due to the use of quinine which will lower the redox potential of tissues at the injection site, which in turn predisposes to anaerobic contamination.

Protection of Medical Personnel (See Chapter 18)

Drug addicts are at increased risk of contracting hepatitis B and the acquired immune deficiency syndrome (AIDS). The pathogenesis and symptomatology of these entities are discussed elsewhere in great detail.[17, 18] Gotta and Sullivan[19] have suggested the following precautions:

- Gowns and gloves should be worn during direct contact with patient's blood, secretions and excretions (including saliva).
- Hand washing is mandatory before and after patient care. Gloves are not a substitute for hand washing.
- Masks should be worn by coughing patients when out of their rooms, by personnel in contact with coughing patients, and by personnel suctioning endotracheal tubes.
- Protective eye wear (eg, goggles) should be worn when splatter of blood, secretions or excretions is possible, such as during bronchoscopy, endoscopy, intubation or extubation.
- Specimens should be transported in impervious containers labelled "Blood Precautions."
- Needles or syringes should be disposable and placed in puncture-proof

containers for disposal by incineration, without any attempt to resheath or bend needles.

- Linens and similar articles should be disposed of, if possible, by incineration.
- Contaminated articles and surfaces should be cleaned with a 1:10 dilution of 5.25% sodium hypochlorite (household bleach) or with phenolic solution.
- Disposable anesthesia circuits should be used.

To the above may be added:
- The entire carbon dioxide assembly should be changed after use for an intravenous drug abuse patient.
- A filter should be placed in the expiratory limb of the circuit. Even though viruses are filterable agents, the filter can trap droplets which could harbor organisms.

Withdrawal

Not uncommonly, a heroin addict will present with symptoms of drug withdrawal. Adverse reactions usually begin 24 to 36 hours after the last opiate injection.

The first manifestations are often perspiration and rhinorrhea, followed by tremors, "muscle twitching," hot and cold flashes and systemic aching. Later symptoms include fever, vomiting, diarrhea, spontaneous ejaculation and orgasm. Involuntary muscle spasms produce kicking movements and the patient often assumes the fetal position. Frank pulmonary edema may develop.

Before induction of anesthesia, the symptoms of withdrawal must be ameliorated. This can be accomplished with methadone. A dose of methadone 20mg, will block the symptoms of severe withdrawal in almost all addicts.

If a lengthy surgical procedure is planned, the possibility of withdrawal symptoms developing during anesthesia must be considered. Signs would include increased airway pressure and pulmonary edema, fever, tachycardia, hypotension, and muscle twitching suggestive of focal or general seizures.

Anesthetic Management

Addicted patients frequently have a very low tolerance for pain. Topical application of preservative-added sterile water (which contains benzyl alcohol 0.9% v/v) provides anesthesia to the skin prior to the insertion of intravenous canulae. The advantage of this technique over lidocaine infiltration is the lack of any burning sensation. Because of repeated patient use, most veins are thrombosed or sclerotic, and cannulation of the sub-clavian or internal jugular vein may be immediately preferable. Multiple unsuccessful attempts at cannulation of peripheral veins result only in deterioration of the anesthesiologist-patient relationship.

Induction with thiopental (dosage adjusted according to state of intox-ication and estimation of hepatic function) is probably preferable to use of etomidate or ketamine. Etomidate has recently been implicated in suppression of adrenal cortical function. The effects on the corticosteroid requirement for the stress of surgery have not been adequately studied.

Isoflurane and nitrous oxide can be used for maintenance of anesthesia. Morphine or methadone should be given if signs of withdrawal become manifest or if the procedure lasts more than six hours.

When used in the presence of narcotics, ketamine has a prolonged action and may result in delayed awakening. The incidence of confusional states is also significant in the postoperative period and may make the diagnosis of hypoxia more difficult.

References

1. *Data from the Drug Abuse Warning Network*, 1982 Annual Data, National Institute on Drug Abuse, pp 22, 37, 47.
2. Goth A.: *Medical Pharmacology*. Toronto, CV Mosby Co, 1984, p 561.
3. Stoelting R.K., Creassor C.W., Martz R.C.: Effect of cocaine administration on halothane MAC in dogs. *Anes Analg Curr Res* 54:422, 1975.
4. McGoldrick K.E.: Anesthetic implications of drug abuse. *Anesthesiol Rev* 7:12–17, 1980.
5. Camargo G., Charlotte C.: Pulmonary function studies in ex-heroin users. *Chest* 67(3):331–334, 1975.
6. Aylett P.: Respiratory function in heroin and methadone addicts. *Br J Addict* 73:171–174, 1978.
7. Solalzi R.W., Ward R.J.: The spectrum of medical liability cases. *Internat Anesthesiol Clinics* 22(1):58, 1984.
8. Stimmel B., Lipski J., Swartz M., et al: Electrocardiographic changes in he-roin, methadone and multiple drug abuse. A postulated mechanism of sudden deaths in narcotic addicts. *Natl Conf Methadone Treat Proc* 1:706–710, 1973.
9. Prystan G.H.: Autonomic responsivity to sensory stimulation in drug addicts. *Psychophysiol* 12:170–178, 1975.
10. Gelb A.M., Mildvan D., Stenger R.J.: The spectrum and causes of liver dis-ease in narcotic addicts. *Am J Gastroenterol* 67:314–318, 1977.
11. Louria D.B.: Medical complications of pleasure giving drugs. *Arch Intern Med* 127:82, 1969.
12. Halpern M.: Deaths from narcotics in New York City. *New York State J Med* 66:2391, 1966.
13. Caldwell T. III: Anesthesia for patients with behavioral and environmental disorders, in Katz R. (ed): *Anesthesia and Uncommon Diseases*. Philadelphia, W.B. Saunders, 1981, p. 683.
14. Schreiber S.N., Liebowitz M.R., Bernstein L.: Limb compression and renal

impairment (crush syndrome) following narcotic and sedative overdose. *J Bone Joint Surg* 54(8):1683–1692, 1972.

15. Pastan R.S., Silverman S.L., Goldenberg D.L.: A musculoskeletal syndrome in intravenous heroin users. *Ann Intern Med* 87:22–29, 1977.
16. Challenor Y.B., Brust J.C.M., Baden M.M.: Complications of addiction to heroin. *Bull NY Acad Med* 49(1):4–18, 1973.
17. Ockner R.K.: Acute viral hepatitis, in Wyngaarden J.B., Smith L.H. (eds): *Cecil Textbook of Medicine*. Philadelphia, W.B. Saunders, 1982, vol 1, pp 781–783.
18. Fauci A.S., Macher A.M., Longo D.L. et al: Acquired immune deficiency syndrome: epidemiologic, clinical, immunologic and therapeutic considerations. *Ann Intern Med* 100:92–106.
19. Gotta A.W., Sullivan C.A.: AIDS and the anesthesiologist. *Sphere* (NYSSA) 36:21–22, 1984.

CHAPTER 4

The Child Undergoing Outpatient Surgery*

Nirmala Balan

Case History. *An apparently healthy three-year-old boy was scheduled for bilateral myringotomy and tube insertion as an outpatient. His mother related that she had been told he had a heart murmur. He had reached appropriate milestones without incident. His main complaint was of frequent upper respiratory infections. He breathed through his mouth and snored in his sleep.*

Introduction

Pediatric anesthesia has emerged as a separate and demanding discipline. This is primarily due to increased physician recognition of the anatomic, physiologic, pharmacologic and emotional differences between children and adults. Outpatient surgery, in particular, has gained acceptance in the pediatric population because it not only reduces the cost of treatment, but it also minimizes emotional disturbances by necessitating less disruption of normal routine and less time spent away from home. In addition, there is a reduced incidence of nosocomial infections. Outpatient surgery in children was first reported in a series of 9000 procedures by Nicoll in 1909, although it did not gain much support until 1970 (Wallace Reed, Phoenix).

The preoperative assessment of pediatric outpatients is based upon sound principles of patient care. However, there are considerations unique to the patient population and to outpatient surgery.

Patient Selection

The selection of appropriate pediatric candidates for outpatient surgery is one of the single most important factors that determines a good outcome.

---

*Reviewed by Dr. Kyoung Suh, Associate Professor of Anesthesiology, Albert Einstein College of Medicine of Yeshiva University, Bronx, New York.

Clearly, the performance of complicated procedures, or simple procedures on sick patients in whom complications are a reasonable expectation, have no place in the outpatient setting. Only healthy ASA I* patients, or patients with well-controlled systemic diseases, such as bronchial asthma and epilepsy, are considered suitable.[4]

All age groups may be considered for outpatient surgery, with the notable exception of the expremature infant (less than 37 weeks of gestation at birth). This restriction should be imposed until the child is at least one year of age; the potential immaturity of temperature control and respiratory and gag reflexes predispose these infants to a significantly higher incidence of postoperative complications, even after minor surgery.[5]

Surgery suitable for outpatient care is associated with minimal bleeding and physiologic derangement. Such procedures include myringotomy, adenoidectomy, orchiopexy, herniorrhaphy and circumcision. Four hours is generally considered the upper limit for outpatient surgery.

Parent selection is an important component of patient selection. The parents must be willing and capable of caring for the child after surgery. They should live within a reasonable distance from the hospital (1 hour driving range). Parents should be provided with written instructions for both pre- and postoperative care and informed about the possibility of overnight hospitalization of their child.

Medical Evaluation

The quality of care given to a day surgery patient should be the same as that for an in-hospital surgical patient and should include a thorough preoperative evaluation. Some principles of the preoperative evaluation apply to all patients in all settings. The anesthesiologist must ascertain that the patient is in the best possible physical condition prior to surgery and assess any real or potential anesthetic-surgical problems. A history of drug allergies should be sought. At this time, a personal or familial history of an untoward response to anesthesia should be determined to assess the possibility of malignant hyperthermia. The patient should be classified according to ASA clinical status. And. the requirements for premedication, if any, should be determined. Informed consent must be obtained from the parents or legal guardian.

Other issues particular to the preoperative assessment of children include: The gestational age of the child at birth must be determined in any patient less than one year of age. If the child has a congenital anomaly, other anomalies should be suspected. If congenital heart disease is present, antibiotics should be administered. The NPO status should be determined

---

*American Society of Anesthesiologists clinical status classification, ASA Class I–V.

TABLE 1. Normal range of pulse rate and blood pressure

Age	Pulse rate (per min)	Blood pressure (mmHg) Systolic	Diastolic
Newborn	120–160	60–90	40–50
1 year	80–160	60–100	40–60
4 years	80–120	70–110	50–70
6 years	75–115	85–115	50–70
10 years	70–110	90–115	55–75

and an overnight fast, including milk and formula feedings, maintained. Clear fluids are permitted up to 4 hours before surgery in children less than 6 months of age and up to 6 hours preoperatively in children less than 3 years of age. Water, glucose water, ginger ale, and apple juice are considered clear fluids. Milk and orange juice are not.

These goals can best be accomplished by first obtaining a detailed history. Since a young child may not be a reliable source for information, the parents should be queried. A consult with the child's pediatrician is also valuable, and previous medical records can yield useful information. A thorough physical examination should also be performed. Vital signs and the height and weight of the patient should be recorded on admission to the day care unit. A careful system review, especially of cardiorespiratory function, is necessary.[6]

Cardiovascular System

Normal cardiovascular parameters differ in infants, children and adults. For example, heart rate in the neonatal period is 120 to 140 beats/minute and progressively decreases to 80 beats/minute by age 12. See Table 1. Neonatal cardiac output is twice that of adults. Blood pressure measurement is especially important in the perioperative period because it correlates well with circulating blood volume. The proper width of the blood pressure cuff should equal two-thirds the length of the patient's upper arm.

Sinus arrhythmia is common in children. Occasionally, the parents may inform the anesthesiologist that their child has a heart murmur. Approximately 30% of children may be found to have an "innocent" or "functional" heart murmur on auscultation.[7] These systolic ejection murmurs, heard along the left sternal border, are designated innocent because they are not related to any demonstrable cardiac abnormality. The mechanism is not understood clearly. These children have normal electrocardiographic and x-ray findings.

If a cardiac murmur is detected in a child by history and/or physical examination, it should be investigated further. A history should be elicited from the parents for evidence of cardiac disease in the child, such as failure to thrive, feeding difficulty, tachypnea, dyspnea, recurrent pulmonary infection and cyanosis. The child's pediatrician should also be consulted. Physical examination of the heart and lungs should be performed, including evaluation of the heart rate, blood pressure, skin perfusion and evidence of congestive heart failure. The murmur may require a more complete evaluation by a pediatric cardiologist and include an electrocardiogram and a chest x-ray.

If the murmur is "innocent," nothing further need be done. If a structural heart defect is noted but the child is thriving well with no evidence of congestive heart failure, anesthesia may be safely administered to the patient on an outpatient basis, with perioperative administration of antibiotics as prophylaxis against infective endocarditis.

Respiratory System

The upper airway of children less than five years of age differs anatomically from that of older patients.[8] The tongue is relatively large, the neck is short and the larynx is located more cephalad. The narrowest part of the airway is subglottic at the level of the cricoid cartilage rather than at the glottis, as in adults.

Young children are more susceptible to postintubation complications for the following reasons[9] (in order of decreasing importance):

- Small size of the larynx. In the adult, 1mm of edema produces only slight hoarseness. In the infant, the same amount of edema reduces the lumen by 75% and produces serious airway obstruction.
- Loose areolar tissue in the submucosa of the subglottic area provides a good trap for edematous fluid.
- The cricoid cartilage forms a complete ring.

Thus, children require a particularly careful preoperative evaluation of the upper airway. At this time, the mouth should also be inspected for the presence of any loose teeth. It may be best to remove loose teeth if the parents' permission can be obtained. At the least, they should be notified of the possibility of dislodgement. A note should be made to this effect in the preanesthetic record.

There are also physiologic differences in the respiratory system of children and adults.[10] The number of alveoli in a full-term newborn is approximately 8% that of an adult. The adult value is reached by eight years of age. Tidal volume, expressed in ml/kg, is the same in both children and adults (6–7ml/kg), but the respiratory rate is higher in children. Alveolar ventilation in the newborn is twice that of the adult: V_A is 60ml/kg/min in adults and 100–150 in the newborn.

Children are therefore more susceptible to developing hypoxemia. This risk is due to a higher metabolic rate (higher oxygen consumption) and a larger closing volume. The uptake of inhalation anesthetic agents is also more rapid in children due to a greater alveolar ventilation and an increased proportion of vessel-rich tissues.

The anesthesiologist should question the parents for any history of croup in the child. If such a history is elicited, appropriate management begins with adequate preoperative hydration. Endotracheal intubation should be avoided if the surgical procedure permits. If the trachea is intubated, a smaller-than-normal sized endotracheal tube is indicated. A small leak of gas should be audible around the tube at $15-20cmH_2O$ peak inspiratory pressure. In the recovery room, the child should receive cool humidified oxygen and be closely observed for stridor, hoarsness, croupy cough and intercostal suprasternal retraction.

A problem that is commonly encountered is the child with the "runny nose." Should the elective surgery proceed or be rescheduled? The first step is to determine the etiology of the runny nose, namely whether it is noninfectious or infectious.

The differential diagnosis for a noninfectious runny nose includes allergic and vasomotor rhinitis. Allergic rhinitis (hay fever) usually presents with persistent sneezing and itching of the eyes and nose. It is not accompanied by fever, and the nasal discharge usually does not become purulent. Antihistamines may produce rapid and relatively complete cure. It is important to question the parents about a history of bronchial asthma, as a runny nose may be a prodrome of an asthmatic attack. Vasomotor rhinitis is a benign process and is precipitated by emotional factors or by temperature changes.

For an infectious runny nose, the differential diagnosis includes acute nasopharyngitis, influenza, laryngotracheitis (croup), bacterial infections (eg, pertussis), and a prodrome of exanthematous diseases such as measles. Acute nasopharyngitis, or the common cold, has an annual incidence of 3 to 6 infections.[11] The etiologic agent is viral, most often the rhinovirus.

Nasopharyngitis in children differs clinically from that encountered among older patients in a number of ways. Colds are more severe in young children; the disease is often more extensive and usually involves the paranasal sinuses and the middle ear, as well as the nasopharynx. It is usually accompanied by fever in children, whereas the illness is usually afebrile in adults. Nasal obstruction, secondary to the nasal discharge, can develop quickly, leading to moderate respiratory distress in small infants with relatively greater dependence on nose-breathing. The viral pathogens tend to impair local defense mechanisms; thus, the child is at risk for secondary bacterial infections. There is a higher incidence and severity of purulent complications, including otitis media, sinusitis, pneumonia and communicability (to staff and other patients).

Because the etiology of nasopharyngitis is so varied and because of potential secondary complications, it has been suggested that an upper respiratory tract infection (URI) precludes elective surgery.[12] However, a recent large study suggested that the administration of halothane to patients harboring an acute uncomplicated upper respiratory tract had the ability to beneficially alter the course of that infection by a reduction in both the prevalence and duration of symptoms. In both in vitro and in vivo studies in animals, anesthesia per se had the ability to change the natural course of a viral infection.[13]

It is often possible to differentiate between allergic rhinitis and a URI by history and physical examination. Emphasis should be laid on the following questions: Is the problem acute, chronic or seasonal? Is the patient's appetite normal or decreased? Is the child as active as usual, or does he have behavioral changes with irritability and lethargy? What is the color and the quantity of the nasal discharge? Is there a history of nasal obstruction, cough, fever and earache? A rectal temperature of more than 38°C (100.4°F) is suggestive of infection.

An elevated white cell count ($>$12,000–15,000/mm^3) with a shift to the left (bands $>$500/mm^3) or neutrophilia ($>$10,000/mm^3) suggests a bacterial infection, while an eosinophil count of more than 500/mm^3 suggests an allergic phenomenon.

If, on the basis of history and physical findings, a diagnosis cannot be made, a chest x-ray should be obtained to rule out pneumonia or atelectasis. Sane and co-workers,[14] in a review of preoperative chest radiographs in 1500 children, found totally unsuspected but significant radiographic abnormalities in 4.7%. Postponement of surgery was deemed necessary in 3.8%. When ordering and interpreting an x-ray, however, problems of radiation, cost and technical difficulties in pediatric patients must be considered. Motion and expiration may confuse the interpretation.

If the chest x-ray is abnormal, surgery should be postponed. A normal x-ray, however, does not eliminate the possibility of intraoperative complication due to increased tracheobronchial secretions, a reduced ability to clear these secretions, and bronchial spasm due to increased airway irritability.

If elective surgery has been postponed due to suspected upper respiratory tract infection, when should it be rescheduled? In young adults, abnormalities in pulmonary function (reduced lung volumes and diffusion capacity) can be demonstrated for 4–6 weeks after an uncomplicated flu-like syndrome, even though clinical symptoms have resolved. McGill and colleagues[15] emphasized the possibility of intraoperative complications such as atelectasis, unexplained fever and large alveolar-to-arterial oxygen gradients in children with subacute URIs. They recommended that a specific history of URI symptoms within one month of surgery be sought in all children prior to general anesthesia. Although the optimal period of recovery from a URI prior to rescheduling elective surgery has not been defined, it is probably wise to wait 4–6 weeks.

Psychological Preparation

An important aspect of preoperative care, especially for children, is psychological preparation.[16] Children coming to the hospital for surgery may experience fear of strangers, separation anxiety from home and parents, and fear of castration and death.[1]

Preschool children are primarily afraid of separation, and it may be difficult to persuade them to act against their will.[5] Older children are more aware of their bodies, and the principal threat facing them is fear of bodily injury and death.[17]

Special problems may be posed because of a previous traumatic anesthesia experience. It has been well documented that an unpleasant hospital experience can leave a more serious and longer lasting effect on the child than on the adult.[18] The two events that have the greatest potential for causing psychological trauma to the child scheduled for surgery are the injection of the preoperative medication during the induction of anesthesia.

Hence, when anesthetizing children, the aim should be not only to keep them alive but also to protect them from psychological insults and to keep them smiling. Measures should be taken to win the child's confidence and to allay anxieties and fears during the preoperative visit and at the induction of anesthesia.

During the preoperative interview, it is essential to establish a rapport with the child, to reassure him and win his confidence. If the patient trusts the anesthesiologist, the chance of an atraumatic hospital experience is improved.

All procedures to be undertaken must be explained to the child in simple terms. Verbal communication is possible with children as young as 3 years of age. The phrase "putting to sleep" or "going to sleep" should *never* be used with a child; this phrase may have been employed by adults to explain the death of a pet or family member. Premedication is no substitute for psychological preparation of the child facing anesthesia and surgery.

Many hospitals use pamphlets or a motion picture to explain the hospital experience to children.[19] Children's hospitals have been the innovators in the field of preoperative psychological preparation, and most are happy to explain their procedure to interested parties.

Inhalation induction becomes smooth and successful when the child is cooperative and accepts the technique. This can be facilitated by using a transparent face mask and allowing the child to take along a favorite toy to the OR or induction room. The presence of parents in the induction room can greatly help to allay the child's anxieties.[20]

All attention should be focused on the patient during induction of anesthesia. The child should be engaged in conversation prior to and during induction. Extraneous noises should be kept to a minimum during this critical period.

TABLE 2. Normal values for hemoglobin and hematocrit

Age	Hgb (g/dl)	Hct (%)
Birth	18–20	55 [45–65]
2 weeks	13–20	50 [42–66]
3 months	9.5–14.5	36 [31–41]
6 months–6 years	10.5–14.0	37 [33–42]
7–12 years	11–16	38 [34–40]
Adults	12–18	44 [37–52]

Laboratory Tests

Appropriate preoperative laboratory analyses should be obtained 7 to 10 days prior to surgery. Most patients in good general health will require only a hematocrit and a urinalysis. Normal hemoglobin and hematocrit values for patients of varying ages are listed in Table 2.

Anemic patients are at increased risk for anesthesia and surgery. The oxygen carrying capacity of the blood is decreased. While a hemoglobin value of 4g/dl is sufficient to meet basal oxygen requirements in an adult, the reserve decreases in anemia. This is more problematic in children because of their greater metabolic rate. Because coronary sinus blood is normally very desaturated, in the presence of anemia adequate oxygenation of the heart can be maintained only by increased coronary blood flow. Anemic patients are therefore at risk of cardiac arrest during anesthesia. This increased risk has been confirmed by Salem et al,[21] who retrospectively studied 73 anesthesia-related cardiac arrests in children.

Therefore, any child with a hemoglobin value less than 10g/dl should have elective surgery postponed. The child should be fully investigated and adequately treated before surgery is rescheduled.

Anemia is not a specific disease but rather a manifestation of an underlying pathologic process. In children, anemia is usually due to a dietary iron deficiency.[22] Restoration of normal hemoglobin in response to iron supplementation is rapid, usually 2–3 weeks. Any dark-skinned child presenting with a low hematocrit should be investigated for sickle cell disease. Hypoxemia due to sickling in the perioperative period can have serious consequences. The parents should be questioned for a family history of sickle cell disease or trait. A sickle prep and hemoglobin electrophoresis can be obtained if indicated.

Anesthetic Management

There are two schools of thought on the use of premedication in children who are to undergo outpatient surgery.[23] Some anesthesiologists avoid routine premedication because it can prolong recovery time. At our institu-

TABLE 3. Common drug dosages for pediatric patients

Agent	Average (mg/kg)	Max (mg)
Atropine	0.01–0.02	0.4
Pentobarbital	2–4	100
Secobarbital	2–4	100
Diazepam	0.1–0.2	10
Droperidol	0.05–0.1	
Morphine sulfate	0.05–0.1	10
Meperidine	1.0–1.5	100

tion, because we do not have provisions for parental presence during the induction of anesthesia, we prefer to administer pentobarbital and atropine. In special situations, such as the child coming for repeated operations or a very apprehensive child, administration of a preoperative tranquilizer is extremely useful. Diazepam suspension may be prescribed orally. Our recommendation is that all children should receive a vagal blocking agent prior to or simultaneous with the induction of anesthesia. Common drug dosages for premedication are listed in Table 3.

A frequent complication of outpatient surgery is nausea and vomiting. The incidence is higher in children than adults. Prophylactic administration of droperidol ($75\mu g/kg$) may help reduce postoperative vomiting.[24] If oral intake of fluids becomes a problem, an antiemetic, such as diphenhydramine 2mg/kg IM or rectally, should be prescribed.

Outpatient pediatric surgery offers several advantages and has become very popular. With careful patient selection and skilled anesthetic and surgical care, it is a safe and economical means of performing a variety of surgical procedures.

References

1. Epstein B.S., Hannallah R.: Outpatient anesthesia, in Gregory G. (ed): *Pediatric Anesthesia*, New York: Churchill Livingstone, 1983, chapter 17.
2. Nicoll J.H.: The surgery of infancy. *Br Med J* 2:753, 1909.
3. Reed W.A., Ford J.L.: The surgicenter: An ambulatory surgical facility. *Clin Obstet Gynecol* 17:217–230, 1974.
4. Steward D.J.: Outpatient pediatric anesthesia. *Anesthesiology* 43:268–276, 1975.
5. Steward D.J.: Preterm infants are more prone to complications following minor surgery than are term infants. *Anesthesiology* 56:304–306, 1982.
6. Hackel A.: Preoperative evaluation, in Gregory G. (ed): *Pediatric Anesthesia*, New York, Churchill Livingstone, 1983, chapter 12.
7. Kaplan S.: Evaluation of the heart and circulation in health and disease, in *Nelson Textbook of Pediatrics*, Philadelphia, WB Saunders Co, 1975, p 1002.
8. Eckenhoff J.E.: Some anatomical considerations of the infant larynx influencing endotracheal anesthesia. *Anesthesiology* 12:401–410, 1951.

9. Koka B.V., Jeon I.S., Andre J.M., et al: Postinduction croup in children. *Anesth Analg* 56:501–505, 1977.
10. Pang L.M., Mellins R.B.: Neonatal cardiorespiratory physiology. *Anesthesiology* 43:171–192, 1975.
11. Eichenwald H.F., McCracken G.H.: Infections of the upper respiratory tract, in *Nelson Textbook of Pediatrics*, Philadelphia, WB Saunders Co, 1975, pp 939–942.
12. Rockoff M.A.: Pre-existing medical conditions in pediatric anesthesia. American Society of Anesthesiologists Annual Refresher Course Lectures, 1982.
13. Tait A.R., Knight P.R.: Anesthesia and the common cold: Why not sleep on it? *Anesthesiology* 65:3A–A492, 1986.
14. Sane S.M., Worsing R.A., Wiens C.W., et al: Value of preoperative chest x-ray examinations in children. *Pediatrics* 60:669–672, 1977.
15. McGill W.A., Coveler L.A., Epstein B.S.: Subacute upper respiratory infection in small children. *Anesth Analg* 58:331–333, 1979.
16. Lockhart C.H.: Preoperative preparation of the child for hospitalization, anesthesia and surgery. American Society of Anesthesiologists Annual Refresher Course Lectures, 1984.
17. Korsch B.M.: The child and the operating room. *Anesthesiology* 43:251–257, 1975.
18. Eckenhoff J.E.: Relationship of anesthesia to postoperative personality changes in children. *Am J Dis Child* 86:587, 1953.
19. Epstein B.S.: Induction of anesthesia in the pediatric patient. American Society of Anesthesiologists Annual Refresher Course Lectures, 1984.
20. Schulman J.L., Foley J.M., et al: A study of the effect of the mother's presence during anesthesia induction. *Pediatrics* 39:111–114, 1967.
21. Salem M.R., Bennet E.L., Schweiss J.F., et al: Cardiac arrest related to anesthesia. Contributing factors in infants and children. *JAMA* 233:238–241, 1975.
22. Pearson H.A.: The Anemias, in *Nelson Textbook of Pediatrics*, Philadelphia, WB Saunders Co, 1975, pp 1116–1118.
23. Rita L., Seleny F.L.: Pediatric outpatient anesthesia premedication versus no premedication and the choice of anesthetic agent. *Anesthesiol Rev* August 1974, p 9–13.
24. Abramowitz M.D., Oh T.H., Epstein B.S.: The antiemetic effect of droperidol following outpatient strabismus surgery in children. *Anesthesiology* 59:579–583, 1983.

CHAPTER 5

The Patient Undergoing Renal Transplantation*

Rhoda Levine

Case History. *The patient is a 27-year-old man scheduled for renal transplantation. He has a history of glomerulonephritis at age 8, with progressive renal failure that has required dialysis for the past 5 years. He is virtually anuric. He undergoes hemodialysis 3 times a week and was last dialyzed 2 days ago. He has been hospitalized several times for placement of A-V fistulae and currently has a functioning Gore-Tex graft in his left arm. He has a 10-year history of hypertension for which he is taking methyldopa. It is now midnight; he ate a full dinner at 8 PM.*

Physical exam reveals blood pressure 160/100; pulse 98/min; respiration 20/min; temperature 37.1°C; weight 150lb; height 5'4". The chest is clear and heart sounds are normal. Thrill is present at the fistula in the left upper extremity. Dentition is intact.

Laboratory findings include: Hgb 8.5g%; Hct 25%; WBC 10,000, with normal differential; PT 11/11.5; PTT 30/29.5; Na^+ 136mEq/L; K^+ 5.2mEq/L; CO_2 18mmHg; BUN 116mg%; glucose 116mg%; creatinine 6.1mg%.

Introduction

Renal transplantation is a 20th century phenomenon. The first transplants were performed in 1902 between dogs. The animals survived several days with their functioning grafts, long enough to be exhibited at scientific meetings. These efforts proved that renal transplantation was technically feasible. In the early 1900s there were several attempts at renal heterotransplantation into humans, all of which failed. The first successful human transplant was performed in Boston in 1947 on a patient with acute tubular necrosis. The transplant functioned for four days, which proved sufficient time for the patient's own kidneys to recover.

---

*Reviewed by Dr. Sherman Levine, Professor of Medicine and Physiology, Albert Einstein College of Medicine of Yeshiva University, Bronx, New York.

TABLE 1. Long-term graft survival in renal transplantation (%)

	1 year	2 years	3 years
Human Transplant Registry			
Cadaver	46	41	40
Parent	66	62	57
Sibling	72	72	68
HLA Identical Sibling	85	78	
Krakauer et al			
Cadaver	56	—	45
Related	76	—	69

The dialysis machine was introduced in Europe in 1948 and came into extensive use in the U.S. in 1950. Patients with chronic renal failure could now be maintained in reasonable metabolic balance for prolonged periods of time. As the medical and psychological problems of chronic dialysis became known, investigators once again turned to transplantation. The first series of human transplants was performed in the early 1950s, but there were no long-term survivors as the process of rejection was not well understood. In 1956, a kidney was successfully transplanted between identical twins. By 1962, it was possible to suppress immune mechanisms with drugs and radiation which permitted successful allotransplantation from an unrelated donor.

According to the 13th report of the Human Transplant Registry,[1] graft survival is optimal when the kidney is donated by a monozygotic twin. Less favorable results are obtained when the donor is a sibling or parent. Cadaver grafts have slightly less than a 50% chance of functioning for one year after transplantation. See Table 1.

Graft survival rates have shown some improvement over the last 10 years. Pooled reports from the Human Transplant Registry, worldwide data, and a recent study in the U.S.[2] indicate improvement in both cadaveric and related graft survival from 1977 to 1981. Long-term patient survival was better in patients whose grafts functioned well than in patients who required dialysis postoperatively. One-year patient survival now approaches 98% in most centers. Deaths are primarily due to sepsis, which is a complication of immunosuppression.

Graft Preservation

A major factor influencing graft survival is the time between removal of the kidney from the donor and restoration of perfusion in the recipient. In transplantation from a live donor, this interval can be kept to a minimum by coordinating the two operations. Where cadaver kidneys are to be used, the organ must be cooled to allow time for tissue typing, transportation in most cases, and surgical preparation of the recipient site.

Initially, donor kidneys were irrigated with cold Collins' solution and placed in a sterile bag in a container of iced slush. Later, machines were designed to perfuse cadaver kidneys with cold electrolyte solution. Pressures and flow rates could then be measured as well as "urine" volume to give some indication of renal function. Poorly functioning kidneys could be identified, more thorough histocompatibility testing could be undertaken, and time made available for selection of the most compatible recipient and optimal preoperative preparation. The outcome of transplantation has remained good with up to 72 hours of perservation in either pulsatile perfusion or cold slush solution. More investigation will be needed, however, as a perfusion-related nephropathy and endothelial damage have been reported in machine perfused kidneys.[3, 4]

Indications for Transplantation

Chronic renal failure (CRF) may be successfully treated with either dialysis (hemodialysis or peritoneal dialysis) or transplantation. Transplantation is often seen as a positive alternative to dialysis. The patient is no longer physically or psychologically dependent on a machine, is more mobile and can return to school or work. Dietary restrictions can be relaxed. There is the expectation that fertility will be restored and libido improved. Children can resume a normal growth pattern. Neuropathy and osteodystrophy should regress and anemia decrease.

But transplantation has disadvantages. There is a minimal but measurable operative mortality and morbidity. Instead of a machine, patients are now dependent on lifelong immunosuppressive medications, with all their potential complications. Additional surgery may be required, eg, for secondary hyperparathyroidism, slipped femoral epiphysis, bowel obstruction. The graft may fail or be rejected.

Most transplant recipients are chronic dialysis patients. Criteria for eligibility for transplantation are formulated by each transplant center. However, patients with severe cardiovascular disease, psychosis unrelated to uremia, and those with renal diseases known to attack the transplanted kidney (eg, oxalosis) are generally considered ineligible. Also, patients with metastatic disease are not good candidates since immunosuppressive drugs decrease the body's defenses against tumors and will hasten growth and spread of the latter.

Pathophysiology

Transplant recipients usually have little or no renal function. Pathophysiologic changes in the patient scheduled for transplantation are related to functions that the kidneys can no longer perform. See Table 2.

TABLE 2. Pathophysiologic changes in the patient
with advanced renal failure

Cardiovascular
Hypertension
Volume overload
CHF
Peripheral edema
Pulmonary congestion and edema

Metabolic
Hyperkalemia
Acidosis

Musculoskeletal
Calcium deficiency
Seconday hyperparathyroidism
Prone to fractures

Neurologic
Peripheral neuropathy
Cerebral edema
Confusion, coma, convulsions

Hematologic
Anemia— ↓ RBC synthesis
          ↑ RBC destruction
          Bleeding

Gastrointestinal
Bleeding
Nausea and vomiting

Immunologic
Prone to infection

Cardiovascular

Volume overload resulting in congestive heart failure, edema, hypertension, and pericardial and pleural effusions are common in patients with end-stage renal disease. Hypertension is often the result of inability to excrete salt and water, but it may be primary and the etiology of the renal failure. Blood pressure is often adequately controlled by dialysis alone; however, antihypertensive medication may be neceasary. These agents alter the responsiveness of the autonomic nervous system both to normal homeostatic stimuli and to administered drugs. Morbidity is increased if hypertension is poorly controlled (diastolic blood pressure >110mmHg).

Antihypertensive therapy should not be discontinued in the perioperative period. Reserpine and guanethidine deplete peripheral catecholamine stores and reduce the response to indirect-acting vasopressors (eg, ephedrine) but increase sensitivity to exogenous norepinephrine. Clonidine and methyldopa are centrally acting α-adrenergic agonists; abrupt discontinuation may cause rebound hypertension, especially in the postoperative period. Several mechanisms have been proposed for the efficacy of β-adrenergic blocking agents (eg, propranolol) in the management of hypertension. In any case and whatever the relationship, decreased blood pressure is accompanied by decreased cardiac output, impairment of norepinephrine release following sympathetic nerve stimulation, and, frequently, by decreased secretion of renin. Patients on chronic β-blocker therapy may be unable to increase their heart rate in response to volume depletion, hypoglycemia, or other sympathetic stimuli. Therefore, a slow, stable heart rate cannot always be regarded as a reassuring sign.

Anephric patients may develop hyponatremia from water overload. This can occur when sodium-containing fluid losses (gastrointestinal, edematous fluid sequestered in traumatized tissue) are replaced only with water. It is best treated by restricting infusion of free water. If the patient is symptomatic (confused, lethargic, convulsing) dialysis is indicated. If no access is available, hypertonic saline can be administered at 50ml/hour up to a total of 200ml. Actual seizure activity is treated with anticonvulsants. Hypernatremia is most commonly the result of water depletion; it should thus be treated by increasing the amount of free water administered to the patient.

Electrolytes and Nitrogenous Wastes

Perioperative hyperkalemia occurs in the presence of large potassium loads, eg, from cellular breakdown and blood transfusion. A serum potassium of 5.5mEq/L is associated with an increased risk of life-threatening arrhythmias. Electrocardiographic evidence of hyperkalemia includes T-wave peaking with modest elevations, loss of P-waves, and widening of QRS complexes. These changes become more pronounced with increased hyperkalemia. As cardiac muscle function is impaired, cardiac output is severely compromised. The most rapid treatment is a slow infusion of 10–20ml 10% calcium chloride. This should be reserved for the patient with severe hyperkalemia (≥7.5mEq/L). Calcium infusion does not alter serum potassium concentrations, but it does decrease the neuromuscular irritability associated with hyperkalemia. ECG monitoring should be continuous, particularly in the patient who is receiving digitalis and who may respond to calcium infusion with an increase in the frequency of digitalis-related arrhythmias (eg, premature ventricular contractions). The effects of calcium infusions are rapid (5 min), but short-lived, and more definitive treatment should be begun immediately. Administration of 50ml 50% glucose with 10 units of regular insulin to transfer potassium intracellularly is indicated for potassium levels in excess of 7.5mEq/L. If acidosis is also present in the normovolemic patient, infusions of sodium bicarbonate at a rate of 1 ampoule (44mEq) per hour for 2 to 3 hours are beneficial. However, the potassium returns to extracellular fluid after several hours. Removal of potassium from the body is accomplished by dialysis or by the use of cation exchange resins administered orally or rectally (eg, Kayexalate®) to slowly exchange sodium for potassium in the gastrointestinal tract.

Hypocalcemia is frequent in patients with advanced renal failure and is secondary to abnormal vitamin D metabolism and decreased intestinal absorption. Calcium levels usually return to normal after several months of dialysis.

Inability to excrete nitrogenous wastes causes confusion, disorientation, and ultimately coma.

Acidosis

Metabolic acidosis is relatively benign at a bicarbonate level of 15mEq/L or greater, although it prolongs the effect of nondepolarizing neuromuscular blocking agents (tubocurarine and pancuronium) and decreases buffer reserve. Acidosis may be treated with sodium bicarbonate (1 ampoule will increase plasma bicarbonate in a 70kg person by about 1mEq/L). However, sodium overload may occur.

Hematologic Status

The anemia of chronic renal disease is caused by decreased erythrocyte synthesis, which in turn is likely due to decreased renal erythropoietin synthesis and shortened erythrocyte life (hemolysis is increased in uremia). Unstressed patients may tolerate hemoglobin levels as low as 5g%; however, oxygen carrying capacity is markedly reduced. Tachycardia often compensates to normalize oxygen delivery to tissues. Peripheral oxygen delivery is impaired because 2, 3-DPG levels do not increase in these patients.[5] However, this effect is probably offset by metabolic acidosis. Perioperative decreases in cardiac output attributable to myocardial depressant drugs (eg, anesthetic agents) or increases in tissue oxygen requirements (shivering and hyperthermia) may severely compromise tissue oxygenation. The anemic patient requires supplemental oxygen.

Although blood transfusion is not without risks (volume overload transfusion reactions, and transmission of hepatitis and AIDS) it is often necessary in the patient scheduled for renal transplantation. Hemoglobin levels of 10g/dl are often necessary to provide adequate oxygen-carrying capacity for transplant surgery.

Preanesthetic Evaluation

Interview

Evaluation of the following areas during the preanesthetic interview is particularly important in the patient who presents for renal transplantation.

TABLE 3. Medications commonly taken by patients
with end-stage renal disease

Antibiotics
Antidepressants
Antihypertensives
Bicarbonate
Digitalis
Diuretics
Immunosuppressives
Ion exchange resins
Steroids
Vitamins

- Previous surgery and/or anesthesia. Any complications related to the renal disease should be documented.
- Medications the patient is taking chronically. Table 3 lists medications commonly involved. Antihypertensive medications and steroids should be continued up to the time of surgery. β-blocking agents should be continued, but the observation that labetalol and halothane may cause severe myocardial depression should be noted.[6]
- Exercise tolerance. An estimate should be made since this is a good indicator of cardiovascular and pulmonary reserve and indicates tolerance to anemia.
- Diabetes mellitus. If the patient has diabetes, it is important to monitor blood glucose and potassium. Life-threatening hyperkalemia in diabetic patients receiving renal transplants has been reported.[7,8]
- Time of last dialysis. Hemodialysis should be performed at least 6–8 hours before surgery to allow equilibration between the intravascular and extracellular fluid compartments. Clotting time should be evaluated before surgery in patients who receive heparin during hemodialysis and should be within normal limits. Patients who receive peritoneal dialysis can continue their exchanges until just prior to the transplant.

Physical Examination

Important issues to consider during the physical exam are listed in Table 4. These include:

- Blood pressure. The recipient's blood pressure should be well controlled. This ensures a smoother anesthetic course and decreases the chance that hypertension will endanger the vascular anastomoses.
- Infection. There should be no evidence of either bacterial or viral infection (eg, URI) since large doses of immunosuppressant agents will be administered postoperatively.
- The location and status of the dialysis access should be evaluated to ensure adequate protection and monitoring during surgery.

TABLE 4. Important areas to be evaluated during the physical examination

---

Blood pressure
Heart rate
Temperature
Dialysis access
Cardiac status
Neuropathies
Fluid status

- A thorough neurological exam should be performed and any preoperative neuropathy documented. The presence of neuropathy may affect the choice of anesthetic technique.
- The state of hydration should be evaluated. Volume status in these patients is variable. Evidence of congestive heart failure (eg, râles, edema) is not uncommon when volume intake has been excessive. On the other hand, volume may be depleted immediately postdialysis. This, plus a labile cardiovascular response to anesthesia, may cause hypotension after induction, especially in the patient who receives inhalation agents or after regional blockade. Therefore, the weight loss during the last dialysis must be known and compared with the "stable" or "ideal" weight.

Laboratory Evaluation

Laboratory evaluation of the patient for renal transplant is outlined in Table 5. An SMA-6 analysis is mandatory. Potassium values should be 3.0–4.5mEq/L. Arrhythmias are more frequent in the presence of both hyper- and hypokalemia. Hyperkalemia is more likely because perioperative events provide a potassium load (eg, blood transfusion, tissue damage, washout of potassium from the graft). Disturbances of serum sodium indicate the necessity for correction in electrolyte replacement during surgery. Acid-base status can be estimated from bicarbonate levels.

The serum calcium concentration should be obtained. Hypocalcemia may decrease myocardial contractility and depress neuromuscular function.

TABLE 5. Laboratory parameters to be measured in the patient with chronic renal failure

---

K^+, HCO_3^-, Na^+
Ca^{++}
BUN, creatinine
Hgb, Hct, Platelets, WBC, bleeding time
Chest x-ray—heart size, vasculature, effusions
EKG—rate, rhythm, K^+ effects

Although BUN and creatinine will be reported, the absolute values of these parameters have little influence on anesthetic management.

Most transplant recipients are anemic. If the patient has been transfused during preoperative dialysis, postdialysis hemoglobin and hematocrit levels may be inaccurate because equilibrium may not be complete for several hours. The degree of acceptable anemia varies; most centers require a clinically tolerated anemia, assessed by the ability to exercise, rather than an absolute number. As patients with end-stage renal disease may have platelet dysfunction, a bleeding time should be recorded. Platelet transfusion is rarely needed.

A chest x-ray should be evaluated for evidence of cardiac failure. The ECG tracing may indicate prior myocardial damage, left ventricular hypertrophy and strain from chronic hypertension or arrhythmias, and can correlate with hyperkalemia.

Anesthetic Management

The amount and type of preanesthetic medication depend on the physical status of the patient, extent of surgery (with or without nephrectomy), duration of surgery, and anesthetic technique. Anticholinergic agents do not alter renal function. Their use depends on the type of anesthesia planned and personal preference of the anesthesiologist.

Barbiturates and opioids can be used in doses that do not cause respiratory or circulatory depression. Tranquilizers such as diazepam are frequently considered "ideal" premedication in patients presenting for renal transplantation. Care should be taken when using droperidol or Innovar®; preoperative confusion has been associated with use of these drugs.[9]

Virtually all currently available anesthetic agents and techniques have been used in the management of patients for renal transplantation. Depending on the preferences of the individual anesthesiologist and any special medical or surgical conditions that may be present, the risks and options for anesthetic management should be explained to the patient to ensure informed consent.

More than 5,000 renal transplant operations are performed in the United States each year. Thanks to improved preservation techniques, the transplant recipient can now be adequately and safely prepared for "urgent" rather than "emergency" surgery.

References

1. The 13th Report of the Human Transplant Registry. *Transplantation Proceedings* 9:9–26, 1977.
2. Krakauer H., Grauman J.S., McMullan M.R., et al: The recent U.S. experience in the treatment of end-stage renal disease by dialysis and transplantation. *N Engl J Med* 308:1558–1563, 1983.

3. Anderson N., Wylie R., Williams G.M.: Structural and metabolic changes in "preserved" renal allografts. *Surg Forum* 24:332–334, 1973.
4. Spector D., Limas C., Frost J.L., et al: Perfusion nephropathy in human transplants. *N Engl J Med* 295:1217–1221, 1976.
5. Lichtman M.A., Murphy M.S., Bayer B.J., et al: Hemoglobin affinity for oxygen in chronic renal disease. The effect of hemodialysis. *Blood* 43:417–424, 1974.
6. Hunter J.M.: Synergism between halothane and labetalol. *Anaesthesia* 34:257–259, 1979.
7. Charters P.: Renal transplantation in diabetes mellitus. *Anaesthesia* 35:199–204, 1984.
8. Hirshman C.A., Edelstein G.: Intraoperative hyperkalemia and cardiac arrest during renal transplantation in an insulin-dependent diabetic patient. *Anesthesiology* 51:161–162, 1979.
9. Zauder H.L.: Anesthesia for patients who have terminal renal disease, in Hershey S.G. (ed): *Refresher Courses in Anesthesiology*. Philadelphia, J.B. Lippincott Co, 1976, Vol 4, pp 163–173.

CHAPTER 6

The Patient with Pheochromocytoma*

Richard B. Patt

Case History. *A 48-year-old Hispanic woman was scheduled for excision of an adrenal pheochromocytoma. Three years prior to admission, she developed brief episodes of diaphoresis and feelings of hot and cold. Because the onset of symptoms coincided with irregular menses, her complaints were attributed to menopause.*

Six months prior to admission, she developed an upper respiratory tract infection, and the bouts of diaphoresis became more pronounced. She also complained of palpitations, blanching of her hands, and dizziness. She was noted to be hypertensive and was treated with methyldopa, which was later discontinued when her hypertension had abated.

A week prior to admission, after a second upper respiratory tract infection, there was increased diaphoresis, palpitations, and hypertension. Hydrochlorothiazide and timolol were prescribed. One hour after taking timolol for the first time, she developed sudden nausea, vomiting, diaphoresis, and dizziness. She was seen in the emergency room, and electrocardiographic findings of sinus tachycardia prompted admission to the coronary care unit.

Symptoms continued, and she remained tachycardic (100–120 beats per minute) and mildly hypertensive (150/100). ECG tracings showed widespread markedly depressed S-T segments and inverted T waves. There was no chest pain, and serial cardiac enzymes were normal. A nuclear ejection fraction was calculated at 27%, and an echocardiogram showed diffuse hypokinesis. She had one episode of supraventricular tachycardia, which responded promptly to 5mg I.V. verapamil.

A 24-hour urine collection was obtained, and catecholamine studies showed: norepinephrine 745μg (normal 20–83μg); epinephrine 257μg (normal <20μg); vanillylmandelic acid 26.9mg (normal <7mg); total metanephrines 7.1mg (normal 0–0.9mg). Plasma catecholamine levels were not

---

*Reviewed by Dr. Ruth Freeman, Associate Professor of Medicine, Gynecology and Obstetrics, Albert Einstein College of Medicine of Yeshiva University, Bronx, New York.

available. Computerized axial tomography revealed a 5cm × 6cm partially necrotic mass in the left adrenal gland, consistent with pheochromocytoma.

The patient was given phenoxybenzamine 10mg twice daily. Dosage was increased to 40mg twice daily, and propanolol 10mg four times a day was added. She was discharged pending surgery. ECG reevaluation 2 weeks later revealed persistent T wave inversion. A repeat echocardiogram showed an ejection fraction of 87%. Ventricular function was normal, but several areas of localized hypokinesis of the lateral wall of the left ventricle persisted. Excision of the pheochromocytoma was scheduled electively.

Pathophysiology

Pheochromocytoma is a catecholamine secreting tumor made up of cells, pheochromocytes, that are ordinarily found in the adrenal medulla. The tumor received its name because it is selectively colored by chromium salts. Pheochromocytes are derived embryonically from the neuroectoderm. They have the capacity to take up and decarboxylate certain biologic amines (the Amine Precursor Uptake and Decarboxylation system, or APUD). Pheochromocytomas, like adrenal carcinoid tumors, are thought to arise because of derangement in this system. The tumors vary in size from 1 to 4000 grams and average about 100 grams.

Histologically, it is difficult to differentiate between the benign and malignant forms of pheochromocytoma. The only certain criterion for malignant disease is the presence of metastases. Clinically, the disease is characterized by hypertension that is either episodic or sustained. In 95% of cases, the tumor is abdominal. Ninety percent are located in the adrenal medulla, and 10% are bilateral. Most of the remainder are found in the sympathetic chain or bladder wall. Twenty percent of patients have functional tumors in multiple sites. Less than 10% are malignant. Malignancy is characterized by local invasiveness, and distant spread. Age range is from infancy to old age. One third of reported cases occur in children. Occasionally it may be familial or part of a constellation of endocrine abnormalities, variously termed Multiple Endocrine Adenopathy (MEA) or Multiple Endocrine Neoplasia (MEN). See Table 1.

There is an increased incidence of pheochromocytoma associated with other neuroectodermal dysplasias, including mucosal neuromas, neurofibromatosis, Sturge-Weber disease, tuberous sclerosis, and Lindau-Van Hippel disease.

The hallmark of pheochromocytoma is hypertension. The hypertension may be persistent or paroxysmal, but only rarely is it absent. Yet, the incidence of pheochromocytoma in the hypertensive population is less than 0.1%. The classic triad of symptoms for pheochromocytoma is headache (characteristically severe and pounding), palpitations (with or without tachycardia) and diaphoresis. In a recent series of 76 patients with

TABLE 1. Stages of multiple endocrine adenopathy (MEA) or multiple endocrine neoplasia (MEN)

MEA/MEN I (Werner's syndrome)	islet cell tumors of the pancreas (Zollinger-Ellison syndrome) parathyroid adenoma or hyperplasia pituitary tumor carcinoid syndrome (no pheochromocytoma)
MEA/MEN II or IIA (Sipple's syndrome)	pheochromocytoma medullary thyroid cancer parathyroid adenoma or hyperplasia
MEA/MEN III or IIB	pheochromocytoma thickened corneal nerves Marfanold habitus alimentary tract ganglioneuromatosis

pheochromocytoma, all but three had one or more of the above symptoms, and in 55 patients at least two symptoms were present.[1] In another series, the absence of these three symptoms in the presence of hypertension ruled out pheochromocytoma in 99.9% of cases.[2] Other symptoms include nausea, vomiting, chest or abdominal pain, tremulousness, anxiety, personality changes, and visual disturbances. Flushing is rare. The symptoms of pheochromocytoma may mimic chronic anxiety or depression.

About 50% of pheochromocytoma patients have sustained hypertension, with or without intermittent exacerbations. Normotension with paroxysmal hypertension is present in about 50% of patients, usually accompanied by the triad of symptoms listed above. In the paroxysmal group, the incidence of attacks varies from several times per month to several times daily. Duration may be minutes or hours (usually less than one hour). Severity of symptoms tends to correlate with the degree of hypertension, and episodes are characteristically followed by fatigue.

Even in the absence of symptoms, pheochromocytoma should be strongly considered in the presence of the following conditions: 1) malignant hypertension; 2) hypertension refractory to treatment; 3) paradoxical hypertensive response to antihypertensive medications; 4) unexplained hypertension during the induction of anesthesia or during surgery; 5) hypertension associated with parturition; 6) hypertension associated with imipramine or desipramine therapy.

Progressive weight loss, hyperglycemia, angina, and cardiomyopathy are frequent associated findings. Orthostatic hypotension has two etiologies: intravascular volume is decreased secondary to a chronic high level of sympathetic tone; and, excessive sympathetic tone prevents further reflex catecholamine-mediated vasoconstriction in response to position changes.

Death from pheochromocytoma is usually due to congestive heart failure, acute myocardial infarction, or intracerebral hemorrhage.

Diagnosis

History provides a high index of suspicion, but definitive diagnosis rests on biochemical confirmation of excess catecholamine production. The most widely used tests are analysis of 24-hour urine collections for excretion of free catecholamines (epinephrine and norepinephrine) and their metabolites (vanillylmandelic acid and total metanephrines). These tests are relatively easy to perform and are readily available. However, collecting reliable specimens on an outpatient basis (especially in pediatric patients) is difficult. Catecholamine analyses correlate with creatinine content from 2- and 4-hour collections and have recently been reported to be as accurate as 24-hour specimens.[3] Accuracy of results is contingent on good renal function and on levels of metabolizing enzymes (monoamine oxidase, catechol-o-methyltransferase) within the tumor.

Of the urinary indices, an abnormally elevated level of total metanephrines correlates best with the presence of pheochromocytoma, and vanillylmandelic acid level is the least sensitive test.[4] In most circumstances, the diagnosis can be confirmed or excluded by urine analysis, but current studies show that urinary tests are less accurate than properly performed serum assays of catecholamines.[5] If results of biochemical testing are equivocal, they may be repeated.

Provocative and suppression tests are used infrequently to diagnose pheochromocytoma because of associated risks, but they may be considered in some patients in whom the results of biochemical testing are repeatedly equivocal. Provocative tests are particularly hazardous because of induction of catecholamine release. They are usually reserved for patients with highly suggestive symptoms and normal or only slightly elevated blood pressure (diastolic pressure ≤ 100 mmHg). The glucagon stimulation test has been found to have fewer side effects than testing with histamine or tyramine, and it is now the most widely used provocative test.

Suppression tests are indicated for normo- or hypertensive patients with elevated levels of catecholamines. Clonidine, which has been used recently with success,[4] lowers blood pressure by a central α_2-adrenergic effect. Ordinarily, increases in plasma catecholamines are mediated by activation of the sympathetic nervous system. In contrast, catecholamine excess in the presence of pheochromocytoma is due to tumor production, and normal storage and release mechanisms are bypassed. Following the administration of clonidine to patients with pheochromocytoma, catecholamine levels remain unaltered, while suppression occurs uniformly in other patients. In both normal and pheochromocytoma patients, clonidine administration will lower blood pressure, and hypotension is a hazard.[5] Prior insertion of an intravenous line is required, and initial treatment of hypotension is with volume expansion. If hypotension is persistent, one of several vasopressors may be used (phenylephrine, metaraminol, dopamine). This test should not be performed in the presence of volume depletion or β-

blockade. Pentolinium has similar effects on plasma catecholamine levels, but it may cause urinary retention, and is not available in the United States.

Preoperative Preparation

Meticulous diagnosis and preoperative preparation are essential for the patient with pheochromocytoma. Morbidity and mortality in undiagnosed, unprepared patients who are undergoing surgery for other procedures is unacceptably high, especially during the induction of anesthesia.[6]

If a pheochromocytoma is identified, familial screening should be carried out. Definitive therapy is surgical excision. Preoperative noninvasive localizing studies, such as ultrasonography or computed tomography, are generally performed. In general, invasive or stressful studies (arteriogram, intravenous pyelography, selective adrenal vein sampling for catecholamines) are avoided because stress may precipitate a hypertensive crisis.[7] These patients are already volume depleted, and the use of highly concentrated dyes, such as those employed for intravenous pyelography, can cause hyperosmolar dehydration and precipitate renal shutdown or a crisis. Consultation with an endocrinologist and preoperative medical preparation are mandatory to insure maximum preoperative cardiovascular stability.

Patients with pheochromocytoma are, as a rule, volume depleted. Elevated plasma catecholamine levels primarily produce α-adrenergic stimulation, and the result is persistent, generalized vasoconstriction and hypovolemia. Alpha-adrenergic blockade is the most accepted form of preoperative intervention. It attenuates catecholamine-induced vasoconstriction and thereby reduces blood pressure and restores normal circulating volume. Reduced hematocrit is an early sign of intravascular volume restoration.

Adequate α-blockade is desirable because preoperative volume repletion and normotension will reduce the risk of intraoperative hypertension. Phenoxybenzamine, a long-acting oral α-adrenergic blocking agent, may be administered in doses between 20mg and 60mg daily, up to 250mg per day. Prazosin, which acts, at postsynaptic α-adrenergic receptor sites and by directly relaxing vascular smooth muscle, is also used.

There is some controversy regarding the degree of α blockade that is optimal and whether these drugs should be administered through the morning of surgery. Complete α-blockade may attenuate the hypotension that usually follows tumor isolation; hypotension at this point is ordinarily interpreted as a sign of complete tumor extirpation. Also, total α-blockade theoretically may block the patient's hypertensive response, which is of diagnostic value in surgical exploration for a second tumor. It has been suggested that α-blocking agents be continued on the day of surgery, but that the dose be reduced or deleted in patients in whom the tumor's location is uncertain or who may have multiple tumors. Prophylactic transfusion of packed red blood cells 12–18 hours preoperatively has been suggested as an alternative method to replete intravascular volume.[8]

Most patients require a minimum of 10–14 days of α-blocking therapy. Desired end results are control of blood pressure, mild orthostasis, resolution of ST-T wave abnormalities, and absent or rare premature ventricular contractions. Epinephrine and, to a lesser extent, norepinephrine are glucagon-like, and the levels associated with pheochromocytoma are sufficient to produce moderate elevations in serum glucose levels via glycogenolysis and fatty acid mobilization. Adequate α-adrenergic blockade blunts this effect and makes intraoperative hyperglycemia less likely.

Cardiomyopathy or myocarditis frequently accompanies pheochromocytoma and is generally attributed to the effects of long-term hyperstimulation by catecholamines. Manifestations include ST-T wave abnormalities, cardiac dysrhythmias, and signs and symptoms of congestive heart failure. ST-T wave abnormalities attributable to myocarditis usually resolve with a 2-week to 6-month course of α-adrenergic blocking therapy.

The case history presented illustrates the salutary effects of preoperative α-adrenergic blockade, increased ejection fraction and exercise tolerance. Persistent tachycardia or dysrhythmias are indications for adjunctive β-blockade. Beta-blockade is contraindicated in the absence of α-blockade. A heart depressed by β-adrenergic blockers may not be able to maintain adequate cardiac output should unopposed α-mediated vasoconstriction from the release of catecholamines result in abrupt increases of systemic vascular resistance and afterload.[9] In the case presented, before the diagnosis of pheochromocytoma had been considered, a single dose of a β-blocker prior to α-blockade resulted in crisis.

Anesthetic Management

Despite optimal preparation of the patient for surgery, the anesthesiologist must anticipate cardiovascular instability, especially during induction, laryngoscopy, tumor manipulation, and clamping of the tumor's venous drainage. Hemodynamic changes are generally due to catecholamine excess, or, in the case of the hypotension seen with surgical isolation of the tumor, depletion. An anesthetic plan should be formulated to minimize sympathetic stimulation, and to deal rapidly and effectively with its sequelae.

The preoperative visit and premedication are essential to relieve anxiety. As was noted earlier, stress can precipitate a hypertensive crisis in a patient with pheochromocytoma.

In addition to standard monitoring, additional modes should include the 5-lead ECG, and intraarterial and pulmonary arterial cannulations to

TABLE 2. Vasoactive and cardioactive compounds that should be available for surgery for a pheochromocytoma patient

Agent	Dose	Preparation
Hypotensive Agents		
Nitroprusside	0.25–4.0μg/kg/min	50mg/250ml D$_5$W (0.02%)
Phentolamine	1–5mg boluses or 0.5–20μg/kg/min	25mg/250ml D$_5$W (0.01%)
Nitroglycerine	0.25–5.0μg/kg/min	50mg/250ml D$_5$W (0.02%)
Trimethaphan	2.5–30μg/kg/min	500mg/250ml D$_5$W (0.2%)
Hypertensive Agents		
Dopamine	2–30μg/kg/min	200mg/500ml D$_5$W (0.04%)
Norepinephrine	0.05–0.15μg/kg/min	4mg/250ml D$_5$W (0.0016%)
Phenylephrine	10μg/min titrated	10mg/250ml D$_5$W (0.004%)
Antiarrhythmic Agents		
Lidocaine	1–2mg/kg	
Propranolol	1–2mg in divided doses	

evaluate changes in hemodynamics, volume status and blood gases. At least 2, large-bore, peripheral intravenous cannulae should be secured for rapid fluid administration. Blood products must be immediately available.

The need for vasoactive compounds should be anticipated, and infusions prepared preoperatively. See Table 2. Sodium nitroprusside is the most widely used antihypertensive agent, although phentolamine, trimethaphan, or nitroglycerine may be substituted. Hypotension unresponsive to fluid administration is treated most frequently with infusions of dopamine or norepinephrine, although phenylephrine or metaraminol preparations may be used. Perioperative cardiac dysrhythmias are not uncommon, and lidocaine, propanolol and a defibrillator (200–300 joules for ventricular fibrillation) should be available.

Certain pharmacologic agents should probably be avoided, including those that induce histamine release (morphine sulfate, tubocurarine), potentiate catecholamines (ketamine), sensitize the myocardium to catecholamines (halothane), increase intraabdominal pressure (succinylcholine) or are vagolytic (pancuronium, gallamine).

Induction is best accomplished with an ultra-short-acting barbituate supplemented with a combination of a volatile anesthetic, fentanyl, and either lidocaine or a benzodiazepine derivative to attenuate hemodynamic responses to laryngoscopy. Atracurium or vecuronium are the relaxants of choice. Despite sensitization of the myocardium to catecholamines, halothane has been widely used for maintenance of anesthesia. Neurolept anesthesia has proven satisfactory. Deep general anesthesia with enflurane or isoflurane is also used commonly, although hypotension is a hazard. The choice of anesthetic agents, per se, is less important than preparedness and a thorough knowledge of the pathophysiology of the disease and the principles of management.

References

1. Gifford R.W. Jr, Kvale W.F., Maher F.T., et al: Clinical features, diagnosis, and treatment of pheochromocytoma: A review of 76 cases. *Mayo Clin Proc* 39: 281–302, 1964.
2. Plouin P.F., Degoulet P., Tugaye A., et al: Le depistage pheochromocytome: Chez quels hypertendus? Étude semiologique chez 2585 hypertendus dont 11 ayunt un pheochromocytome. *Nouv Presse Med* 10:869–72, 1981.
3. Kaplan N.M., Kramer N.J., Holland O.B., et al: Single voided urine, metanephrine assays in screening for pheochromocytoma. *Arch Intern Med* 137:190–3, 1977.
4. Bravo E.L., Gifford R.W. Jr: Pheochromocytoma: Diagnosis, localization, and management. *N Engl J Med* 311:1298–1303, 1984.
5. Bravo E.L., Tarazi R.C., Gifford R.W., et al: Circulating and urinary catecholamines in pheochromocytoma. *N Engl J Med* 301:682–6, 1979.
6. Desmonts J.M., le Houelleur J., Remond P., et al: Anaesthetic management of patients with pheochromocytoma: A review of 102 cases. *Br J Anaesth* 49:991–998, 1977.
7. Rouby J.J., Gory G., Gaveau T. et al: Dangerous rise in pulmonary wedge pressure following aortography in a patient with pheochromocytoma. *Anesth Analg* 59:154–6, 1980.
8. Dereo G.A. Jr, Stewart B.H., Tarazi R.W. Jr: Preoperative blood transfusion in the safe surgical management of pheochromocytoma: A review of 46 cases. *J Urol* 111:715–21, 1974.
9. Maddern P.J., Davis N.J., McGlew I., et al: Pheochromocytoma: Aspects of management. *Anaesth Intens Care* 4:156–8, 1976.

CHAPTER 7

The Patient with Known or Suspected Malignant Hyperthermia*

Anna Stanec

Case History. *A 6-year-old white male was scheduled for elective strabismus repair. During preanesthetic evaluation in the preadmission testing clinic (PAT) he was evaluated for general anesthesia as an ASA I patient for same-day surgery. Premedication consisting of atropine and meperidine was ordered. Later that day, the mother telephoned and told the anesthesiologist on call that she had forgotten to tell the doctor in the PAT about her sister's son (8 years old) who had had an abnormal reaction to anesthesia three years earlier. The cousin was scheduled for a tonsillectomy in another hospital, but due to this reaction, the surgery was cancelled. She was not sure what investigation followed, but was told that she had to inform the anesthesiologist about this episode each time she or her children were scheduled for surgery. She had never received general anesthesia. She had two more children, one of whom (age 10) had uneventful anesthesia for a hernia repair one year ago. Her parents had never had any anesthesia as far as she knew, except for local anesthesia at the dentist's office.*

Introduction

The syndrome of malignant hyperthermia (MH), a pharmacogenetic myopathy of humans and swine, has been increasingly recognized over the last two decades. Since the syndrome was first fully described in 1960,[1] it has become identified as a common cause of anesthesia-related death in the United States.

MH is primarily a disease of children and young adults and occurs more commonly in males. The incidence is estimated at 1 per 15,000 anesthetics in the pediatric population and 1 per 50,000 anesthetics in adults.[2] The overwhelming majority of MH episodes in MH susceptible (MHS) indi-

---

*Reviewed by Dr. Gerald Gronert, Professor of Anesthesiology, Mayo Clinic, Rochester, Minnesota.

viduals occur during anestheisa. Awake episodes triggered by stress are common in MHS swine but rare in man.[3] Postoperative episodes in the recovery room after an uneventful anesthetic may occur. An accurate estimation of the incidence of MH episodes outside of the operating room is not known, nor are the causes of these episodes.

The sudden occurrence of an MH crisis in an apparently healthy surgical patient with resultant death or serious residual complications raises the legal issue of medical malpractice. Obtaining a thorough family and personal anesthesia history and continuous monitoring of temperature, heart rate and blood pressure during general anesthesia meet the minimum standard of care. Routine application of these measures permits early recognition of the syndrome, which is the key to successful treatment. Increased awareness among anesthesiologists of the catastrophic consequences of an unrecognized MH episode has contributed to a dramatic decrease in perioperative mortality among MHS patients from 60%–70% two decades ago to 5%–10% now.

Pathophysiology

The presenting symptoms during an MH crisis result from a hypermetabolic state in skeletal muscle. This state can be triggered by the depolarizing muscle relaxant succinylcholine or by potent halogenated inhalation anesthetics. The important early clinical manifestations of a developing MH episode are sudden unexplained tachycardia or arrhythmia, skeletal muscle rigidity, unstable blood pressure, tachypnea, central venous desaturation, hypercarbia and lactate accumulation with respiratory and metabolic acidosis. Thus, a presumptive diagnosis of MH can be made before significant temperature rises occur.

MH susceptibility is based upon a hereditary predisposition, transferred as an autosomal dominant trait with variable expressivity of one or more genes.[4] There are regional variations in the incidence of MH due to genetic pooling. Since some MHS persons are never anesthetized or exposed to pharmacologic triggering agents, the number of susceptible individuals in the general population may be higher than generally recognized. Some genetic carriers do not develop the MH syndrome on exposure to anesthetics. Therefore, a history of an uneventful anesthetic course does not preclude MH susceptibility. The critical combination of factors that prevents or causes development of an MH episode in an MHS individual on the day of surgery is not known.

The development of the MH syndrome leading to an MH crisis may be dramatically rapid and alarming, or it may have a slower onset with symptoms masked by some pharmacological agents or other circumstances. Factors such as excitement and emotional or physical stress prior to anesthesia may predispose MHS patients to a crisis.

Review of the literature indicates that the exact etiology and pathophysiology of MH remain unclarified, despite years of intensive investigation.[5, 6] The cause of the sudden rise in intracellular calcium of skeletal muscle after exposure to triggering agents has not been identified. Some of the suggested mechanisms include abnormal accumulation of calcium in the sarcoplasmic reticulum, toxic accumulation of calcium in the mitochondria, weakened cellular membranes, increased activity of the sympathetic nervous system, and abnormal cAMP metabolism. It has been proposed that MH is an acute stress syndrome of man.[7] However, it is not established whether the role of the sympathetic nervous system in the development of an MH episode is primary or secondary to the stress of an MH crisis.[6]

Preanesthetic Evaluation

Since MH is an anesthesia-related disease, it is incumbent upon the anesthesiologist to care for MHS individuals. The primary goal is to assure that patients who have been identified as MHS are not frustrated in obtaining proper surgical and anesthetic care.

Identification of MHS patients can be difficult. While MH is under intensive investigation and many noninvasive screening tests are being studied, there are limited circumstances where a diagnosis can be made without performing a muscle biopsy; in addition, muscle biopsy results can be equivocal.

The preoperative assessment and preparation of patients with known or suspected MH includes verification of family and personal anesthetic history, interpretation of screening and diagnostic tests, and organization of preanesthetic management including the prophylactic administration of dantrolene sodium.

Family and Patient History

Several important events short of an anesthetic catastrophe should be sought in the family and patient histories, and all information should be recorded in the patient's chart. First is a history of survival of a typical MH episode, which may or may not be documented by clinical and laboratory findings. Clear documentation of a typical MH episode may be used to make a presumptive clinical diagnosis. The details of the family history (family tree), including the severity of MH episodes and the outcome of affected individuals, should be known. This information can be obtained from anesthesia records, if they are available, or from the treating anesthesiologist.

A history of masseter muscle rigidity in response to succinylcholine should also be sought. This paradoxical response to succinylcholine is an early sign of MH susceptibility. The coincidence of positive muscle biopsy and masseter muscle rigidity is estimated to be 60% to 65%.[8,9] Elevated levels of serum creatine phosphokinase (CPK) usually accompany masseter rigidity.

Second is a history of any type of muscle disease or weakness. Approximately 30% to 40% of individuals with various muscle diseases may develop MH or an abnormal reaction to succinylcholine. The most common associated muscle abnormalities are muscle cramps; excessively developed skeletal muscles; and localized muscle weakness, such as ptosis, strabismus, kyphoscoliosis, inguinal hernia, and club foot.

A history of severe, painful and persistent cramps in the calf or other skeletal muscles that are not related to exercise is suggestive of MH susceptibility. Approximately 70% of individuals who suffer such cramps and who have additional MH-related risk factors, including elevated CPK levels, are MHS. Muscle cramps can be sufficiently severe to affect life style.

Specific disorders that are associated with MH include Duchenne's muscular dystrophy, central core disease, osteogenesis imperfecta, myotonia congenita, King-Denborough syndrome, Schantz-Janpel syndrome, lymphoma, sudden infant death syndrome, and neuroleptic malignant syndrome.

A history of unexplained fever during or after anesthesia is suggestive of MH. Approximately 50% to 60% of these patients are MHS. Although the majority of MHS individuals tolerate exercise well, in some patients exercise may induce flushing and fever. Any history of this should therefore be investigated. Awake and exercise-related MH episodes are rare.

A history of sudden, unexplained cardiac arrest in a family member that occurred outside the operating room or during anesthesia should be further investigated.

A retrospective differential diagnosis of episodes suggestive of MH is important. A description should be obtained from the patient or the parents and, by a process of elimination, other causes of tachycardia, fever and hypermetabolism can be excluded. The best way to establish a clinical diagnosis is by obtaining the facts from the physicians involved in previous episodes and from anesthesia records.

Screening and Diagnostic Tests

Currently, there are no reliable noninvasive tests for the diagnosis of MH susceptibility in man. The only accepted diagnostic tests are the pharmacologic, halothane-caffeine contracture tests, which are performed on skeletal muscle strips in vitro.[10]

Estimation of serum CPK was the most commonly used screening test for MH susceptibility, but it is not diagnostic since many MH patients have normal CPK levels. In addition, serum CPK can be increased by diverse causes. CPK may only be considered to indicate MH susceptibility if it is elevated on at least three consecutive occasions in a patient from a known MH family. Elevated CPK values with no family history of MH have no predictive value. If other causes of elevated CPK can be elminated, the correlation with MH is estimated to be 60% to 70%.

A positive response to dantrolene is not necessarily diagnostic of MH. Dantrolene decreases body metabolism and heat production by approximately 40%. Thus, many conditions that can mimic MH may also be improved by dantrolene administration.

The in vitro halothane-caffeine contracture tests are the most reliable diagnostic tests for MH. These tests require a sample of viable muscle, usually vastus lateralis, which is exposed to caffeine and/or halothane. Muscle contracture is evoked by lower caffeine concentrations in MH individuals, and in response to halothane, MH muscle demonstrates a significant abnormal contracture.

Indications for referral to an MH center for a diagnostic muscle biopsy are: a history of an anesthesia-related death in the family, an unclear anesthesia-related death that is highly suspicious for MH, fever during or after anesthesia, masseter muscle rigidity after succinylcholine, elevated CPK levels in the absence of other causes, and postoperative myoglobinuria.

There are, however, problems with the contracture tests and their interpretation. Muscle must be tested as soon as the biopsy is performed, so patients must travel to an MH center. Thus, some patients may be unwilling to undergo biopsy. The number of institutions that perform the contracture tests is very limited; there are fewer than 10 in the United States. Results between laboratories are not directly comparable since testing protocols differ. An obvious abnormal contracture to halothane and/or caffeine is clearly a positive test, but some overlap occurs and false-positive or -negative result may be obtained. Also, biopsy is generally not recommended for children younger than 5 years of age.

It has been suggested that patients with an occurrence of masseter muscle rigidity after halothane or succinylcholine should be considered MHS until proven otherwise.[8,9] Consultation should be obtained for patients with this history or any other unclear situation after preliminary screening procedures.

The referral contact is Malignant Hyperthermia Association of the United States (MHAUS), Box 3231, Darien, CT 06820. In an emergency, the 24-hour, MH-Crisis telephone hotline is (209) 634-4917 (Index Zero, MH consultant list). This is made available by the Medic Alert Foundation International. Medic Alert bracelets are normally issued to individuals who are diagnosed positive at an MH center. For the patient who, for whatever reason, does not have the clinical or laboratory diagnosis confirmed by the caffeine and/or halothane contracture tests, the anesthesiologist should suggest that he wear a Medic Alert bracelet. However, an MHS individual should be encouraged to live a normal life with the same activities as before the presumptive or conclusive diagnosis was made.

Preanesthetic Management

There are two basic options in treating the MHS patient whose diagnosis is not confirmed: postpone the surgery and obtain more information, or treat the patient as MHS. The decision depends upon the urgency of the surgical procedure and the expertise of the anesthesiologist in dealing with the MH syndrome. An anesthesiologist who is unfamiliar with MH should refer the case to a medical center.

The final decision is made after discussion with the patient or the parents. Adequate time should be allowed for the family to make this decision. The option of referral to an MH center or to the nearest medical center where anesthesiologists may be more familiar with caring for MHS individuals should be presented. Actual anesthetic management, monitoring procedures and the choices of regional versus general anesthesia for a particular surgical procedure and the risks should be explained in detail.

Once surgery has been decided upon, it is important to psychologically prepare the patient. Stress may be a factor in the occurrence of an MH episode. Elimination of anxiety may prevent or modify the development of an MH episode even if genetic predisposition exists. The anesthesiologist should therefore both reassure and educate the patient about the anesthesia for MHS patients. The anesthesiologist should also convey confidence about the ability to successfully treat any problems that may arise.

In addition to psychological preparation, the patient should be well sedated with agents that have antianxiety effects. Anticholinergic and opioid drugs should be avoided. A history of current medications or drug abuse should be obtained prior to ordering preoperative medications so that the potential for drug interaction can be minimized.

Surgery for MHS patients must be performed in an operating room where potent halogenated anesthetics have not been used for at least 12 hours. A vapor-free, clean anesthesia machine must be used. The vaporizer should be emptied and air or oxygen flow continued for several hours prior to use.

The results of baseline laboratory tests, such as CPK, lactate, arterial blood gases and pH, SGOT, SGPT, glucose, electrolytes, and if available ionized calcium, should be obtained and charted. It is important that MHS patients be well hydrated prior to anesthesia.

Arrangements must also be made for postoperative management in the recovery room. This includes availability of monitoring devices, cooling measures and dantrolene for intravenous use. Some MHS individuals develop an MH episode for the first time in the recovery room, which may occur several hours after an uneventful anesthetic course.

Dantrolene Sodium (Dantrium)

Current recommendations for MHS patients include pretreatment with intravenous dantrolene. If MH susceptibility cannot be verified, dantrolene pretreatment may not be required, but dantrolene must be available in the OR and recovery room. If the history is suspicious for MH and there is no time for further investigation, pretreatment is indicated.

Dantrolene is a direct-acting skeletal muscle relaxant.[11] It probably interferes with the release of calcium ions from the sarcoplasmic reticulum. Thus, its site of action is beyond the neuromuscular junction. Since the absorption of dantrolene after oral administration in humans is incomplete and slow, various oral pretreatment schedules have been used in the past.[11,12] However, MH episodes after oral dantrolene pretreatment have been reported.[13,14] In addition, the side effects produced by effective oral doses require preoperative hospitalization. Thus, intravenous dantrolene pretreatment is the most effective preventive measure. Still, monitoring and cooling measures must be available for all patients.

The recommended prophylactic intravenous dose of dantrolene prior to induction of anesthesia is 2.5mg/kg by slow injection. Each vial contains 20mg dantrolene sodium and 3000mg mannitol adjusted to approximately pH 9.5 when reconstituted with 60ml sterile water for injection without a bacteriostatic agent. Use of water that contains a bacteriostatic agent will cause the dantrolene to precipitate.

Adequate supplies of dantrolene and sterile water for injection, as well as personnel to mix the solutions, must be available if an MH episode should arise. This point is extremely important. Intravenous dantrolene should be injected within 5–10 minutes from the time a clinical and/or laboratory diagnosis of an MH episode is made; speed is of the essence in a rapidly developing MH episode.

Each 20mg vial of dantrolene must be reconstituted with 60ml sterile water for injection and the vial shaken until the solution is clear. For an average 70kg patient, 7–10 vials of dantrolene must be prepared. Unaided, it can take the anesthesiologist 20–30 minutes to prepare 7–10 vials of dantrolene solution. Mixing of the dantrolene should thus commence early when an MH episode is suspected. Additional personnel to mix the powder will be necessary.

Anesthetic Management

It is essential that a "safe" anesthetic technique be used in all survivors of an MH episode and in members of families who have exhibited this syndrome. Unclear cases should be referred to an MH center for diagnostic muscle biopsy testing.

The anesthetic technique of choice for MHS individuals is local, regional, spinal, or epidural anesthesia, where applicable. Either the amide or ester type of local anesthetic may be used. It should be remembered, however, that regional techniques do not protect MHS patients from developing an MH episode. If the administration of large volumes of drug is anticipated, the agent of choice is probably an ester-type local anesthetic.

Recently Berkowitz and Rosenberg safely used an amide-type local anesthetic for femoral block in MHS patients.[15] Small volumes of amide-type local anesthetics may also be used for procedures in the dental office where the longer duration of action is advantageous.

For general anesthesia the neuroleptanalgesic technique is recommended utilizing diazepam, droperidol, fentanyl, barbiturates, nitrous oxide/oxygen, and vecuronium, atracurium or small doses of pancuronium. Continuous monitoring of temperature, acid-base status, ECG and blood pressure is essential. Monitoring of end-tidal carbon dioxide with a capnograph and the arterial hemoglobin oxygen saturation with a pulse oximeter is recommended.

In the management of MHS obstetric patients, reassurance of normal pregnancy and labor is probably the most important factor. For delivery, epidural or spinal anesthesia is recommended. Routine dantrolene pretreatment is not required in MH patients who are asymptomatic during the course of pregnancy and labor, but dantrolene must be available in the obstetric suite since both the mother and the newborn may require it. In patients who develop early clinical or laboratory signs of MH during labor, intravenous dantrolene pretreatment is indicated prior to general or regional anesthesia. The safety of dantrolene in pregnant women has not been established. However, the risk of rapid development of an MH crisis in the mother outweighs that of placental transfer of dantrolene.

Drugs that are considered to be safe, those that are contraindicaed and those that remain controversial are listed in Table 1. Theoretically, all drugs with the ability to raise intracellular calcium could be detrimental,

TABLE 1. Use of anesthetic agents and other drugs in malignant hyperthermia susceptible patients

"Safe" drugs	Contraindicated drugs	Controversial drugs
Nitrous oxide	All potent inhalation	Tubocurarine
Barbiturates	anesthetics	Ketamine
Diazepam	Depolarizing muscle	Large volumes of amide-
Midazolam	relaxants-succinylcholine,	type local anesthetics
Tranquilizers	decamethonium	Phenothiazines
Droperidol	Digitalis preparations	Antidepressants
Fentanyl		Catecholamines
Sufentanil		Sympathomimetic agents
Morphine		Belladona alkaloids
Nondepolarizing muscle		Anticholinesterase agents
relaxants-pancuronium,		
vecuronium, atracurium		
Local anesthetics		
Magnesium sulfate		
Phenytoin		
Propanolol		
Calcium blockers		
Corticosteroids		
Procainamide		

TABLE 2. Malignant hyperthermia emergency protocol*

---

1. Stop anesthesia and surgery, hyperventilate with 100% oxygen.
2. Administer IV dantrolene sodium 2.5mg/kg and further doses up to 10mg/kg as needed to control the clinical symptoms.
3. Simultaneously start cooling by cold saline IV solutions and other routes.
4. Correct acidosis (1–2mEq/kg bicarbonate) and hyperkalemia (10–50 units of insulin in 10–50ml of 50% D/W).
5. Monitor: ECG, temperature (skin and rectal), urinary output, arterial and central venous pressure.
6. Maintain urine output at a minimum of 2ml/kg/hour. Administer furosemide 0.5–1mg/kg if needed.
7. Change anesthetic tubing and soda line, if halogenated inhalation agents were used.
8. Administer IV procainamide 7mg/kg for persistent arrhythmias.
9. Determine and follow: arterial or venous blood gases and pH, serum potassium, sodium, calcium, lactate, CPK, SGPT, SGOT, LDH, clotting factors and myoglobin.
10. Observe the patient in an ICU setting for 24–48 hours.
11. Monitor body temperature since hypothermia may develop after vigorous treatment of MH crisis.
12. When the patient's condition has stabilized, continue IV dantrolene 1mg/kg per 6 hours for at least 48 hours.

---

*From information provided by the Malignant Hyperthermia Association of the United States (MHAUS) and Norwich-Eaton Pharmaceuticals.

and all drugs that lower intracellular calcium may be beneficial, regardless of the mechanism. Both effects should occur in a dose-dependent manner.

Treatment of an MH crisis is outlined in Table 2. Many anesthesiologists have never seen an MH episode. Nevertheless, every practitioner must be prepared to detect a developing episode early and treat it immediately, since one may occur in a patient seen tomorrow.

Controversial Issues

There are many unanswered questions about MH, but the main controversial issue for the clinician is the interpretation of the results of the caffeine and halothane contracture tests.[16, 17] The questions raised are:

- What is the significance of a positive muscle biopsy in the absence of a positive personal anesthetic history?
- What is the significance of a negative muscle biopsy in the presence of a positive personal anesthetic history?
- What is the significance of a negative muscle biopsy and a negative personal anesthetic history in an individual from a family with a positive history of MH susceptibility?

The majority of anesthesiologists will treat all of the above cases as susceptible and avoid exposure to triggering agents. Thus, regardless of the results of muscle biopsy tests, only "safe" anesthetic techniques are used.

References

1. Denborough M.A., Lovell R.R.H.: Anaesthetic deaths in a family. *Lancet* 2:45, 1960.
2. Britt B.A., Kalow W.: Malignant hyperthermia: A statistical review. *Can Anaesth Soc J* 17:293–315, 1970.
3. Gronert G.A., Thompson R.L., Onofrio B.M.: Human malignant hyperthermia: awake episodes and correction by dantrolene. *Anesth Analg* (Cleve) 59:377–378, 1980.
4. Ellis F.R., Cain P.A., Harriman D.G.F.: Multifactorial inheritance of malignant hyperpyrexia susceptibility (MHS). *Br J Anaesth* 49:514–515, 1977.
5. Britt B.A.: Etiology and pathophysiology of malignant hyperthermia. *Fed Proc* 38:44–48, 1979.
6. Gronert G.A.: Malignant hyperthermia. *Anesthesiology* 53:395–423, 1980.
7. Wingard D.W.: Malignant hyperthermia—acute stress syndrome of man, in Henschel E.D. (ed): *Malignant Hyperthermia: Current Concepts*, New York, Appleton-Century-Crofts, 1977, pp 79–95.
8. Flewellen E.H., Nelson T.E.: Halothane-succinylcholine induced masseter spasm: Indicative of malignant hyperthermia susceptibility. *Anesth Analg* 63:793–797, 1984.
9. Ellis F.R., Halsall P.J.: Suxamethonium spasm. A differential diagnostic conundrum. *Br J Anaesth* 56:381–384, 1984.
10. Rosenberg H., Reed S.: In vitro contracture tests for susceptibility to malignant hyperthermia. *Anesth Analg* 62:415–420, 1983.
11. Britt B.A.: Dantrolene (review article). *Can Anaesth Soc J* 31:61-75, 1984.
12. Gronert G.A.: Puzzles in malignant hyperthermia. *Anesthesiology* 54:1–2, 1981.
13. Fitzgibbons D.C.: Malignant hyperthermia following preoperative oral administration of dantrolene. *Anesthesiology* 54:73–75, 1981.
14. Ruhland G., Hinkle A.J.: Malignant hyperthermia after oral and intravenous pretreatment with dantrolene in a patient susceptible to malignant hyperthermia. *Anesthesiology* 60:159–160, 1984.
15. Berkowitz A., Rosenberg H.: Femoral block with mepivacaine for muscle biopsy in malignant hyperthermia patients. *Anesthesiology* 62:651–652, 1985.
16. Gronert G.A.: Controversies in malignant hyperthermia. *Anesthesiology* 59:273–274, 1983.
17. Nelson T.E., Flewellen E.H., Gloyna D.F.: Spectrum of susceptibility to malignant hyperthermia: diagnostic dilemma. *Anesth Analg* 62:545–552, 1983.

CHAPTER 8

The Spinal Cord Injured Patient*

Michael Domurat

Case History. *A 26-year-old woman with a history of heroin abuse dived into a shallow swimming pool and struck her head on the bottom. She immediately complained of difficulty in appreciating sensation in her legs, changing paresthesias and neck pain. She was able to move all extremities. Prior to transport to the hospital, her neck was stabilized in a cervical collar. In the emergency room, cervical x-ray demonstrated a C5–C6 dislocation. Shortly after admission, she was unable to move her lower extremities. Skeletal tongs were inserted and traction applied but the dislocation could not be reduced. Emergency exploration and stabilization of her neck was then undertaken.*

Physical examination showed an undernourished patient of weight 100 lbs, pulse 58 bpm and regular, blood pressure 90/60, respiratory rate 35/ minute. Rhonchi were present at both lung bases. Neurologic status was conscious with changing sensory and motor levels.

Laboratory examinations yielded the following data: Hct 29%, Hgb 9.8gm, WBC 18,500. SMA-6 was within normal limits. Arterial blood gas data on room air were: PaO_2 66mmHg, $PaCO_2$ 35mmHg, pH 7.35.

Introduction

Spinal cord injury (SCI) occurs in the United States at an approximate incidence of 10,000 per year and accounts for less than 1% of all trauma cases.[1] It is an injury common to young men: 80% of all SCI occurs in individuals who are younger than 40 years of age, and nearly 50% of victims are in the 14–24 year old age range.[2] Mortality from SCI is 47.1% compared with an overall mortality of 6.7% for all trauma victims. The average health care cost from time of injury to time of death for nonsurvivors exceeds $300,000 per patient.[3]

---

*Reviewed by Dr. Stephen Weitz, Associate Professor of Neurosurgery, Albert Einstein College of Medicine of Yeshiva University, Bronx, New York.

Vehicular-related accidents, diving injuries, sports injuries and gunshot wounds account for most cases of injury to the spinal cord. The mobile areas of the spine are most susceptible to spinal cord trauma. Nearly 50% of SCIs occur in the C4–C7 region, 13% in T3–T6, and 18% in T10–T12.[4]

In addition to the SCI and the resultant disruption of neural activity distal to the site of injury, trauma to other organs may also require emergency surgery. The anesthesiologist must be aware of the consequences of disrupted neural activity on multiple systems during the acute phase of injury and the subsequent recovery period. The chronicity of the disease and its impact on multiple systems presents an anesthetic challenge. The anesthesiologist should be familiar with the pathophysiology of each phase of spinal cord injury and recovery, be prepared to evaluate the degree of dysfunction, and plan appropriate anesthetic management.

Pathology

Potential recovery from SCI is dependent upon three factors: 1) the extent of initial cord injury; 2) prevention of further trauma during rescue, transport and hospitalization; and 3) avoidance of hypoxia and systemic hypotension, which may further compromise neural function.[5 (p376)]

In most cases, trauma itself does not produce immediate anatomic transection of the spinal cord. Neural disruption results from microvascular injury produced by the forces of trauma, which trigger a series of events producing disruption of neural activity distal to the area of injury.[6] Vascular injury and bleeding into the grey matter is accompanied by edema of the white matter and may extend one or two segments above and below the site of injury. Edema of the cord may compromise blood flow, causing lactic acidosis and ischemia. It has been postulated that further insult may be contributed by release of norepinephrine and other vasoactive peptides.

The injury can be minimized if proper therapy is initiated early in the posttraumatic period. Reduction of posttraumatic compression, fluid resuscitation to restore perfusion pressure, and maintenance of optimal arterial oxygen saturation are essential interventions. Although corticosteroids and mannitol are frequently given to reduce cord edema, their efficacy has not been established.

The period of time following SCI is divided into acute, intermediate and chronic phases. Characteristic pathophysiologic changes unique to each phase dictate different preanesthetic assessment and management.

Acute Phase of SCI (0–4 weeks)

Initial assessment of the SCI patient includes evaluation of respiratory and circulatory status. Patency of the airway must be maintained as well as adequate perfusion and oxygenation to the cord to prevent further hypoxic damage.

SCI patients must be assumed to have a cervical fracture until proven otherwise. During the period of initial assessment, the patient is immobilized on a stiff board with the spine in a neutral position and stabilized by means of sandbags. The head is taped in a fixed position, or traction tongs can be applied to the skull.

Intubation of the trachea is necessary in the obtunded, apneic patient in whom there may be abolition of protective airway reflexes. Oral intubation should be performed only after the neck is immobilized and stabilized. Awake nasotracheal intubation performed "blindly" or with a fiberoptic laryngoscope may be necessary in the patient with an unstable cervical fracture.

The extent of neural disruption should be established, and radiographic studies of the involved areas of the spine should be undertaken. A lateral x-ray of the neck is essential to rule out a cervical spine fracture. CT scan may help define the areas of injury when plain x-ray films are equivocal. Any other suspected areas of trauma should also be evaluated.

Spinal Shock

Spinal shock and pulmonary insufficiency are the predominant pathophysiologic changes in the acute phase of SCI. Spinal shock is characterized by generalized depression of neural activity distal to the spinal cord lesion, accompanied by the loss of descending facilitory impulses from the higher centers, particularly the corticospinal tract. Loss of cerebral facilitation of voluntary motor function manifests as flaccid paralysis. Depression of spinal reflexes results in gastric and bladder distension, absent deep tendon reflexes and paralytic ileus.

Loss of neural activity and the resulting denervation of muscle predispose the patient to hyperkalemia when succinylcholine is administered during anesthetic induction. Although the potential for a hyperkalemic response has been thought to develop within 1 week of injury, it may persist 6 months or more. The denervated muscle becomes supersensitive, and the entire cell behaves like the end-plate in response to a depolarizing muscle relaxant.[7] Some physicians recommend that, in the absence of any major muscle destruction or burn, succinylcholine may be safely given within the first 24–48 hours postinjury. We feel that the newer, shorter-acting, nondepolarizing muscle relaxants are more appropriate since the exact onset of the hyperkalemic response has not been clearly demonstrated. Cooperman demonstrated that the maximal response occurred between 4 weeks and 5 months postinjury.[8] Furthermore, the response is not reliably attenuated by pretreatment with a nondepolarizing muscle relaxant.

Injury to the cord above the level of T6 results in vasodilation and postural hypotension due to loss of sympathetic tone below the site of injury. Lesions in the region of T1–T4 eliminate sympathetic innervation of the sinoatrial node and allow vagal effects to predominate on the heart rate.

Vagal tone and resulting bradycardia may be further accentuated by stimulation of the nasal, oral or tracheal mucosa. Asystole has been reported after attempts at tracheal intubation. Pretreatment with atropine 0.4mg intravenously prior to tracheal intubation or suctioning is effective in preventing reflex bradycardia.

The SCI patient presenting with hypotension may have hemorrhagic shock from concurrent multiple trauma. However, the presence of an abnormal heart rate is not reliable in differentiating the cause of hypotension. Although tachycardia usually accompanies hemorrhagic shock, bradycardia may indicate either neurogenic etiology or accompanying volume depletion.

Electrocardiographic changes consistent with subendocardial ischemia have been demonstrated in clinical and experimental cord transections at C5–C6.[9] Other EKG changes include sinus pauses, shifting sinus pacemaker, atrial fibrillation, multifocal PVCs, ventricular tachycardia and ST-T wave changes consistent with increased levels of catecholamines.[5]

Systolic blood pressure commonly stabilizes at 90–100mmHg, which is considered adequate for cord perfusion in the supine position. However, loss of sympathetic tone and the compensatory mechanism for postural changes may jeopardize cord perfusion during repositioning and periods of operative blood loss. Spinal cord perfusion pressure should be adequately maintained with judicious volume loading using crystalloid or colloid solutions or blood replacement. Atropine 0.4mg may be given to correct bradycardia.

If hypotension persists despite reasonable fluid administration, the judicious use of vasopressors to replace the loss of neurogenic vasoconstriction will usually promptly restore the blood pressure to normal. Patients in the acute phase of injury have a marginal capacity to respond to volume stress and are therefore prone to the development of pulmonary edema; placement of a central venous catheter or pulmonary artery catheter is essential for optimal volume resuscitation prior to surgery. Urine output should also be a guide to volume administration and be optimally maintained at 0.5–1.0ml/kg/hr. Blood loss must be adequately replaced to achieve a preoperative hematocrit of at least 30%.

The SCI patient should be regarded as having a full stomach. A nasogastric tube should be placed because of the high risk of aspiration. Protracted vomiting may predispose the patient to metabolic alkalosis and hypokalemia. Serum potassium may be further depleted by loss into the distended paralytic intestine and alteration in aldosterone secretion.

Hypercalcemia and hypercalciuria may manifest as early as 10 days postinjury; the etiology is increased tissue mobilization as a result of the flaccid paralysis of voluntary muscle and reduced muscular activity accompanying spinal shock. Serum calcium levels of as high as 16mg% have been reported.[10] Cardiac conduction disturbances may appear when the serum calcium exceeds 12mg%. Prolongation of the PR interval, widening of the

QRS complex and shortened QT interval are the major manifestations. Treatment of hypercalcemia is hydration with normal saline to lower serum calcium by dilution. Sodium also inhibits renal reabsorption of calcium. Concomitant use of furosemide reduces the risk of overhydration and further enhances renal elimination of calcium.

Respiratory Dysfunction

Injuries of the cervical and high-thoracic segments of the spinal cord are associated with varying degrees of respiratory dysfunction. The most common cause of death after cervical cord injury is acute respiratory failure.

During the first 24–48 hours postinjury, the patient may require surgical intervention for reduction of extremity fractures, stabilization of unstable vertebral fractures, or intrathoracic, intra-abdominal or intracranial procedures. However, if at all possible, emergency surgery planned during the first 24–48 hours postinjury should be delayed in order to maximize the patient's ventilatory reserve. Measures should include intermittent positive pressure ventilation, chest percussion, postural drainage and assisted cough. The presence of preexisting lung disease should be established and treated.

Lesions at C2–C4 generally result in complete apnea and the patient is dead on admission. Partial lesions at this level produce sleep apnea. These patients generally hypoventilate even when awake. They are at greatest risk of developing sleep apnea during the first 5 nights post-cord insult.[11] It is most likely a manifestation of a defect in the medullary ventilatory center secondary to edema and ischemia from lower cord trauma that extends in a cephalad direction. Occasionally it may be the result of a gunshot wound to the neck. Patients at risk of developing sleep apnea require constant surveillance during this vulnerable period; nursing supervision and the use of a sleep apnea monitor are recommended to provide adequate protection. Treatment requires intubation and assisted ventilation.

Lesions at the level of C4–C5 result in a major loss of diaphragmatic movement and gross impairment of ventilation. C5–C6 lesions are accompanied by reduced ventilation secondary to partial loss of diaphragmatic movement.

If the lowest uninvolved segment is at or below C6, diaphragmatic innervation is intact but ventilation is reduced because of intercostal paralysis. This may reduce the tidal volume by 60% if rib cage expansion is abolished. In addition, vital capacity may initially be only 30% of the predicted value. Because of decreased vital capacity, inspiratory capacity and expiratory reserve volume, the patient is unable to cough and clear secretions from the upper respiratory tract. In addition, the acute SCI patient may have aspirated stomach contents and a ventilation-perfusion mismatch may exist.

Evaluation of pulmonary function includes chest x-ray to exclude rib fracture, pneumothorax, atelectasis and aspiration. Arterial blood gas measurement should be a part of the preoperative evaluation of respiratory function. Arterial carbon dioxide content ($PaCO_2$) serves as a reliable indicator of alveolar ventilation; arterial oxygen (PaO_2) reflects the degree of ventilation–perfusion ($\dot{V}/\dot{Q}$) mismatch. In one study of 11 patients with spinal cord injury, during the first week postinjury the average PaO_2 of 35/47 arterial blood gas measurements was less than 80mmHg. Four of the 11 patients had PaO_2 values of less than 65mmHg.[12] Atelectasis and pulmonary vasoconstriction secondary to catecholamine release is the most likely explanation for the development of $\dot{V}/\dot{Q}$ mismatch.

Vital capacity is a reliable indicator of respiratory function. It serves as a guide for further respiratory support and as a means of evaluating recovery of respiratory function. Improvements in forced expiratory volume and functional residual capacity have been demonstrated over time; values may even approach 60% of predicted.[12] Factors contributing to improved pulmonary function include: decreased cord edema, decreased use of respiratory depressant drugs, improved diaphragmatic function and strength, and strengthened accessory muscles of respiration.

Other Systems

Patients with cord transections above T6 become poikilothermic. In a warm environment the patient loses the ability to lower body temperature; oxygen demand may be increased and inadequately met in the patient with compromised pulmonary function. An ambient temperature of 21°C (69.8°F) has been shown to be optimal in stabilizing body temperature at an acceptable level.[5 (p382)] Oxygen consumption was also decreased by nearly 20%.

Elevated body temperature may indicate an ongoing infectious process. Peritonitis is often masked by lack of pain and abdominal rigidity. Additional laboratory studies may be indicated to help pinpoint the source of infection. Whenever an SCI patient's body temperature is elevated, poikilothermia should be eliminated as a source.

More than 25% of spinal cord injury patients suffer from gastrointestinal bleeding which may be further exacerbated by the use of steroids. These patients are often given trials of antacids or cimetidine to prevent steroid and stress-induced gastrointestinal ulceration. Cimetidine has been shown to inhibit hepatic monooxygenase function, perhaps by its binding to microsomal cytochrome P-450.[13] The metabolism and elimination of many drugs—diazepam, propranolol, phenytoin, warfarin-type anticoagulants, lidocaine, theophylline and chlordiazepoxide—may be impaired during concommittant cimetidine therapy. Anemia may also be present as a result of gastrointestinal erosion.

Cessation of intestinal persistalsis, often lasting 3–5 days, may accompany spinal shock; intraabdominal and retroperitoneal hemorrhage may prolong the period of paralytic ileus. The resulting increase in intraabdo-minal pressure secondary to bowel distention may further compromise an already limited respiratory reserve. This also predisposes the acutely in-jured patient to vomiting and aspiration of gastric contents.

The bedridden SCI patient is highly susceptible to venous stasis, and pulmonary embolus is a leading cause of death within the first month after injury. Compression stockings, low-dose heparin and stabilization of the spine to allow early ambulation are prophylactic measures.

Intermediate Phase of SCI

The onset of the intermediate phase of recovery from SCI develops approx-imately one month after injury. It is characterized by the resolution of spinal shock and the appearance of autonomic hyperreflexia. This is a con-dition in which afferent somatic sensory and visceral impulses arising from below the level of the lesion enter the isolated spinal cord and elicit a massive sympathetic response from the adrenal medulla and sympathetic nervous system. The sympathetic response is no longer modulated by the normal inhibitory impulses arising from the brainstem and hypothalamus.

Autonomic hyperreflexia manifests in 85% of spinal cord transections above the T5 level in which splanchnic outflow remains intact. Afferent impulses originating from bladder or bowel distention, childbirth, man-ipulations of the urinary tract or surgical stimulation are transmitted along the pelvic, pudendal or hypogastric nerves to the isolated spinal cord. Vasoconstriction occurs below the lesion; reflex activity of carotid and aortic pressure sensors produce vasodilation above the lesion, which is often accompanied by bradycardia, ventricular arrhythmias and even heart block. The anesthesiologist must be aware that the potential for this com-plication arising during surgery is maximal 4 weeks after injury; although it gradually subsides, it may reoccur after many years.[3]

The hyperkalemic response to succinylcholine extends into this period, as does hypercalcemia from prolonged immobilization. The risk of ven-ous thromboembolism also increases as the duration of immobilization lengthens.

Chronic Phase of SCI

Renal function may deteriorate in the SCI patient because of repeated infections and stone formation secondary to hypercalciuria. Ascending pyelonephritis and chronic renal failure result in loss of serum protein, sodium and potassium. In addition, serum BUN and creatinine become elevated. Preoperative evaluation of electrolytes, protein, BUN and creati-nine are essential; efforts must be made to restore these values to within normal limits before undertaking any elective surgery. Urinary tract infections should be resolved with appropriate antibiotic therapy.

Compounding protein and electrolyte abnormalities is the negative nitrogen balance into which the SCI patient enters almost immediately after injury. In addition to skeletal muscle wasting, visceral wasting may also ensue secondary to inactivity and/or denervation. Wasting of the diaphragm is potentially dangerous to a patient who may rely entirely on diaphragmatic activity for breathing.

As patients enter the chronic stage of SCI, they become more susceptible to limb fractures during periods of movement and positioning for surgery. Muscle spasm and contractures are seen when spinal shock resolves and may present technical difficulties to locating intravenous sites and positioning for surgery. Physical therapy with passive range of motion should be initiated soon after injury to prevent contractures. Throughout all stages of recovery from spinal cord injury, the anesthesiologist should be aware of the potential for underlying depression, anger and denial, as well as drug dependence. Such psychological problems are often overlooked when treating SCI patients for their more obvious, physical injuries.

References

1. Albin M.S.: Resuscitation of the spinal cord. *Crit Care Med* 6:270, 1978.
2. Young J.S., Burns P.E., Bowen A.M., et al: *Spinal cord injury statistics. Experience of the Regional Spinal Cord Injury Systems*, Phoenix, Arizona, Good Samaritan Medical Center, 1982.
3. Cottrell J.E., Newfield P., Giffin J.P., et al: Spinal cord injury, in, Cottrell J.E., Newfield P. (eds), *Handbook of Neuroanesthesia: Clinical and Physiologic Essentials*, Boston, Little Brown & Co, 1983, p 339.
4. Ransohoff J., Flamm E.S., Demopoulos H.B.: Mechanisms of injury and treatment of acute spinal cord trauma, in, Cottrell JE, Turndorf H (eds), *Anesthesia and Neurosurgery*, St. Louis, CV Mosby Co, 1980, pp 361–386.
5. Kopaniky D.R., Frost E.A.M.: Management of spinal cord trauma, in, Frost E.A.M. (ed), *Clinical Anesthesia in Neurosurgery*, Boston, Butterworth, 1984, pp 375–396.
6. Dohrmann G.J., Wagner F.C. Jr, Bucy P.C.: The microvasculature in transitory traumatic paraplegia: An electron microscopic study in monkey. *J Neurosurg* 35:263, 1971.
7. Gronert G.A., Theye R.A.: Pathophysiology of hyperkalemia induced by succinylcholine. *Anesthesiology* 43:89, 1975.
8. Cooperman L.H.: Succinylcholine-induced hyperkalemia in neuromuscular disease. *JAMA* 213:1867, 1970.
9. Greenshoot J.H., Reichenbach D.: Cardiac injury and subarachnoid hemorrhage: A clinical pathologic correlation. *J Neurosurg* 30:521, 1969.
10. Maynard F.M., Imai K.: Immobilization hypercalcemia in spinal cord injury. *Arch Phys Med Rehab* 58:16, 1977.

11. Tenicela R., Rosomoff H.L., Fiest J., et al: Pulmonary function following per-cutaneous cervical cordotomy. *Anesthesiology* 29:7, 1968.
12. Ledsome J.R., Sharp J.M.: Pulmonary function in acute cervical cord injury. *Am Rev Resp Dis* 124:41, 1981.
13. Henry D.A., MacDonald I.A., Kitchingman G., et al: Cimetidine and raniti-dine: comparison of effects of hepatic drug metabolism. *Br Med J* 281:775, 1980.

CHAPTER 9

The Patient with Juvenile Laryngeal Papillomas*

Ashok Kumar

Case History. *A 5-year-old child was scheduled for elective excision of laryngeal papillomas, first diagnosed one year previously following the onset of stridor. This was the sixth admission for the same surgical procedure. The boy had developed normally and appeared healthy except for mild hoarseness. Laboratory examinations were all within normal limits.*

Pathophysiology of Juvenile Laryngeal Papillomas

Laryngeal papillomas of juvenile type are benign tumors that are thought to be of viral etiology (warts). They cause symptoms, such as hoarseness, cough, stridor and airway obstruction, that make them indistinguishable from other laryngeal lesions.[1] The diagnosis is suspected from physical appearance at direct laryngoscopy and confirmed by biopsy.

Papillomas may occur at any age, but they develop most commonly at one year. They may be found anywhere in the respiratory tract, but 90% of the lesions are on the vocal cords. Because papillomas undergo spontaneous regression, evaluation of therapy is difficult.

Papillomas are probably viral in origin; about 50% of the afflicted children are born to mothers with documented genital warts at the time of delivery. There is an increased incidence of skin warts among family members. Intranuclear papoviral-like particles have been demonstrated clinically.

The main sign is stridor, which is produced by airflow during respiration through an obstructed airway. The sounds may be harsh or soft, musical, high or low pitched depending on the type, site and extent of airway narrowing and speed of airflow.

Stridor due to laryngeal papillomas may be inspiratory or expiratory. The abnormal sound is caused by two factors: narrowing in the larynx by

---

*Reviewed by Dr. Dinesh Mehta, Associate Professor of Otolaryngology, Albert Einstein College of Medicine of Yeshiva University, Bronx, New York.

the tumor causing increased airflow and turbulence; narrowing of the extrathoracic trachea from dynamic compression during inspiration. When the laryngeal tumor causes severe narrowing or "fixed obstruction," stridor will be present during inspiration and expiration.

The cornerstone of therapy at present is palliative, rather than therapeutic, surgery. This has been attempted with various modalities including electrocautery, ultrasound, cryosurgery, and laser surgery.

The goals of surgery are to maintain a patent airway and good voice tones, and to avoid tracheostomy, which is associated with a higher incidence of "seeding" in the trachea and bronchi. Children require repeat microscopic endoscopy at frequent intervals for direct visual inspection and reduction of tumor mass. The laser has gained widespread acceptance for papilloma excision because of bloodless precise removal of papillomas with minimal trauma to underlying structures. Hence, the danger of laryngeal stenosis is greatly reduced and, with remission of the papilloma, the functional integrity of the larynx is well maintained.

Laser

The medical applications and uses of the laser have increased greatly over the last 20 years.[2] Currently, lasers are used for cauterization, tumor destruction and for bloodless surgery.

The close cooperation of physicists, engineers and physicians has led to the application of lasers in medicine. It is a prime example of the value of clinical application of basic science discoveries.

The safe use of a new medical instrument such as the laser requires that personnel be aware of the background principles and hazards involved. Laser is a form of electromagnetic radiation, and strict adherence to safeguard against health hazards is essential.[3]

Laser is an acronym for Light Amplification by Stimulated Emission of Radiation. The precursor of laser was the Maser, an acronym coined by Nobel laureate C.H. Townes, Microwave Amplification by Stimulated Emission of Radiation. In 1958, work was extended from microwaves to the visible light spectrum and led to the construction of the first ruby laser in the Bell Telephone Laboratories. The output of the early laser was not precisely controlled until the technique of "Q" switching permitted all the energy of radiation to be stored in the laser and released in pulses. The use of lasers in space technology led to further developments that have been incorporated into the present-day lasers seen in the operating room. See Figure 1.

Characteristics

Lasers can be generated from solids, liquids or gases with resultant radiation of different wavelengths and biomedical properties. See Table 1. The

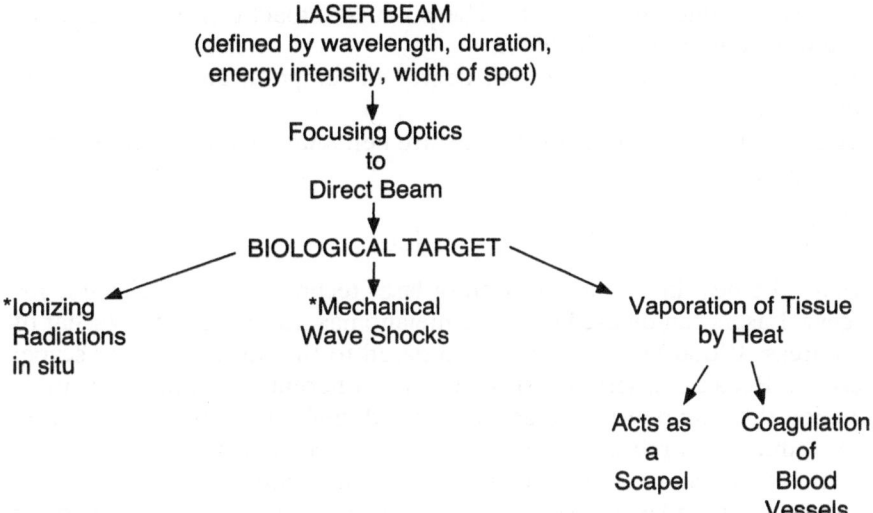

FIGURE 1

material used to generate the laser defines depth of vaporization and damage of tissue.

Atoms of elements that can be excited to emit light waves are contained in the laser in long narrow tubes with mirrors at either end. External energy is provided initially to excite some of the atoms. The light wave emitted by these few atoms is amplified by stimulating other atoms to emit. This gives rise to a beam or wave which develops tremendous energy by reflection between the mirrors. Finally, the radiation wave emerges from the partially reflective mirror as an intense directional beam of light.

Laser beams have unique properties compared to other light-wave beams. This is because all other light or radiation is comprised of wave emissions from individual atoms that are independent of other excited atoms.

Well-described laser characteristics include:

• A near single frequency of low band-width, ie, an almost pure monochromatic beam.

TABLE 1. Currently used laser sources.

Solids	Gases
Ruby (red beam)	Carbon dioxide (invisible beam)
Neodymium–glass	Helium–neon (red beam)
Yttrium–aluminum–garnet (YAG)	Argon (blue-green beam)
Neodymium YAG	Krypton
	Nitrogen

- Precisely defined wave fronts. The point of impact can be the same as the wavelength, eg, 0.000069cm.
- Enormous intensity and a high degree of temporal and spatial coherence.
- High plane of polarization and tremendous electromagnetic field strength.

Applications

Perhaps the best-known application of laser technology to medicine is for surgery. Lasers can be used to excise melanomas, tumors and the eschar of burn areas. Blood loss is reduced compared to that during regular scapel excision. Because lasers are a source of coherent and monochromatic radiation that can be focused accurately with high intensity, they are used in procedures that require precision. The laser accomplishes tissue excision by vaporization and at the same time seals small blood vessels. The use of a microscope with a laser ensures a bloodless operative field with controlled depth of tissue removal. The carbon dioxide laser, for instance, emits an invisible wave of 10.6 microns, which is absorbed within 0.2cm of tissue surface.

In dermatology, lasers have been used for many years to remove tattoos, to bleach birth marks and to remove skin tumors and hemagiomatas. In ophthalmology, lasers are used for diagnosis of early cataracts and for photocoagulation in several conditions, eg, retinal detachment. Other diagnostic uses include the application of laser spectroscopy to microanalytic techniques, Pap smears, and immunofluorescent techniques.

Laser radiographs appear superior to conventional x-rays, and uses that are under investigation include breast tumor imaging and occlusion of hemangiomas. An argon laser blood counter can determine CBC, WBC, Hct, and can calculate mean corpuscular volume and hemoglobin concentration. Lasers are also being investigated in caries prevention in dentistry.

Laser fiberoptic transmission constitutes another entire area of potential applications. Laser fiberoptic transmission can be an effective vehicle for mass communication in examination of patient records, test results, and in medical teaching. A helium-neon laser beam communication system has been used in the Cleveland Hospitals for central anesthesia monitoring in the operating suite.

Laser Safety Program

Development of a laser safety program is most important prior to intraoperative use of the laser. The laser can ignite any combustible material, and as such, it is a fire hazard. Any tissue the laser is focused on will be vaporized, whether it is diseased or healthy. In addition, contact with the laser, like all radiation, should be avoided. There is no known acceptable or safe dose. There may be biological effects from scattered or reflected radiation. The long-term effects on the genetic system are unknown, as are the effects during pregnancy.

Area control is essential to a safety program. Laser devices should be in isolated, low-traffic areas, locked in cabinets and used only by authorized personnel. Adequate ventilation and scavenging systems should remove all by-products as the dangers of inhalation or dissemination of viral, bacterial or tumor tissue has not been determined.

A good suction system should be available to remove smoke and vaporized tissue which might otherwise disseminate virus particles to the respiratory tract of the operating room personnel or within the patient. Surfaces in the room should be minimally reflective. Warning signs and light alarms should be posted at the entrances.

A laser safety officer should head the safety program, which must include plans for emergency treatment of laser radiation and personnel education programs.

Eye protection is one of the most significant aspects of the safety program. The lens of the eye can focus the laser beam and cause retinal burns. Eye safety can be afforded by use of goggles, which must have high optical density and be specific for the laser wavelength in use. The goggles must be worn continuously during laser use and must fit the forehead and temple to enclose the globe of the eye. The carbon dioxide beam is invisible, and a visible tracer light is incorporated to enable the surgeon to select the target area. The axis of the visible tracer and laser beam should be aligned prior to use.

Skin exposure may lead to acute or chronic burns. Sterile gloves are adequate, but black leather gloves are preferred if the hands are close to or in the field of the laser beam. Other areas should be draped with cloth (wet if possible). Laser beams undergo scattering and can be reflected like x-ray radiation. Hair, flammable hair preparations, scrubbing solutions, and some anesthetic agents are a direct fire hazard.

Electrical hazard exists because the initial excitation of the atoms requires high-energy currents and electrical circuits. This adds to the existing hazards of electrical apparatus already in the operating room.

Laser measure and knowledge of the magnitude of laser output levels are an absolute prerequisite to controlled use. The present methods of measuring high-energy laser beams and standardizing are far from ideal and subject to error. Energy density is defined by the total energy (joules) and spot size (cm^2) but this does not take into account the pulse duration of the beam nor does it give an indication of the biological effect.

Patient Protection

Laser hazards to the patient arise from damage to normal tissue or from fires. The patient's eyes should be covered with wet gauze. If a misdirected or reflected beam strikes unprotected normal tissue, it too is vaporized.

The risk of fire is highest with use of flammable anesthetics or when the endotracheal tube is within the laser field.[4] Commercial endotracheal tubes (red rubber or plastic) are combustible. Both oxygen and nitrous oxide support combustion.

There are a number of approaches to reduce the risk of ignition of the endotracheal tube. The simplest is use of an anesthetic technique that does not require endotracheal intubation. Jet venturi ventilation (proximal ventilation) may be provided from catheters incorporated in the operating laryngoscope. Although these techniques theoretically compromise control of the airway and ventilation and have a potential risk of gastric distention, large studies have documented minimal complications.

When endotracheal intubation is necessary, the tube may be protected by a nonflammable material.[5] Aluminum foil has been used, but sharp edges may damage the tracheal muscosa. Airway obstruction by broken pieces has been described.[6] In addition, reflection of the laser beam off the metallic surface causes burning of healthy tissue. Combustible tubes may be wrapped with muslin, which requires continuous soaking. Red rubber tubes have been reported as the least likely to burn vigorously, and they do not produce dangerous vapors immediately on laser contact. The cuff is inflated with saline as a further protective measure. However, the red rubber cuffs exert high pressures and the tubes must be resterilized. It is important to note that the blue barium sulfate stripes on the PVC tubes ignite more rapidly than the rest of the tubing.

Endotracheal tubes made of flexible metal rings are less likely to ignite, but they may cause pressure damage to the larynx and are cumbersome for suctioning.[7] A new tube made of silicone with a coating of aluminum oxide (Laser Shield®, Xomed, Jacksonville, FL) is available. It may be excessively rigid if used for nasal intubation.[8]

Oil-based lubricants should be avoided on all endotracheal tubes and endoscopes.

Use of helium as the carrier gas reduces the rise in temperature around the site of laser exposure, which prevents endotracheal tubes from reaching a temperature of spontaneous ignition. However, the protective effect of helium diminishes rapidly when the power outlet reaches a level greater than 10 watts. Periodic calibration by a competent specialist is, therefore, required.

Anesthetic Management

The anesthetic plan is determined by the symptoms of the laryngeal papillomas and the extent of treatment previously rendered. At the first endoscopy, the extent of pathology is unknown and there is the potential for airway obstruction during induction. At subsequent endoscopies the risk is lowered, but the ability to perform emergency tracheotomy must still be available. Patients with a tracheotomy (a diminishing group) are relatively easier to manage from an airway point of view.

Anesthetic exposures are often multiple. All patients are anxious, and preoperative communication and establishment of rapport are crucial to allow inhalation induction or intravenous cannulation. Premedication drugs must achieve sedation without danger of compromising the airway. Belladonna drugs are a prerequisite.

Both inhalation (excluding flammable agents) and intravenous techniques have been used. Ketamine anesthesia should be avoided as laryngospasm can occur. The vocal cords or target area must be relaxed and immobile.[9] Small movements may cause the surgeon to misdirect the beam, and damage to normal tissue may result. Short-acting neuromuscular blocking agents, such as succinylcholine, atracurium or vecuronium, should be used.

Continuous suction removes vaporized tissue which would otherwise create a fog. Alveolar ventilation should be monitored, ideally by mass spectrometry, because of the small size of the endotracheal tubes used. Because air leaks around the endotracheal tube are common, end-tidal nitrogen levels are not insignificant. ECG monitoring is essential; an audible alarm is necessary because the room is darkened during laser surgery.

Vagal reflexes can originate from surgical pharyngeal stimulation. Multiple doses of succinylcholine or the use of halothane may also give rise to cardiac arrhythmias. Atropine and intravenous lidocaine should be readily available. A large dose of steroids is given intraoperatively to attenuate edema formation in the vocal cords. At the conclusion of the procedure spontaneous respiratory efforts may be misdiagnosed as partial airway obstruction, as the small internal diameter of the endotracheal tube presents significant airway resistance.

Postoperatively, the area around the field should be checked for accidental burns, especially in the trachea, pharynx, and tongue. Airway integrity must be carefully monitored.

References

1. Strong M.S., Vaughan C.W., Cooperhand S.R.: Recurrent respiratory papillomatosis: management with CO_2 laser. *Ann Otol Rhinol Laryngol* 85:508–516, 1976.
2. Goldman L., Rockwell R.J. Jr: *Laser in Medicine*, New York, Gordon & Breach Science Publishers Inc., 1971.
3. Goldman L.: Laser medical instrumentation. *Medical Instrumentation* 10(2): 125–129, 1976.
4. Snow J.C., Norton M.L., Saluja T.S. et al: Fire hazard during CO_2 laser microsurgery on the larynx and trachea. *Anesth & Analg* 55:146–147, 1976.
5. Kumar A., Frost E.: Prevention of fire hazard during laser surgery. *Anesthesiology* 54(6):350, 1981.

6. Hermens J.M., Bennett M.J., Hirshman C.A.: Anesthesia for laser surgery. *Anesth & Analg* 62:218–229, 1983.
7. Norton M.L.: New endotracheal tube for laser surgery of the larynx. *Ann Otol Rhinol Laryngol* 87:554, 1978.
8. Vitkun S., Sidhu U.S., Lagade M.R.G. et al: Intranasal trauma caused by sharp edged laser resistant endotracheal tube. *Anesthesiology* 62:834, 1985.
9. Snow J.C., Kripke B., Strong M.S. et al: Anesthesia for carbon dioxide laser microsurgery on the larynx and trachea. *Anesth & Analg* 53:507–512, 1974.

CHAPTER 10

The Patient with Aortic Valvular Disease*

Irene Osborn

Case History. *A 56-year-old man with a history of noncritical aortic stenosis and aortic insufficiency was admitted to the hospital with a 2-week complaint of spiking fevers, arthralgia, and neuralgia. The patient had had a dental procedure 6 weeks prior to admission, for which antibiotic prophylaxis had been given. His hospital course was significant for positive blood cultures for Staph epidermidis and he was treated with appropriate antibiotics. He began to improve but soon developed substernal chest pain, diaphoresis, and shortness of breath. The electrocardiogram showed prolongation of the P-R interval without ischemic changes. The diagnosis of acute aortic insufficiency was confirmed by echocardiogram, and the patient was scheduled for aortic valve replacement.*

Past medical history included rheumatic fever as a child with no history of cardiac decompensation. The patient had only one previous hospitalization, for cellulitis 6 months prior to admission. He denied hypertension, diabetes mellitus or other systemic illnesses. He smoked 2 packs of cigarettes per day and reported an allergy to penicillin.

Physical examination revealed a slightly obese male in mild distress, alert, oriented and cooperative. Vital signs were: blood pressure 110/65; pulse 96/min; respiratory rate 22/min; weight 225 lbs; height 6 ft. Chest examination revealed coarse rôles in both bases, slightly increased on the left side. The heart had regular rhythm with a grade III/VI systolic ejection murmur at the left sternal border, and a low-pitched diastolic murmur. The abdomen was soft and nontender; lower extremities were unremarkable.

Laboratory findings included the following: serum chemistries were within normal limits; Hct 36%; PT, PTT and platelets were within normal limits. The chest x-ray showed cardiomegaly and congestive heart failure. Electrocardiogram revealed a sinus rhythm of 80/min with a normal axis; left ventricular hypertrophy; P-R interval 0.28mm, QRS 0.08mm; and Q waves in leads V_1 through V_4.

---

*Reviewed by Dr. Yasu Oka, Professor of Anesthesiology, Albert Einstein College of Medicine of Yeshiva University, Bronx, New York.

Further noninvasive studies revealed: aortic valve area 1.0cm²/m² (normal = 2.6–3.5cm²/m²); left ventricular ejection fraction 0.52 (normal = 0.62– 0.85). Due to the patient's critical condition and the urgent nature of the surgery, no cardiac catheterization was performed.

Aortic Stenosis

Aortic stenosis (AS) is a chronic disorder that may be caused by rheumatic disease. It may also be secondary to congenital bicuspid valve disease. Isolated AS is the most common cardiac valvular lesion.[1] Idiopathic calcific AS occurs most often in the elderly. The pathological process is considered to be degenerative, and the aortic valve progressively becomes calcified and obstructed.

The primary pathology is obstruction to left ventricular ejection. Increased pressure overload of the ventricle occurs with an increase in left ventricular mass (concentric hypertrophy). This leads to reduced ventricular compliance and contractility. Increased systolic wall tension is characteristic of AS.

The hypertrophied left ventricle is extremely vulnerable to ischemia because of increased myocardial oxygen consumption as well as decreased coronary blood flow. See Figure 1. Increased myocardial work is primarily due to the generation of increased wall tension, which is very oxygen costly and therefore likely to cause ischemia. Late changes in AS include decreased left ventricular contractility with dilatation and, ultimately, a decrease in stroke volume and cardiac output.[2]

An asymptomatic period (up to 50 years or more) is seen initially when AS occurs without other valvular pathology. See Figure 2. Sudden death

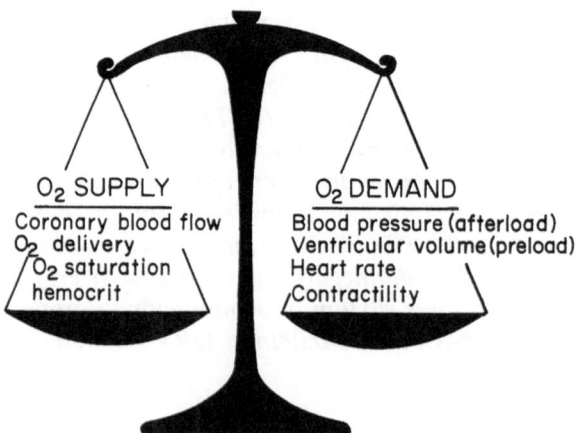

FIGURE 1. Myocardial oxygen balance. Adapted by permission from Kaplan J.A.: *Cardiac Anesthesia*. Orlando, Florida, Grune & Stratton, 1979.

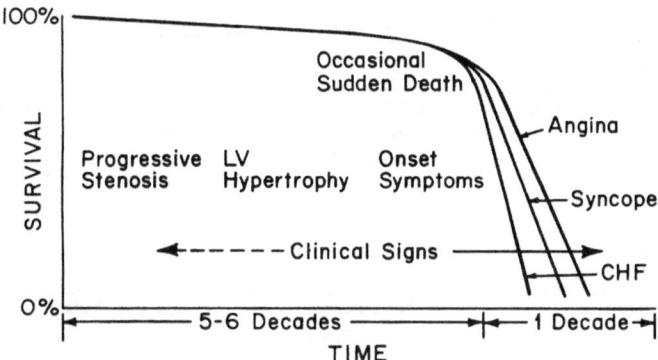

FIGURE 2. Natural history of aortic stenosis. From *Cardiac Anesthesia* by Thomas J. Conahan III. Copyright ©1982 by Addison-Wesley Publishing Company, Inc. Reprinted with permission.

may occur in previously asymptomatic patients. The frequency of sudden death is estimated to be 0.4% per year during the first three decades; thereafter, it increases with age.

Angina, syncope, and congestive heart failure are the most common symptoms of the disease and signify the onset of its severity. Bacterial endocarditis is found in approximately 1% of patients and causes a significant increase in mortality.[3]

During evaluation, the electrocardiogram should be examined to note rhythm and possible presence of junctional bradycardia. Tachycardia is the hazard most likely to precipitate an imbalance between myocardial oxygen supply and demand. The best indicator of the severity of AS is the calculated valve area. Cardiac index and pressure measurements should also be examined. An ejection fraction of less than 50% indicates impairment of myocardial contractility.

Aortic Insufficiency

Aortic insufficiency (AI) may be either acute or chronic. Acute onset may be secondary to infective endocarditis, trauma, or aortic aneurysm. Chronic AI can be caused by rheumatic disease, hypertension, syphilis, or less common diseases such as Marfan's syndrome.

The basic hemodynamic abnormality in AI is a decrease in effective stroke volume. This is due to diastolic regurgitation of part of the total stroke volume from the aorta back into the left ventricle. Chronic AI results in left ventricular volume overload with resultant increased myocardial fiber length. This produces eccentric hypertrophy (increase in both chamber size and wall thickness).

Baseline myocardial oxygen requirements are increased in AI because of the very large increase in ventricular mass. Simultaneously, myocardial

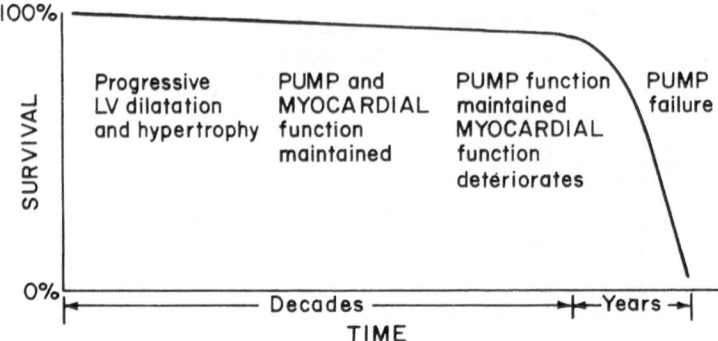

FIGURE 3. Natural history of chronic aortic regurgitation. From *Cardiac Anesthesia* by Thomas J. Conahan III. Copyright ©1982 by Addison-Wesley Publishing Company, Inc. Reprinted with permission.

oxygen supply is compromised by a reduced coronary perfusion pressure (CPP = diastolic BP − LVEDP).

In spite of these changes and even though calculated myocardial work may be twice normal, myocardial ischemia is uncommon in chronic AI. Imbalances between myocardial oxygen demand and supply rarely occur because myocardial fiber shortening accounts for most of the increase in cardiac work.

It is important to distinguish chronic AI from acute AI. Cardiomegaly and wide pulse pressure are commonly observed with chronic AI. Signs and symptoms of pulmonary venous hypertension and a narrow pulse pressure are associated with acute AI. The natural history of chronic AI is that of a long asymptomatic period during which the left ventricle undergoes progressive enlargement. See Figure 3. Symptoms, classically those of left ventricular failure, usually appear only after the onset of irreversible changes in myocardial contractility.[5, 6]

In combined AS and AI there can be significant regurgitant flow through small orifices because of the relatively high diastolic pressure gradient from aorta to left ventricle. Because of the regurgitant flow, left ventricular end diastolic pressure (LVEDP) increases. Left ventricular diastolic and systolic tension increase greatly, so that hypertrophy and left ventricular mass are greater than in pure AS. For these reasons, symptoms of pulmonary congestion and myocardial ischemia occur at a larger aortic valve area than in pure AS. The critical valve area for severe stenosis is approximately $0.9 cm^2/m^2$ when significant aortic regurgitation is present; it is about $0.5 cm^2/m^2$ in pure aorta stenosis.[2]

Preoperative Evaluation

The preoperative assessment should focus on the cardiac disease process as well as its effects on the other body systems.

History and Physical Examination

Emphasis should be placed on the history of symptoms and their progression. The patient's baseline level of activity should be determined. On examination, signs of congestive heart failure must be carefully evaluated: enlarged heart, râles, S_3 gallop, peripheral edema, pulsatile and enlarged liver. Symptoms of chronic AI may be observed, such as wide pulse pressure, "water hammer" pulse, head bobbing, and diastolic thrill.[4]

The hazard of anesthesia in patients with congestive heart failure is magnified because of greatly reduced myocardial reserve and cardiac output. Pulmonary congestion and the presence of pleural effusions foster severe ventilation/perfusion defects with increased pulmonary shunting and dead space ventilation. The reduced cardiac output can promote changes in depth of anesthesia and concomitant alterations in cardiovascular dynamics and critical organ perfusion during anesthetic induction. These latter changes have been seen following even small variations in inspired concentrations of inhalation agents or minimal doses of intravenous drugs.[10]

Adequate therapy for congestive heart failure can rarely be accomplished in a few hours. If time is available, medical therapy should include bed rest, a low-salt diet, vigorous diuresis, adequate digitalization, potassium supplementation, and pharmacologic therapy for control or conversion of serious dysrhythmias.[10]

Laboratory Examination

Electrocardiograms will reveal evidence of coexisting coronary artery disease (ST segment depression or T-wave inversion or flattening) as well as a previous myocardial infarction (diminished R-wave voltage with preceding abnormal Q waves). Moreover, they will demonstrate the presence of atrial contraction and the degree of left and right ventricle hypertrophy. Chest x-ray will confirm clinical disease findings and evaluate any underlying pulmonary disease.[9]

The echocardiogram can demonstrate specific valvular abnormalities and dysfunction. It can also quantitate cardiac chamber enlargement and ventricular ejection fraction. It is particularly useful for identifying valvular abnormalities such as mitral stenosis.[8]

Angiographic studies with injection of contrast material in the left ventricle are helpful in defining the size of the left ventricular cavity, the thickness of the wall, the size of obstruction, the degree of deformity and mobility of the aortic cusps, and the presence of accompanying mitral regurgitation. The grading of valvular stenosis requires measurement of both flow and pressure gradients across the valve in question. These gradients may appear deceptively low if the patient is hypovolemic and/or has a low cardiac output. For AI, the data of most importance are left ventricular ejection fraction and LVEDP.

Monitoring

The degree of sophistication of monitoring should be determined by the hemodynamic status of the patient. The electrocardiogram, including a continuously displayed V_5 lead, should be used in all patients. This is particularly important in patients who are vulnerable to ischemia. Direct measurement of arterial blood pressure is essential for all patients; arterial catheterization also facilitates the monitoring of arterial blood gases.

Temperature and urinary output determinations are important for management. The perioperative insertion of a pulmonary artery catheter is certainly indicated. Although central venous pressure should reflect directional changes in left atrial pressure, there may be significant differences between right- and left-sided pressures in those patients with less compliant ventricles. Knowledge of the wedge pressure will help the anesthesiologist maintain adequate intravascular volume.[9] In addition, determination of aortic diastolic pressure allows maintenance of this parameter in order to ensure adequate stroke volume.[9]

Anesthetic Management

Any premedication should be administered with caution. In general, a moderate amount of sedation with intravenous supplementation in the operating room is well tolerated. Undue anxiety may provoke tachycardia, which must be avoided.

For patients with AS, sinus rhythm is essential since the noncompliant ventricle requires a high ventricular volume (up to 40% of output is supplied by the force of atrial contraction). Hypotension can seriously jeopardize myocardial blood flow. Patients with AI can tolerate a faster heart rate (80–90/min) which maintains stroke volume and reduces ventricular size. A gentle reduction in afterload will also augment cardiac output. In acute AI, the failing right ventricle may be the limiting factor in successful management.

The choice of specific anesthetic agents and techniques depends in large part on the individual anesthesiologist's skill and experience. The principles discussed apply also to patients with aortic valvular disease undergoing noncardiac surgery. The essential concept is careful titration of drugs to obtain the best anesthetic and surgical conditions while maintaining hemodynamic stability.[3]

References

1. Jackson J.: Valvular heart disease, in Thomas S. (ed): *Manual of Cardiac Anesthesia*. New York, Churchill Livingston, 1984, pp 231–267.
2. Chambers D.A.: Acquired valvular heart disease, in Kaplan J. (ed): *Cardiac Anesthesia*. New York, Grune & Stratton, 1979, pp. 220–232.

3. Reves J.G.: Anesthesia for acquired cardiac disease. Annual American Society of Anesthesiologists 1984 Refresher Course Lectures, 123.
4. Schlandt R.C.: Altered cardiovascular function of rheumatic heart disease and other acquired valvular disease, in Hurst J. (ed): *The Heart*. New York, McGraw Hill, 1974, pp. 967–971.
5. Rappaport E.: Natural history of aortic and mitral valve disease. *Am J Cardiology* 35:221, 1975.
6. Morganroth J., Perloff J.K.: Acute severe aortic regurgitation. *Ann Intern Med* 87:223, 1977.
7. Geer R.T.: Anesthetic management of patients with cardiac disease, in Wollman & Greenhow (ed): *Surgical Clinics of North America*, Philadelphia, W.B. Saunders, 1975, p 903.
8. Leidtke A.J. Determinants of cardiac performance in severe aortic stenosis. *Chest* 69:192–200, 1976.
9. Thomas S.J., Lowenstein E.: Anesthetic management of the patient with valvular heart disease, in Philbin D. (ed): *International Anesthesiology Clinics*, Boston, Little Brown & Co, 1979, 17:75–87.
10. Garman J.K., Fogdall R.P.: The Prebypass Period, in Ream A.K. & Fogdall (ed): *Acute Cardiovascular Management*, Philadelphia, J.B. Lippincott, 1982, pp 406–12.

CHAPTER 11

The Patient in Diabetic Ketoacidosis*

Richard B. Patt

Case History. *A 55-year-old diabetic man was admitted to the emergency room in a semicomatose state, with gangrene of both feet. His diabetes had been managed with diet alone until 2 years prior to admission, when tolbutamide was added. There was no history of myocardial insufficiency or hypertension, nor was the patient taking other medications. There was a 4-month history of bilateral lower extremity pain, with discoloration and skin changes, progressing to gangrene. The patient had continually refused to be admitted to the hospital and was treated symptomatically at home. On the night before admission he had been vomiting, and in the morning he was noted to be unresponsive.*

In the emergency room the patient was pale, diaphoretic, and responsive only to noxious stimuli. The pulse was thready at 110 beats per minute, blood pressure was 100/60, and respiratory rate was 40 per minute. The lungs were clear, and the patient's breath was noted to have a distinct fruity odor. There was dry gangrene involving the inferior third of the right leg, and wet gangrene of the ankle on the left. Two peripheral veins were cannulated, blood and urine samples were obtained, and the patient was transferred to the OR for emergency bilateral amputation.

The surgical team was anxious to operate immediately, reasoning that only by eliminating the septic foci would the patient's metabolic abnormalities be reversed. Consultation between anesthesia and surgery personnel resulted in transfer to the recovery room for a brief period of resuscitation and stabilization.

In the recovery room, normal saline in aliquots of 250cc was administered, while urine output and CVP were monitored. Initial CVP was 0–1cmH$_2$O. Urinalysis revealed 2 + ketones. Precordial ST-T wave depression of 2mm resolved gradually as fluid was administered.

Initial laboratory values were as follows: glucose 640, Na$^+$ 134, K$^+$ 3.2,

---

*Reviewed by Dr. Harry Shamoon, Associate Professor of Medicine, Albert Einstein College of Medicine of Yeshiva University, Bronx, New York.

Cl^- 90, HCO_3^- 12, BUN 32, Hct 48%, WBC 23,000. After 4 liters O_2/ minute was delivered by facemask, the following values were obtained: PaO_2 54, $PaCo_2$ 55, pH 6.95, HCO_3^- 12, BE 12. Chest x-ray revealed no acute pulmonary disease.

The stomach was decompressed with nasogastric suctioning and the trachea was intubated easily without sedation or topical anesthesia. At FlO_2 = 0.5, the lungs were mechanically ventilated with an 800cc tidal volume at a rate of 16 breaths per minute. In the course of resuscitation, $PaCO_2$ and PaO_2 were normalized, and the pH was raised to 7.34 following the administration of 50mEq bicarbonate in divided doses.

The hyperglycemia and acetonuria were treated with intravenous boluses of crystalline insulin, and a continuous infusion at 10 units/hour. The infusion plus 40 units of insulin, followed 1 hour later by 20 units, reduced serum glucose to 350mg% and eliminated acetone from the urine. Hourly aliquots of 20mEq potassium phosphate in 100cc normal saline raised extracellular potassium to 3.4mEq/L. A urine output of 1cc/kg/hour was established with 4 liters of normal saline over 2 hours, by which time the CVP was raised to 5cmH$_2$O, the pulse had slowed to 100 and BP was 110/60. Gradually the patient began to make purposeful motions, and respond to verbal contact.

Definitions

An accepted classification of patients with diabetes mellitus designates the insulin-dependent patient as type I and patients not dependent on insulin as type II. Type I patients were formerly referred to as "juvenile" or "brittle" diabetics. Patients tend to be young, with a history of onset of diabetes in childhood. They are frequently underweight, and are prone to bouts of diabetic ketoacidosis (DKA).

Type II patients are generally older, obese, and are relatively resistant to developing DKA. When these patients are cooperative, diabetes can usually be controlled with weight loss, diet, and oral antihyperglycemic agents. With advanced disease, or when stressed, type II patients may require insulin.

Distinct etiologies and mechanisms have been suggested for each type of diabetes. Viral-initiated autoimmune destruction of panceatic beta cells with absolute insulin deficiency is the proposed mechanism for type I diabetes, although there is clearly familial predisposition.[1] Type II diabetes tends to be more easily traced to genetic factors. Although type II diabetes is characterized by gradual diminution of beta cell function, the more important cause of pathology is decreased sensitivity to insulin activity, partly due to a reduction in the number of insulin receptors. Resistance to circulating insulin seems to play as important a role as absolute deficiency of insulin.[1]

Pathophysiology

Classically, stress, in the form of infection, trauma, pregnancy or a high-carbohydrate diet, increases insulin requirements and places the diabetic patient at risk for developing DKA. Medications that can increase insulin requirements include corticosteroids, thyroid preparations, oral contraceptives and thiazide diuretics. The development of DKA may provide the first indication of overt diabetes in a patient with previously latent disease.[2]

DKA is encountered less frequently than in the past, probably due to better surveillance and maintenance of diabetes, and earlier and more aggressive intervention. In patients who do present with DKA, peripheral microvascular disease is frequently present. Infection, abscess or gangrene of an ischemic or insensitive lower extremity is the most common surgical condition requiring anesthetic intervention.

The patient with diabetic ketoacidosis can be regarded as being in acute metabolic failure, in the same sense as the patient in acute cardiac or renal failure. Diabetics are generally in a state of chronic failure, usually compensated for by medications and diet. There is still considerable debate whether the failing end organ is the beta cell population of the pancreas or the peripheral insulin receptor; but the end result is abnormal carbohydrate, fat, and protein metabolism. Regardless of the inciting factor, the primary defect is an inadequate level of circulating insulin.

Insulin is required for glucose to enter cells, where metabolism can occur. In addition, insulin is crucial for the regulation of hepatic glucose output. The absence of sufficient insulin activity results in concurrent intracellular glucopenia, extracellular glucose excess, and an increase in glucose output by the liver. The cells' predicament is not unlike that posed in Coleridge's *The Rhyme of the Ancient Mariner:* "Water, water everywhere, and not a drop to drink." Despite an (excessively) rich extracellular milieu, transmembrane passage of glucose is limited by insulin lack. These two manifestations of insulin deficiency trigger the other derangements that contribute to the syndrome of DKA.

Intracellular deficiency of carbohydrate substrate leads to breakdown of fats and proteins for energy. The beta-oxidation of free fatty acids into ketone bodies causes acidosis. Glucose mobilization and underutilization results in hyperglycemia which, with elevated plasma ketone levels, promotes an osmotic diuresis, causing dehydration, hypokalemia, and hyponatremia. Body stores of sodium, potassium, calcium, and magnesium are mobilized and further depleted as body base is drawn from the tissues to bind ketones for urinary excretion. As ketone levels exceed the renal ability for clearance, intoxication and neurologic symptoms ensue.

Fluid and electrolyte losses are compounded by vomiting. Acidosis and electrolyte abnormalities predispose to cardiac arrhythmias. Compensatory hyperventilation (Kussmaul respiration) imposes an added energy expenditure. Hemoconcentration and dehydration progress. If these derangements continue unchecked, circulatory collapse, renal failure, stupor, coma, and death follow. Patients prone to developing DKA may already have diabetes-related damage to renal and cardiovascular systems, and may be taking a variety of medications, all of which alter the disease course.

Management

In general, emergency surgery should not be undertaken in a patient in acute DKA until some measure of preoperative stability has been achieved. The neuroendocrine response to the stress of trauma, surgery, and anesthesia includes increases in plasma ACTH, cortisol, epinephrine, norepinephrine, renin, aldosterone, ADH, growth hormone and glucagon. Production of insulin, and thyroxine fall.[3] Hormonal effects result in: 1) increases in hepatic efflux of glucose due to glycogenolysis and gluconegensis; 2) inhibition of cellular uptake of glucose; 3) lipolysis, with formation of acetoacetic acid, β-hydroxybutyric acid and acetone; 4) protein catabolism, with increased urea formation; 5) inhibition of insulin release; and 6) peripheral resistance to insulin.[4] In the presence of compromised beta cell function, compensatory insulin secretion and activity are inadequate to counter elevations in blood sugar.

Teleologically, these responses to injury promote cardiovascular and overall stability by restitution of blood volume through salt and water conservation, and provision of additional substrate to meet increased metabolic demands by carbohydrate mobilization, lipolysis, and protein breakdown. However, in the type I diabetic, metabolic response is out of proportion to the degree of insult. In the case of DKA, activity that is ordinarily homeostatic impairs, and eventually dominates, the patient's overall condition.

Preoperative preparation should be carried out with specific and realistic goals in mind, so that surgery will not be unduly delayed. Abscess and infection are not correctable by conservative management alone. Antibiotic therapy should be instituted, but as long as infective processes remain active, the patient's metabolic derangements will be relatively resistant to therapy. Once the surgical problem is resolved, medical management becomes more effective. After surgery, there is a transition from a state of insulin resistance to insulin sensitivity (reverse-stress phenomena), and iatrogenic hypoglycemia must be avoided.

Preanesthetic Assessment

No single therapeutic regimen has been adopted to correct DKA in the patient with surgical emergency, in part because it is now an uncommon situation. Variability in the nature and severity of metabolic derangements, the urgency of surgery, and the degree of underlying disease make a "cookbook" approach to treatment undesirable. Therapy is directed toward rehydration, electrolyte and acid-base balance, and a return to glucose utilization. The first step toward treatment is establishing a diagnosis and an accurate assessment of the various derangements by history, physical, and laboratory examinations.

History

A prior history of diabetes is present in 90% of patients with DKA,[5] which should generate a high index of suspicion. Unlike hypoglycemic coma, DKA develops gradually, usually over several days. The picture is of progressive illness, with increasing thirst, polyuria, weakness, malaise, anorexia and weight loss. Nausea and vomiting, oliguria, and confusion leading to coma are later signs. An inciting factor may or may not be present, and there may be a history of diminished intake of exogenous insulin.

Physical Examination

The patient appears ill, and may be confused or stuporous. There are signs of dehydration, including dry mucous membranes, decreased skin turgor, sunken eyes, a weak and thready pulse, and decreased blood pressure with orthostasis. Aerophagia is common, with a Kussmaul pattern of respiration (deep, regular, sighing breaths). Acetone on the breath may be mistaken for the odor of alcohol or overlooked entirely. Temperature tends to be normal or subnormal. Fever suggests concurrent infection.

Laboratory Examination

The diagnosis of DKA can be rapidly confirmed by testing of the urine and blood with reagent strips (Dextrostix®, Ketostix®, Chemstrip®) or tablets (Acetest®) shows strongly positive results. If positive for ketones, alcoholic ketosis and starvation should be considered, especially if a history of diabetes is absent. Alcoholic ketosis involves recent excessive alcohol intake and starvation superimposed on chronic alcoholism. It is rarely accompanied by significant hyperglycemia; the hypoglycemia occasionally seen usually responds to intravenous glucose administration. In contrast, in nonketotic hyperosmolar coma there is hyperglycemia, but ketosis is absent.

Once the presence of excessive ketones and glucose has been verified by reagents, blood samples can be drawn and treatment instituted immediately. Serum glucose and acetone, bicarbonate and the pH of arterial blood quantitate the severity of the ketoacidosis. While measurement of plasma ketoacids is technically possible, tests are not generally clinically available. Bicarbonate concentration and pH are better indicators of ketosis than the qualitative ketone test, since the nitroprusside reaction only measures

TABLE 1. Properties of insulin preparations

Insulin preparation	Onset (hr)	Peak activity (hr)	Duration (hr)
Regular (crystalline)	1	2–4	5–7
NPH (isophane)	2	6–12	24–28

acetoacetate and acetone. Elevations in BUN, osmolality and hematocrit help to estimate the dregree of dehydration. Osmolality can be measured in the laboratory or calculated approximately:

$$Osmolality = \frac{2 \ ([Na] + [K]) + [BUN]}{2.8 \times [Glucose]} \times 18.$$

Abnormally high BUN and creatinine levels may signal acute or chronic renal failure. Serum potassium is frequently elevated initially, reflecting a shift from the intra- to extracellular compartment induced by acidosis. Intracellular and total body deficiencies of potassium must eventually be replaced, and serial potassium levels will help determine the proper timing for replacement.

Therapy

If possible, surgery should be postponed for 8–12 hours to correct major fluid, electrolyte, and acid–base derangements. Rarely, urgency of surgery dictates more precipitous resuscitation. Various insulin regimens have been advocated in these situations. Characteristics of commonly used insulin preparations are outlined in Table 1.

Traditionally, large doses of crystalline insulin (100–200 units or more) were given by a combination of intravenous and subcutaneous routes, and repeated as needed.[2] Current practice dictates that insulin be administered intravenously for more predictable absorption, especially when cardiovascular collapse and shunting away from the periphery are present.

Crystalline insulin has a half-life of only 5 minutes in vivo,[6] and insulin receptors become fully saturated at moderate plasma levels. Consequently, therapy is geared towards giving insulin in smaller intravenous doses at more frequent intervals, or by continuous infusion. If ketoacidosis is severe, a moderate bolus of intravenous insulin (20–50 units) is given initially. Approximate recommended dosages are given in Table 2. Continuous infusion of 1–10 units of crystalline insulin per hour has been reported to be effective.[7] Loss of insulin to the wall of the container and tubing is not a practical problem.[8] A combination of infusion and small boluses of insulin may be the best approach, since a higher dosage schedule will provide treatment for the rare patient with insulin resistance.[9] At a maximum insulin effect, blood sugar falls by 100–200mg/dl/hr, with more

TABLE 2. Sliding scale insulin dose

Urine test for glucose	Dose of soluble insulin (units)
2% ++++	20
1% +++	16
½% ++	10
¼% +	6
0% −	0

rapid reductions secondary to rehydration.[10] Precipitous falls may induce cerebral edema from osmotically induced fluid shifts.[11] Once serum glucose falls to 300mg/dl a maintenance infusion of a dextrose-containing solution should be initiated to avoid hypoglycemia.

Extracellular fluid deficit is commonly 10% of body weight (6–10 liters).[11] Replacement is with normal saline, as renal loss of sodium is considerable and not accurately reflected by serum levels. Hypotonic solutions predispose to cerebral edema.[11] Strict records of fluid intake and output should be recorded, and catheterization of the urinary bladder is mandatory. Urine output may be a misleading gauge of adequacy of fluid replacement due to osmotic diuresis, making measurement of cardiac filling pressures a useful adjunct.

Once urine output is reestablished, serial serum potassium levels determine the need for potassium replacement. Potassium can be administered safely at rates of 20–40mEq/hr. Hypophosphatemia is frequently present, and some potassium may be administered as potassium phosphate.[12] Phosphate treatment is not essential, however.

Metabolic acidosis is usually partially compensated by respiratory alkalosis, until exhaustion supervenes. Bicarbonate therapy should be withheld unless serum pH is below 7.15, when bicarbonate may be administered cautiously. Adverse effects of bicarbonate therapy include cardiac arrhythmias from shifts in potassium and an increased affinity of oxygen for hemoglobin, with decreased availability to tissues.

Finally, through all phases of management it should be recognized that the diabetic patient may have varying degrees of renal impairment, autonomic neuropathy, and generalized vascular disease. Preexisting systemic disease should be evaluated and taken into consideration.

References

1. Cahill G.F.: Diabetes mellitus. In, Beeson P.B., McDermott W., Wyngaarden J.B. (eds): *Cecil Textbook of Medicine*. 15th ed. Philadelphia, W.B. Saunders, 1979, p 1974.
2. Marble A., Steinke J.: Physiology and pharmacology in diabetes mellitus. *Anesthesiology* 24:442, 1963.

3. Gann D.S.: Endocrine and metabolic responses to injury. In, Schwartz, S.I. (ed): *Principles of Surgery*. 3rd ed. New York, McGraw Hill, 1979, pp 1–63.
4. Vallance-Owen J., Dennes E., Campbell P.M.: Insulin antagonism in plasma of diabetic patients and normal subjects. *Lancet* 2:336, 1958.
5. Berkow R. (ed): Disorders of carbohydrate metabolism: diabetes mellitus. *The Merck Manual of Diagnosis and Therapy*. 14th ed. Rahway, N.J., Merck Sharp and Dohme Research Laboratories, 1982, p 1042.
6. Maw D.S.J.: The emergency management of diabetes mellitus. *Anesthesia* 30:520, 1975.
7. Page M.M., Alberti K.G.M.M. et al: Treatment of diabetic coma with continuous low-dose infusion of insulin. *Br Med J* 2:687, 1974.
8. Petty C., Cunningham N.L.: Insulin adsorption by glass infusion bottles, polyvinylchloride infusion container and intravenous tubing. *Anesthesiology* 40:400, 1974.
9. Foster D.W.: Diabetes mellitus. In, Petersdorf R.G. et al (eds): *Harrison's Principles of Internal Medicine*. 10th ed. New York, McGraw Hill, 1983, p 671.
10. Moorthy S.S.: Metabolism and nutrition. In Stoelting R.K., Dierdorf S.F. (eds): *Anesthesia and Coexisting Disease*. 1st ed. New York, Churchill Livingstone, 1983, p 488.
11. Felig P.: Current concepts: diabetic ketoacidosis. *N Engl J Med* 290:1360, 1974.
12. Keller U., Berger W.: Prevention of hypophosphatemia by phosphate infusion during treatment of diabetic ketoacidosis and hyperosmolar coma. *Diabetes* 29:87, 1980.

CHAPTER 12

The Morbidly Obese Patient*

Werner Pfisterer

Case History. *A 32-year-old morbidly obese male was admitted for gastric bypass. Height was 177.5cm (5'11"), weight 204kg (449lb); ideal weight was 77.5kg. The patient had been overweight since childhood and had a 150lb gain over the past 2 years. Multiple attempts at dieting were unsuccessful. Previous medical, surgical and social history were unremarkable. The only complaints were dyspnea on one-flight exertion and lack of self-esteem.*

Physical examination was significant only for morbid obesity. Vital signs were: BP 135/85 (large cuff); HR 80/min; respiratory rate 18/min. Laboratory studies were normal and included coagulation profile and urinalysis. Chemistry studies revealed elevated fasting glucose, 160mg%, and slightly elevated liver enzymes. ECG and chest x-ray were normal. A cardiac stress test could not be performed because of treadmill weight restrictions. Pulmonary function testing showed a moderate restrictive pattern. Arterial blood analyses on room air showed: pH 7.39; PCO_2 38; PO_2 71.

Introduction

The word "obese" is derived from the Latin *obedere*, to devour, ie, flesh is consumed by fat. The *Guinness Book of World Records*[1] lists four men who have been documented as weighing more than 1000lb; the heaviest weighed 1400lb.

Obesity is uniquely limited to man and to animals kept by man. It is often secondary to custom-oriented rather than appetite-oriented feeding patterns.[2] Many factors are involved in the pathology of obesity, which eventually results in impaired vital functions, life-threatening complications and significantly reduced lifespan.

Positive caloric balance is the common denominator in obesity. Socio-

---

*Reviewed by Dr. Paul Goldiner, Professor and Chairman, Department of Anesthesiology, Albert Einstein College of Medicine of Yeshiva University, Bronx, New York.

logic, psychologic, pathologic and, more rarely, physiologic factors play ill-defined and controversial roles in the etiology. However, relations between extent of obesity and sex (female > male), income (low > high), and social class (low > high) do exist.[3] Moderate corpulence affects one fifth of the U.S. population and is on the rise, reducing lifespan by 5–20 years.[4]

Definitions

The definitions and determination of obesity and morbid obesity have evolved empirically. Obesity exists when the fat/total body weight ratio exceeds normal with respect to the age and sex of the individual. The upper limit of normal for 18-year-olds is 18% above ideal weight for males, and 25% above ideal for females. This upper limit increases with age, so that by 30 years, 25% above ideal for males and 30% above ideal for females reflect normal increases in fat/lean weight ratios.[5]

Fat/lean body ratio measurements are made by body densitometry, body fat or water content calculated by isotopic and chemical dilution techniques, and measurement of the naturally occurring radioactive isotope of potassium (K 40). Although accurate, these methods of measurement are considered research tools as they are time consuming and the instrumentation is cumbersome. More practical means of assessing obesity include use of retrospective insurance company mortality statistics.[4] Standard tables indicate that normal weight is modified by age, build, height, and sex: overweight is defined as up to 20% above predicted weight. Morbid obesity is greater than twice predicted weight.

Anthropometric methods, which involve body weight-to-height ratios, are probably of the greatest clinical utility in obesity assessment. Largely through the efforts of Billewicz et al,[6] the Body Mass Index (BMI) has gained popularity as the most useful and accurate formula for assessment of obesity. The formula is as follows:

$$BMI = Wt \text{ in kg}/(Ht \text{ in m})^2.$$

Values of BMI less than 25 indicate nonobesity, overweight = 26–29, and obese $\geq$30.[7] Keys and associates have substantiated the usefulness of the BMI in determination of obesity.[8] Advantages of the use of BMI include maximal correlation with adiposity, minimal correlation with height, and ease of calculation.

The Broca index is the most useful indicator of morbid obesity. To derive the Broca index, ideal body weight is first calculated:

$$\text{Ideal Body Weight in kg} = \text{Height in cm} - 100.$$

Individuals whose weight in kilograms is more than twice ideal body weight are considered morbidly obese by the Broca index. Morbidly obese patients can be divided into two separate and functionally distinct groups:

TABLE 1. Characteristics of simple and complex morbid obesity

Simple morbid obesity	Complex morbid obesity (OHS)
Normal $PaCO_2$, pH and pulmonary vascular resistance	Including Pickwickian and sleep-apnea syndromes
No evidence of cardiac failure	Obstructive and familial blunted CO_2 response
Normal or slightly increased alveolar-arterial oxygen difference	Alveolar hypoventilation
Gainfully employed	Hypercarbia
	Hypoxia and pulmonary hypertension predisposing to cor pulmonale

simple morbid obesity; and complex morbid obesity or obesity hypo-ventilation syndrome (OHS). See Table 1.

The famous "boy Joe" in whose dubious honor the name of the Pick-wickian syndrome was coined, was, according to Burwell's description, 61 years old, 5'5" (162.5cm) and 263lb (119.5kg).[9] Although not strictly mor-bidly obese (according to the Broca Index, (162.5−100) 2 = 125kg), boy Joe did exhibit other characteristics of complex morbid obesity necessitat-ing his precipitous removal to the Brigham Hospital by friends, for "falling asleep" on a "full house" during a poker game. As originally described by Burwell, the Pickwickian syndrome consists of marked obesity, somno-lence, twitching, cyanosis, periodic respiration, right venticular hypertro-phy and right ventricular failure. It affects 5–10% of the morbidly obese population.

Risk Factors

Severe obesity is hazardous and carries significant risks even without surgery or anesthesia. (Boy Joe failed to collect on a winning hand!) Peo-ple who are 30–40% above their BMI have a 90% higher mortality rate. Drenrick's study[10] found a 12-fold increased mortality rate among very obese men 25–34 years of age and a 6-fold increase in those 35–44 years of age over a 17-year period. Cardiovascular disease was the most common cause of death in this population.

The incidence of cardiovascular disease is greater in obese patients, 30% higher than that observed in nonobese North Americans. Also, the incidence of associated pathology is higher in the obese than nonobese populations, and may include cerebrovascular disease, hypertension, coronary artery disease, diabetes mellitus, cholelithiasis, thromboem-bolic-venothrombotic disease, abnormalities of lipoprotein and cholesterol metabolism, and cirrhosis. The increased mortality and social stigma have led many severely obese patients to seek medical help.

Therapy

Attempts at weight reduction include appetite suppression by behavioral and/or chemical means, various diets coupled with exercise programs, and finally more drastic, mandibular wiring techniques and anatomical surgical rearrangement. All forms of therapy have inherent difficulties, a variable success rate, and possible complications and failure.

Criteria for gastric surgery include positive Broca index, previous serious attempts at weight loss, good health (except for diabetes or hypertension), age less than 50 years, and psychiatric stability. Best results are seen in patients who have demonstrated previous short-term weight loss by dieting. The two most common types of gastric reduction operations are gastric bypass (food passes from a stomach pouch directly into the jejunum) and vertical banded gastroplasty (food goes through a two-compartment stomach into the duodenum).

The benefits of surgical alteration include weight loss, improved physiologic status (more efficient cardiopulmonary function, increased glucose tolerance, improved lipid profile), and normalized body image and social activity. Complications are divided into acute problems (vomiting, epigastric pain, intestinal obstruction, peritonitis, wound infection, and subphrenic abscess) and chronic difficulties (more frequent after intestinal bypass, which can cause nutritional deficiencies of water-soluble vitamins resulting in encephalopathy and polyneuropathy; exacerbation of hepatic damage; and postoperative cholelithiasis). Careful preoperative assessment and prudent anesthetic management are essential.

Pathophysiology

Metabolic

The pathophysiology of morbid obesity is complex.[2, 11] Considerations of metabolic needs are vital to provide appropriate care for the morbidly obese patient.

Total body metabolism is the chief factor controlling cardiac output and minute ventilation in the otherwise healthy morbidly obese patient. Although the metabolic rate per se is essentially normal, total metabolism increases in linear relation to weight and surface area. Doubling in weight means a doubling of oxygen consumption and carbon dioxide production, with the respiratory quotient remaining normal. Maintaining twice normal minute ventilation and cardiac output even at rest severely reduces already compromised cardiopulmonary reserve. Any physical activity or additional demands, such as fever, further increases the metabolic demand and may cause cardiopulmonary decompensation.

Pulmonary

Changes in respiratory mechanics, respiratory muscle function, and lung volumes result in pulmonary dysfunction, which increases respiratory work and cost of breathing in proportion to the airway pressure–tidal volume product. Excessive airway soft tissue may cause obstruction during anesthetic induction. Compliance of the chest wall is markedly decreased because of torso weight, although lung compliance is usually normal. Thus, total compliance is low, creating a frequency-dependent pattern and less efficient ventilation despite increased energy expenditure.

Abdominal contents are displaced upward in the supine position impairing diaphragmatic function and further decreasing breathing efficiency. Numerous studies to date of diaphragmatic function have been unable to demonstrate intrinsic muscle impairment on biopsy but indicate, via electromyography, increased electrical activity during quiet breathing.[11]

There is marked reduction in functional residual capacity and almost no detectable expiratory reserve volume. While the vital capacity is reduced (especially with increasing age), the inspiratory reserve may be unchanged. The closing volume remains normal as the functional residual capacity decreases, and early small-airway closure results in hypoventilation of dependent lung units, reduced ventilation/perfusion ratio and decreased arterial oxygen content (PaO_2).

The increase in venous admixture can be attenuated by judicial application of PEEP. However, because of coincident fall in cardiac output, oxygen availability falls as PEEP is increased above 15cm H_2O.[12] In one study, large tidal volumes (1000–1200ml) with superimposed PEEP (10–12cmH_2O) in patients of mean weight 154kg did not improve PaO_2. Discontinuation of PEEP resulted in significant improvement in PaO_2.[13] PEEP application should therefore be titrated against frequent PaO_2 measurement.

Probably the only nonnegative lung volume change seen in young and otherwise healthy obese patients is the decrease in dead space/tidal volume ratio (due to an increase in tidal volume). This helps to increase the efficiency of carbon dioxide elimination. Sustained weight loss promotes significant pulmonary changes resulting in decreased carbon dioxide production and alveolar ventilation while oxygen tension, expiratory reserve volume, and functional residual capacity increase.

Cardiovascular

Cardiovascular aberrations are numerous in morbid obesity and are in part related to the abnormal pulmonary condition. The combination of increased metabolic needs and chronic hypoxemia yields a chronically elevated cardiac output. Blood volume and red cell mass are elevated because of hypoxemia and the perfusion needs of the fat organ. Hypertrophy of the left ventricle follows the chronic increase in output and, in the presence of systemic hypertension, predisposes to failure during minimal stress. Pulmonary hypertension related to chronic hypoxemia commonly results in right ventricular hypertrophy and failure in response to the increased workload (primarily in the OHS patients). Increased stroke volume and cardiac output add to total body oxygen consumption, and increased systolic and diastolic pressures result despite normal systemic vascular resistance.[14] Increased hematocrit, decreased fibrinolytic activity with an increase in fibrinogen level, and decreased physical activity predispose the massively obese patient to venothrombosis and thromboembolic disease (23% nonobese versus 48% obese).

After considerable weight loss, oxygen consumption is reduced, producing significant cardiovascular changes. Pre- and post-weight loss cardiac catheterization and chest x-rays revealed significant decreases in the arteriovenous oxygen gradient, cardiac output, systemic arterial pressure, total blood volume, stroke volume at rest, and cardiothoracic ratios.[15]

Gastrointestinal

Gastrointestinal considerations in the obese include production of larger volumes of more acidic gastric fluid and a higher incidence of hiatal hernias. The linear relation between intra-abdominal pressure and weight predisposes the obese patient to a greater risk of regurgitation and aspiration.

Fatty liver infiltration, due to intracellular triglyceride accumulation, predisposes to hepatic dysfunction and is a major cause of postoperative death in the massively obese if postoperative nutritional support is inadequate. Studies on hepatic biotransformation of volatile anesthetics in the obese suggest enhanced oxidation-reduction metabolism and increased levels of serum ionic fluoride. The exact etiology, mechanism, and relationship to possible viscerotoxicity or hepatorenal dysfunction are unclear.[11] The effects of obesity on drug disposition and metabolism continue as fertile ground for investigation. Increased cardiac output and blood volume together with reduced body water–muscle mass/total body weight are thought to alter drug distribution in the obese. Increased lipid solubility of volatile anesthetics, however, produces neither delayed awakening nor prolonged recovery time in obese subjects.[11] Increased cumulative requirements of pancuronium in the obese patient have been observed; etiology remains obscure so monitoring of neuromuscular function is most important in quantitating dose requirements. Pharmacokinetic and dynamic study of metocurine in the obese demonstrated a 1.1 minute increase in elimination half-life for each percent weight above ideal body weight (linear). Significantly slower recovery from neuromuscular blockade resulted. Plasma clearance (ml/kg/min.) under anesthesia was almost 50% slower in the obese vs. non-obese despite normal preoperative renal function.[16] Needle electrodes are most accurate in measurement of neuromuscular blockade as ulnar surface electrodes overestimate and periorbital surface electrodes underestimate block, particularly in obese patients Drugs with high lipid solubility, ie, benzodiazepines and most recently sufentanil, are distributed into a larger volume.[17] The kinetic data from this study suggests that dosage regimens should be based on total body weight.

Preoperative Evaluation

During the preanesthetic visit, cardiopulmonary reserve and psychologic profile can be assessed. Reduced cardiopulmonary reserve must be suspected and investigated if questioning reveals reduced or recent change in exercise tolerance or angina, or dyspnea on exertion. Increased risk is incurred if the patient smokes, has an abnormal sleeping pattern, or is more than 50 years old. Psychologic attributes associated with obesity include passive dependence, low self-esteem, vulnerability to depression, and distorted body image. Psychologic support during the preanesthetic visit is important to enhance patient motivation.

The physical examination must focus on vital signs, fat distribution, thrombophlebitis, and signs of decompensation (edema, jugular venous distention, râles or rhonchi). Of particular importance is airway assessment. Because of the increased risk of aspiration, awake intubation is a reasonable choice if a difficult airway is anticipated. Mucosal bleeding is common as the mucosa is engorged, making oral intubation and especially nasal intubation more difficult. Special note should be made of the presence of intertriginous infection which may warrant prophylactic antibiotic or antifungal therapy.

Laboratory studies can vary widely depending on the type of obesity (simple or complex). The ECG must be checked for signs of ischemia, hypertrophy (right or left), ventricular strain, or atrial enlargement. Chest x-ray may reveal cardiomegaly, pulmonary congestion, elevated diaphragm, or infiltrates. Blood gas analyses in the supine position will usually show a mild hypoxia in simple morbid obesity, and in complex obesity hypercarbia will also be present. Pulmonary function tests may be necessary to measure the extent of restrictive and/or obstructive disease. Liver function tests in the morbidly obese usually reveal mildly elevated SGOT or SGPT levels; if accompanied by abnormal serum albumin or prothrombin time, or greater than 30-unit elevation of transaminase enzymes, other etiology must be sought. Hemoglobin and hematocrit should be measured to assess the presence of polycythemia. Glucose levels must be maintained close to normal, which may be difficult because of insulin resistance. Electrolytes, especially potassium, must be monitored, particularly during insulin and diuretic therapy and in the postgastric bypass patient.

Appropriate drug dosages for obese patients are calculated by lean body mass rather than on a mg/kg basis. Premedication should be light to moderate, and given intramuscularly. A real risk of awareness under anesthesia exists if an intravenous technique is chosen. Use of a cerebral function monitor displaying a spectral edge might be a practical means of assessing anesthetic depth.

The order for replacement blood should be made according to the surgical order schedule. Revision may be necessary if a lipectomy is undertaken since blood loss may become extensive. No different specific recommendations for the obese versus the normal patient have been made regarding maintenance or replacement fluids.

Although regional anesthesia has been used successfully in obese patients, proper needle placement may be more difficult resulting in less predictable levels of anesthesia which may further impair marginal pulmonary reserves. The need for heparin prophylaxis or preexisting backache would preclude the use of subarachnoid block in some obese patients. For intra-abdominal surgery, a combined endotracheal general anesthetic with basal narcosis is best so that ventilation is controlled and the cardiac depressant effects of volatile agents are minimized.

Proper monitoring equipment for the morbidly obese patient includes ECG, temperature probe, oversized blood pressure cuff, and Foley catheter. Needle electrodes are most accurate for determining neuromuscular blockade as ulnar surface electrodes overestimate and periorbital surface electrodes underestimate block, especially in obese patients. Arterial cannulation provides frequent blood gas analyses and continuous blood pressure monitoring for extensive surgery. If marked fluid shifts are anticipated, a central pressure monitor is recommended. Difficulty with insertion of intravenous and monitoring catheters as well as unwieldy patient positioning should be expected.

Finally, anticipated postoperative therapy should be explained to the patient and preliminary provision made in the anesthetic plan for careful postanesthetic care. In particular, consultation with the respiratory therapist and patient education in the use of incentive spirometers as well as semi-Fowler's position are essential.

References

1. McWhirter N.: *Guinness Book of World Records*, Bantam Books, New York, 1985.
2. Bendixen H.H.: Morbid Obesity, ASA 1978 Annual Refresher Course Lectures, Lecture No. 6.
3. Stunkard A., d'Aquili E., Fox S., et al: Influence of social class on obesity and thinness in children. *JAMA* 221:579–584, 1972.
4. Metropolitan Life Insurance Co. Statistics. New Weight Standards for Men and Women. *Statistics Bulletin* 40:3–6, 1980.
5. Bray G.A.: *The Obese Patient*. W.B. Saunders, Philadelphia 1976, pp. 5–43.

6. Billewicz W.Z., Kemsley W.F.F., Thomson A.M.: Indices of obesity. *Brit J Prevent Soc Med* 16:183–8, 1962.
7. Bray G.A., Jordan H.A., Sims E.A.H.: Evaluation of the obese patient. An Algorithm. *JAMA* 235:1487–91, 1976.
8. Keys A., Fidanza F., Karvonen J.M., et al: Indices of relative weight and obesity. *J Chron Dis* 25:329–43, 1972.
9. Burwell C.S., Robin E.D., Whaley E.D.: Extreme obesity associated with alveolar hypoventilation, Pickwickian syndrome. *Am J Med* 20:811–18, 1956.
10. Drenrick E.J., Gurunonjapps S.B., Selzer F., et al: Excessive mortality and causes of death in morbidly obese men. *JAMA* 255:443–5, 1980.
11. Brown B.R. (ed): *Anesthesia and the Obese Patient*. Contemporary Anesthesia Practice Series, F. Davis, Philadelphia, 1982, Vol. 5.
12. Santesson J.: Oxygen transport and venous admixture in the extremely obese. *Acta Anaesth Scand* 20:387–94, 1978.
13. Salem M.R., Dalal F.Y., Zygmunt M.P., et al: Does PEEP improve intraoperative arterial oxygenation in grossly obese patients? *Anesthesiology* 48:280–81, 1978.
14. Chiang B.N., Periman L.V., Epstein F.H.: Overweight and hypertension. *Circulation* 39:403–21, 1969.
15. Alexander J.K., Peterson K.L.: Cardiovascular effects of weight reduction. *Circulation* 45: 310–18, 1972.
16. Schwartz A.E., Matteo R.S., Ornstein E., et al: Pharmacokinetics and dynamics of metocurine in the obese. *Anesthesiology* 65:A295, 1986.
17. Schwartz A.E., Matteo R.S., Ornstein E., et al: Pharmacokinetics of sufentanil in the obese. *Anesthesiology* 65:A562, 1986.

CHAPTER 13

The Patient with Myasthenia Gravis*

John Prinscott

Case History. *A 24-year-old Hispanic female was admitted for elective thymectomy. Four months previously, the patient had noticed drooping of her eyelids, followed by progressive generalized weakness that was worse in the evening and affected the arms more than the legs. She also complained of difficulty in swallowing, intermittent slurred speech and occasional diplopia.*

Although an edrophonium test was negative, electromyography was positive for myasthenia gravis (MG). Vital capacity was 2.21, increasing to 2.6L after administration of pyridostigmine. The patient had taken pyridostigmine 60mg orally 3 times daily for 1 month prior to this admission. A review of the family history revealed that her sister had died at age 17 years from respiratory arrest, 1 year after being diagnosed as having MG.

Physical examination showed a well-developed female; height 152cm; weight 55kg; bilateral eyelid weakness, which was more pronounced on the right side; and decreased motor strength in both arms (4/5). Urinalysis and blood chemistries were within normal limits: Hct 36%; Hgb 12g/dl; sickle cell trait documented.

Introduction

Although myasthenia gravis (MG) has been identified for over a century, only recently has the pathophysiology of the disease been elucidated. MG was first described in 1879 by W.H. Erb,[1] who studied three patients, and again by Jolly in 1895.[2] The first description of MG in the United States was in 1897 by Collins.[3] In 1953, neonatal MG was reported by Strickroot et al.[4] MG manifests as a fluctuating weakness of voluntary muscles. It is divided into three types: the most common is adult myasthenia, followed by neonatal myasthenia, and a congenital phenomenon that occurs in 1–2% of cases.

---

* Reviewed by Dr. Hideo Nagashima, Professor of Anesthesiology, Albert Einstein College of Medicine of Yeshiva University, Bronx, New York.

TABLE 1. Adult myasthenia gravis classified by symptomatology. From Osserman[5].

Group 1	ocular MG
2-a	mild generalized MG; slow onset; frequent ocular involvement
2-b	moderate generalized MG with some bulbar symptoms
3	acute fulminating MG progressing in weeks or months to severe bulbar symptoms
4	late severe MG; marked bulbar symptoms and severe generalized weakness

Neonatal MG occurs in 10–15% of offspring of myasthenic mothers. Some 66% of these babies exhibit signs and symptoms of the disease within the first few hours of life, and 78% within the first three days. Common abnormalities include poor sucking and swallowing, hypotonia, weak movements, feeble crying and respiratory difficulties. There is no relationship between neonatal MG and the severity of MG in the mothers. Congenital MG presents before the age of two years in patients whose mothers do not have MG. The symptoms, bilateral ptosis and opthalmoplegia with generalized weakness, are usually present at birth.[4] The following discussion focuses primarily on adult MG. See Table 1.

The most frequent complaint of myasthenic patients is diplopia;[5] ptosis, the second most common sign, may be missed if it is mild. Ptosis may be unilateral or bilateral and characteristically may shift from side to side. Dysarthria is an early symptom of bulbar involvement, followed by difficulties in chewing and swallowing leading to weight loss. In advanced MG, the most frequent bulbar sign is facial weakness. In 15–20% of myasthenic patients, the chief complaint is extremity weakness; the arms are affected more frequently. Although respiratory muscle weakness may prompt the patient to visit a physician, this is rarely the first symptom.

The incidence of MG is 2–3 times greater in females than in males in the 10–40 year age group; onset after age 40, however, is more common in males.[6] MG is thought to affect 2–4 persons per million U.S. population, although the incidence may be higher since MG is believed to be a frequently missed diagnosis.[7]

Pathophysiology

MG is a disease of neuromuscular transmission. Histologically, there is widening of the synaptic space at the neuromuscular junction and degeneration of the junctional folds. There is also a decreased density of acetylcholine (ACh) receptors on the postsynaptic membrane.[8] The amount of ACh released by the presynaptic membrance, however, is either normal or increased as a compensatory mechanism. Atrophy affected skeletal muscle occurs in approximately 10% of patients.[9] The decrease in ACh-receptor density postsynaptically permits fewer muscle fibers to be activated by a nerve impulse. When the ACh receptors are decreased to less than 25% of normal, single muscle fibers become unresponsive to ACh. In both normal and myasthenic patients, upon repeated nerve stimulation, less, ACh is released. This fact, coupled with the decreased ACh-receptor density, results in progressive failure of muscle contraction with repeated nerve stimulation.

MG is an autoimmune disease. About 30% of patients with MG have antibody to a striated muscle antigen. This percentage increases to 95% in patients with MG and a thymoma. Between 85–90% of patients with MG have IgG antibody to the ACh receptor, which causes degradation of the receptors and the decreased density on the postsynaptic membrane.[10]

Thymomas, which are found in less than 0.1% of the general population, occur in 9–16% of patients with MG; 30–40% of patients with a thymoma have MG. Consistent findings, even in the absence of thymoma, include thymitis with germinal cell hypertrophy. Approximately two thirds of patients with MG without thymoma who undergo thymectomy have gradual improvement of the disease over the first two years postoperatively. Best results occur with thymectomy performed within the first three years of the diagnosis and between the ages of 10 to 40 years.[11]

Diagnosis

The diagnosis of MG is made by testing muscle strength postexercise and demonstrating weakness rather than fatigue. Most patients with generalized MG have a reduced vital capacity, which is also found in 40% of patients with ocular involvement only. This usually is accompanied by a decrease in forced maximum inspiratory flow, which diminishes the ability to cough and can predispose the patient to respiratory infection. Maximum breathing capacity is reduced out of proportion to the decrease in vital capacity.[12, 13] Exacerbation of MG has been shown to occur in the presence of infection, stress (both physical and mental), hyper- or hypothyroidism, and certain drugs.[14, 15]

MG has a variable course of progression as more muscle groups are involved. Although the clinical presentation of MG is unique, the diagnosis may be overlooked if the syndrome is not considered. A history of intermittent weakness and easy fatigability is characteristic. Muscle groups should be tested for strength after a period of exercise in order to elicit weakness (fatigue is a subjective symptom).

Electrophysiologic testing most commonly consists of supramaximal stimulation of a nerve at low rates (1–3/sec) with application of surface electrodes to the muscle. With repeat stimulation of the nerve there is a decrement in the muscle action potential (fatigue) and decreased post-tetanic facilitation.[16] Typically, the circumflex humeral (deltoid innervation), ulnar or median nerves are used for testing.

Diagnosis can also be confirmed by pharmacologic testing, such as documented improvement in muscle weakness after anticholinesterase administration. The most specific test is isolation of ACh antibody. Other tests include single-fiber electromyography, stapedius-reflexometry, nystagmography and curare testing.[17] Curare testing, either generalized or regional, is usually reserved only for patients in whom other diagnostic testing is inconclusive. The test has potentially dangerous side effects and is seldom used.

A systemic curare test consists of the administration of 0.5–1mg intravenous increments of curare to elicit an exacerbation of myasthenic weakness with less than one tenth the normal curarizing dose. Muscle function, including vital capacity, is assessed 5 minutes after each dose. An anesthesiologist should be available during this test because of the potential for respiratory arrest.[18] With the regional curare test, a tourniquet is applied to both arms to prevent systemic absorption. A dose of 0.2mg curare dissolved in 20ml saline is given intravenously in one arm, and 20ml saline alone is given in the other arm. Muscle function is examined 7, 11 and 16 minutes later by dynamometry and ergography.[19] The disadvantage of the regional curare test is that only the muscles of the selected limb are tested, even though these muscles might not be as sensitive to curare as other muscle groups affected by MG. Advantages include safe administration of a confirmatory diagnostic test.

Treatment

Anticholinesterases are the drugs of choice in the treatment of MG, and several are available. See Table 2. Pyridostigmine bromide is the most commonly employed. After oral administration, the onset of action is within 15–30 minutes, and peak action is at 1–2 hours. Duration is 3–4 hours. Oral pyridostigmine is available in three dosages: 10mg, 60mg, and 180mg. Common total daily dosages range from 30–120mg given 3–6 times per day. Pyridostigmine is also available as a syrup (12mg/ml) or as a 5% solution.

The dosage of anticholinesterase medication for MG must be adjusted to

TABLE 2. Anticholinesterase medications available in U.S. for the treatment of myasthenia gravis

Drug	Trade name	Oral dose (mg)	Parenteral dose (mg)	
			I.V.	IM
Neostigmine	Prostigmin	15	0.5	0.5–1.0
Pyridostigmine	Mestinon	60	2	3–4
Ambenonium	Mytelase	6	not available	

the individual patient. First, the optimal intravenous dose is determined, and then this amount is converted to the oral equivalent. Optimal dosage should be confirmed by the edrophonium test. Patients who are receiving adequate anticholinesterase therapy will show no real improvement in muscle function following edrophonium administration.[20]

Ephedrine may enhance the beneficial effect of anticholinesterase therapy in MG. Anticholinesterase agents are also frequently combined with adrenal corticosteroids or immunosuppresive drugs.[16] Steroid therapy is usually with prednisone on an alternate day schedule for patients whose disease is not adequately controlled by anticholinesterases or thymectomy. Steroids may be given perioperatively to compensate for the delay in the therapeutic effect of thymectomy and because of a reported synergistic effect.[21] Beneficial effects have also been reported by combining thymectomy with radiation therapy and/or plasmapheresis.

Perioperative Management

Preoperative laboratory data for MG patients should include arterial blood gas analyses and pulmonary function tests. Special attention must be given to serum glucose and electrolytes in patients maintained with steroid preparations, since prolonged therapy may induce fluid and electrolyte disturbances, and hyperglycemia or glycosuria. For example, hypokalemia, which can increase the muscle weakness of myasthenic patients, must be corrected. Preoperative sedation should be light in order to minimize any chance of respiratory embarrassment.

It is recommended to continue anticholinesterase therapy in patients who are dependent on these drugs for normal daily activity; in patients with only mild symptoms, however, these medications should be discontinued on the morning of surgery.[22] Anticholinesterase therapy can be restarted in the recovery room after clinical examination of the patient, especially with regard to bulbar and respiratory function, and testing of hand grip strength with a dynamometer. In an unconscious patient, a nerve block monitor may be used. Neostigmine 0.5–1mg IM can be given every two to three hours until medication can be absorbed orally, at which time pyridostigmine can be restarted. Because the beneficial effect of thymectomy can be delayed from several weeks to several years postoperatively, it is necessary to reassess the dosage for a prolonged postoperative period. All patients with MG should be monitored postoperatively in an ICU setting.

Many patients with MG receive steroids. Sudden preoperative withdrawal of these agents can cause an increase in myasthenic weakness and the complications of adrenal insufficiency, such as intraoperative hypotension and cardiovascular collapse. Because of anticipated surgical stress, the usual dosage of steroids should be supplemented perioperatively.

Most of the literature regarding preoperative assessment of myasthenic patients concerns patients scheduled for thymectomy, which does not require muscle relaxation. A retrospective analysis by Leventhal, Orkin, and Hirsh[23] of 24 patients who underwent thymectomy enabled the authors to devise a scoring system to determine which patients will require postoperative ventilatory support. The predictive accuracy is 91%. Patients were given halothane or enflurane by endotracheal tube without muscle relaxation. Eight of the 24 patients required postoperative ventilatory support. A score of greater than or equal to 10 points by the following criteria predicted the need for ventilatory support:

- duration of MG ≥ 6 years—12 points
- other respiratory disease—10 points
- pyridostigmine > 750mg/day—8 points
- vital capacity ≤ 2.9L—4 points

Postoperative mechanical ventilation of all patients with MG has also been recommended.[24] Under these circumstances, anticholinesterase medications are discontinued 12–24 hours preoperatively and restarted gradually in the postoperative period.

Many patients with MG are scheduled for an operative procedure which requires muscle relaxation. When feasible, regional anesthesia is a good choice in these patients since complete muscle relaxation can be obtained with spinal or epidural anesthesia. If general anesthesia is indicated, however, adequate relaxation can be accomplished with deep inhalation anesthesia with a halogenated agent, such as isoflurane.

Because of the decreased postsynaptic ACh-receptor density, MG patients are extremely sensitive to nondepolarizing muscle relaxants and are resistant to depolarizing blocking agents such as succinylcholine. However, it should be noted that a phase II block with succinylcholine has been found to occur earlier with slower recovery.[22] In addition, anticholinesterase medications inhibit pseudocholinesterase and acetylcholinesterase. Thus, metabolism of succinylcholine is decreased.

The dose of pancuronium to produce 95% twitch depression is diminished by a factor of four in myasthenic patients.[25] Addition of halothane causes an eightfold increase in sensitivity to pancuronium.[26] Atracurium in reduced dosage has been used successfully.[27] Whenever possible muscle relaxants should be avoided, but there is no absolute contraindication to their usage.

If a local anesthetic is given to an MG patient taking anticholinesterase medication, amide-linked agents such as lidocaine are preferable since they are not dependent on pseudocholinesterase for metabolism. Trimethaphan is also metabolized by pseudocholinesterase and should not be used as a hypotensive agent.

Exacerbation of MG can occur secondary to surgical stress with the subsequent development of a myasthenic crisis. During crisis, patients have decreased responsiveness to anticholinesterases. This situation must be differentiated from a cholinergic crisis which is secondary to an anticholinesterase overdosage.[28] In both situations, there is an increase in muscle weakness which may involve the respiratory musculature and thereby necessitate respiratory support. A small dose of edrophonium (10mg intravenously) will improve strength in a patient with myasthenic crisis but will have little or negative effect in a patient with cholinergic crisis. With either crisis there are autonomic signs such as salivation and sweating, but mydriasis occurs with myasthenic crisis while miosis occurs with a cholinergic crisis. A myasthenic crisis should be suspected in a stressed patient with progressive weakness. Vital capacity, pulmonary function, heart rate and blood pressure should be monitored in these patients rather than arterial blood gases. In both myasthenic and cholinergic crises it is best to withhold anticholinesterase medications while providing mechanical support of ventilation. Plasmapheresis is indicated in the treatment of myasthenic crisis. In some situations a mixed crisis can arise with over-treatment of a patient with anticholinesterase drugs during a myasthenic crisis.

References

1. Erb W.: Zur Casuisik de bulbaren Lahmugen. 3 Ueber einen neuen wahrscheinlich bulbaren Symptomencomplex. *Archiv für Psychiatric und Nervenkrankheiten* 9:336, 1879.
2. Jolly F.: Ueber Myasthenia gravis pseudoparalytica. *Berliner Klinische Wochenschrift* 32:1, 1895.
3. Collins J.: Asthenic bulbar paralysis. *Internal Med Magazin* 5:203, 1897.
4. Strickroot F.L., Schaeffer R.L., Bergo H.E.: Myasthenia gravis occurring in an infant born of a myasthenia mother. *JAMA* 120:1207, 1942.
5. Osserman K.E.: Studies in myasthenia gravis—review of a twenty year experience in over 1200 patients. *Mt Sinai J Med* 38:538, 1971.
6. Schwab R.S., Leland C.: Sex and age in myasthenia gravis as critical factors in incidence and remission. *JAMA* 153:1270, 1953.
7. Kurtzke J.F.: Epidemiology of myasthenia gravis, in Schoenberg BS (ed): *Advances in Neurology*, New York, Raven Press, 1978, Vol 19, pp 545–566.
8. Drachman D.B., Kao I., Pestronk A., et al: Myasthenia gravis as a receptor disorder. *Ann NY Acad Sci* 274:226, 1976.
9. Oosterhuis H., Bethlem J.: Neurogenic muscle involvement in myasthenia gravis. *J Neurol Neurosurg Psychiatry* 36:244, 1973.
10. Oosterhuis H.: Immunopathology, in Oosterhuis H. (ed) *Myasthenia Gravis*, New York, Churchill Livingstone, 1984, pp 104–130.
11. Oosterhuis H.: The thymus and myasthenia gravis, in Oosterhuis H. (ed): *Myasthenia Gravis*, New York, Churchill Livingstone, 1984, pp 51–76.
12. Osserman K.E., Foldes F.F., Genkins G.: Myasthenia gravis, in Cheymol J. (ed): *International Pharmacological Therapeutic Sections 14*. Oxford, Pergamon, 2:561, 1978.
13. Ringguist I., Ringguist T.: Respiratory mechanisms in untreated myasthenia gravis with special reference to the respiratory forces. *Acta Med Scand* 190:499, 1971.

14. Oosterhuis H.: Clinical aspects, in Oosterhuis H. (ed): *Myasthenia Gravis*, New York, Churchill Livingstone, 1984, pp 21–50.
15. Kennedy F.S., Moersch F.P.: Myasthenia gravis. A clinical review of 87 cases observed between 1915 and the early part of 1932. *Can Med Assoc J* 37:216, 1937.
16. Drachman D.B.: Myasthenia gravis. *N Engl J Med* 2:136, 1978.
17. Oosterhuis H. The diagnosis, in Oosterhuis H. (ed): *Myasthenia Gravis*, New York, Churchill Livingstone, 1984, pp 142–158.
18. Rowland L.P., Aranow H., Hoefer P.F.A.: Observations on the curare test in the differential diagnosis of myasthenia gravis, in Viets H.R. (ed): *Myasthenia Gravis*, Springfield, Illinois, C.C. Thomas, 1961, pp 411–434.
19. Foldes F.F., Klonymus D.H., Maisel W., et al: A new curare test for the diagnosis of myasthenia gravis. *JAMA* 203:649, 1968.
20. Foldes F.F., Nagashima H.: Myasthenia gravis and anesthesia, in Oyama T. (ed): *Endocrinology and The Anaesthetist*, New York, Elsevier, 1983, pp 171–203.
21. Heisner J.C., Rutherford R.B., Ringle S.P.: Thymectomy for myasthenia gravis. A changing perspective. *Arch Surg* 117:533, 1982.
22. Miller J., Lee C.: Muscle diseases, in Katz J., Benumof J., Kadis L.B. (eds): *Anesthesia and Uncommon Diseases*, Philadelphia, W.B. Saunders Co, 1981, pp 530–561.
23. Leventhal S.R., Orkin F.K., Hirsh R.A.: Predicting postoperative ventilatory need in myasthenia. *Anesthesiology* 53:26, 1980.
24. Miller R.D., Savarese J.J.: Pharmacology of muscle relaxants and their antagonists, in Miller R.D. (ed): *Anesthesia*, New York, Churchill Livingstone, 1986 pp 889–943.
25. Blitt C.D., Wright W.A., Peat J.: Pancuronium and the patient with myasthenia gravis. *Anesthesiology* 42:624, 1975.
26. Miller R.D., Way W.L., Dolan W.M., et al: The dependence of pancuronium and d-tubocurarine-induced neuromuscular blockades on alveolar concentrations of halothane and Forane. *Anesthesiology* 37:573, 1972.
27. Osserman K.E., Kaplan L.I.: Studies in myasthenia gravis: Use of edrophonium chloride in differentiating myasthenia from cholinergic weakness. *Arch Neurol Psych* 70:385, 1953.

CHAPTER 14

The Head-Injured Patient*

Elizabeth A.M. Frost

Case History. *A 20-year-old healthy, Caucasian male had been drinking with friends when a brawl broke out. He was struck on the head with a bottle and appeared to be momentarily dazed. However, he continued fighting until police intervention terminated the disturbance. In the police van, his silence was initially attributed to alcoholic overdose and to cocaine ingestion. On arrival at the police station he could not be roused. He was transferred immediately to the emergency room.*

Physical examination showed a well-nourished, comatose patient; pulse 132bpm, and regular; blood pressure 180/100; respiratory rate 40/min. Chest sounds clear. Breath smelled of alcohol. A large stellate wound in the frontotemporal area was bleeding profusely. Right pupil was larger than left. He withdrew his arms to painful stimulation. Glasgow Coma Scale 6. Arterial blood gas data on room air were PaO_2 68mmHg; $PaCO_2$ 24mmHg; pH 7.5.

Introduction

Head trauma accounts for one third of all admissions to emergency units. Most head injuries occur and present to the emergency room between 4 PM and midnight. The frequency is highest on Friday and Saturday evenings.

The annual incidence of head injury in the United States is approximately 0.2%.[1-5] Males outnumber females by three to one.[3-5] Younger age groups are especially affected; in New York, 39% of head injuries occur in patients under 15 years of age.[6]

In most communities, traffic accidents account for over 50% of injuries; in some urban areas, however, violence and falls predominate. Alcohol consumption has been associated with over 50% of fatal vehicular accidents.[7] Detectable blood alcohol levels have been found in more than 50% of head injured patients in emergency rooms.[8,9]

---

*Reviewed by Dr. K. Tabaddor, Associate Professor of Neurosurgery, Albert Einstein College of Medicine of Yeshiva University, Bronx, New York.

The annual mortality rate from head injury is estimated at 0.03%.[10] About 60% of deaths occur before the patient receives medical assistance. As many as 40% of fatalities can be avoided if medical aid is available within 10 minutes.

In a review of 116 patients who were able to speak following head injury but who subsequently died (a clinical situation encountered in 38% of deaths), Rose and Jennett[11] concluded that in 75%, one or more avoidable factors were present; and, in at least 54%, these factors (hypoxia, hypotension, delay in treatment, sepsis, seizures, and iatrogenic complications) contributed to death. Respiratory obstruction is the primary, preventable cause of death.

Types of Head Injuries

Many types of insults affect the intracranial contents. Head injury is not a homogeneous disease. Therapy and prognosis depend on the pathology.

Injury to Brain Coverings

Depressed skull fractures under lacerations are considered compound and should be repaired surgically within 24 hours to minimize infection.[12] Bony fragments should not be manipulated in the emergency room, as they may be tamponading a lacerated vessel or dural sinus. Similarly, penetrating objects which are still in place should be protected from any movement during transportation and removed under controlled conditions in the operating room.

Missile Injuries

Civilian gunshot wounds are usually caused by relatively low-velocity bullets. The bursting fracture of the skull results from a high-pressure wave transmitted from the brain.[13] Epidural, subdural or intracerebral hematomas may result in up to 50% of cases.[14] In the absence of a hematoma, devitalized brain tissue may act as a mass lesion and cause extremely high levels of intracranial pressure (ICP) within a few hours.[15] Surgery is aimed at debridement and evacuation of blood clots. The major contaminant is *Staphylococcus* and appropriate antibiotic therapy should be started.[16]

Epidural Hematoma

Traumatic epidural hematoma, usually the result of an automobile accident, is an infrequent complication of head injury. It is associated with laceration of middle meningeal vessels or dural sinuses. Patients are usually young adults (15–20 years). The clinical course with arterial bleeding is one of rapid deterioration following a lucid interval. Clinical signs of tentorial herniation with ipsilateral third cranial nerve palsy are often present. In rapidly deteriorating conditions, treatment should not be delayed pending radiologic evaluation. Venous epidural hemorrhages develop more slowly, and time for more complete diagnostic testing may be available.

Subdural Hematoma

The most common cause of subdural hematoma (SDH) is trauma, but it may occur spontaneously (coagulopathies, aneurysms, and certain neoplasms). It is considered acute if the patient is symptomatic within 72 hours, subacute if the time interval is 3–15 days, and chronic if symptoms develop after 2 weeks. Acute SDH is the most common intracranial hematoma of traumatic origin requiring surgical evacuation. A lucid interval may occur. Subacute and chronic SDH are usually observed in patients over 50 years of age. A history of head trauma may be absent. Clinical presentation varies from focal signs of brain dysfunction to a depressed level of consciousness or development of an organic brain syndrome. ICP is usually elevated, although this symptom may not be observed in chronic situations.

Intracerebral Hematoma

Coup and contracoup injuries usually produce cerebral contusion and intracerebral hematomas. The development of delayed intracerebral hematoma has a poor prognosis.

Preanesthetic Care

Although only about 20% of head injured patients require operative intervention, the anesthesiologist is frequently required to assist in emergency care. As the initial brain injury is not amenable to treatment, therapy is aimed at prevention of further brain damage and establishment of an optimal physiologic environment to maximize recovery.

Respiratory Assessment and Care

Patients who are unconscious after head trauma may have an impaired airway either because of mechanical obstruction from foreign bodies, such as vomitus or dentures, or failure to control anatomical structures, such as tongue or pharynx. Severe head injury can obtund laryngeal and pharyngeal reflexes and depress the cough reflexes. Since gastric motility frequently ceases immediately after any stress or trauma, regurgitation and silent aspiration may occur, especially in an inebriated patient. Fractures of the face or the base of the skull may compromise the airway by edema, blood, or bony displacement.[17]

TABLE 1. Criteria in the diagnosis of respiratory insufficiency

If one or more of these criteria exist, the diagnosis of respiratory insufficiency is made.

Respiratory rate	< 40/minute; > 10/minute
Respiratory pattern	irregular
Vital capacity	< 15ml/kg
Maximal inspiratory force	> −20cmH$_2$O
Dead space ventilation (VD/VT)	> 0.5
Pulmonary shunt	> 15%
PaCO$_2$	> 45mmHg; < 25mmHg

Following head injury, all patients are considered hypoxic until proven otherwise. Transient respiratory arrest at the time of head injury may cause diffuse microatelectases, which may result in large areas of poorly ventilated lung. Other, less well-defined factors may result in the opening of anatomic arteriovenous anastomoses with redistribution of flow following head trauma. A regional decrease in compliance and/or an increase in resistance, sometimes secondary to changes in surfactant or pulmonary congestion, may cause ventilation perfusion mismatch.

Pulmonary shunt greater than 15% is highly correlated with poor outcome.[18] The oxygen requirement of the injured brain is increased; thus, adequate cerebral oxygenation is a priority. Early recognition and prompt aggressive treatment of respiratory dysfunction are of major importance in initial care. Causes of respiratory dysfunction include neurogenic damage, intoxication, fluid overload, disseminated intravascular coagulopathy, fat embolism, and thoracic trauma.

One study examined outcome in 197 severe head injury patients, half of whom were intubated and ventilated within one hour of injury, and the other half after that time. Mortality in the first group was 22.5%, and 38.4% in the second group (p=0.001).[17] Prior studies had considered intubation "early" if it occurred within 6 hours after injury. Not only does early intubation improve survival, but the definition of "early intubation" must be held more critically to short times, ie, less than one hour.

Intubation and ventilatory support should be provided if one or more of the criteria listed in Table 1 are present. It is better to intubate a patient who has marginal respiratory insufficiency and can be extubated after a few hours than to lose an otherwise salvageable victim because of massive aspiration or because expanding cerebral edema has caused brain stem compression.

Controlled respiration not only improves oxygenation but allows regulation of arterial carbon dioxide content (PaCO$_2$). While optimal values of PaCO$_2$ in head injury have not been determined, excessive hypocarbia (PaCO$_2$ < 25mmHg) may cause deleterious cerebral vasoconstriction. The resultant respiratory alkalosis shifts the oxygen dissociation curve to the left and oxygen is less available to the brain. On the other hand, hypercarbia may cause severe intracranial hypertension.

TABLE 2. Glasgow Coma Scale

Best verbal response	
None	1
Uncomprehensible sound	2
Inappropriate words	3
Confused	4
Oriented	5
Eyes open	
None	1
To pain	2
To speech	3
Spontaneously	4
Best motor responses	
None	1
Abnormal extensor	2
Abnormal flexion	3
Withdraws	4
Localizes	5
Obeys	6
Total Coma Scale	15

Diffuse head injury in adults is often characterized by cerebral hypoperfusion. Decreasing flow further by hyperventilation may be inappropriate. In children, after any severe head injury, hyperemia may occur. In these circumstances, increasing ventilation may be most beneficial. Thus, a means of determining cerebral blood flow (CBF) is desirable. Radioisotope scans are ideal but are generally not available on an emergency basis. Flow can be approximated by the following equation:

$$CBF = AVDO_2 \times CMRO_2,$$

where $AVDO_2$ = arteriovenous oxygen difference and $CMRO_2$ = cerebral metabolic rate for oxygen.

The $CMRO_2$ has been shown to correlate fairly accurately with the Glasgow Coma Scale evaluation. (See Table 2.) Arteriovenous oxygen difference can be estimated by subtracting oxygen content in the jugular bulb from the PaO_2 in the radial artery. Jugular bulb samples are obtained from a catheter passed through a Tuohy needle inserted in the internal jugular vein.

Normal oxygen difference across the brain is 6–7vol%. Differences of 10 or more indicate an exteme decrease in CBF. Therapy should then center on attempts to increase flow, ie, decrease hyperventilation and administration of diuretic agents to decrease brain edema. Values below 6 suggest that intracranial pressure may be safely decreased by increasing ventilation, reducing $PaCO_2$ and thus constricting cerebral vessels.[19]

Securing an impeccable airway takes priority in any patient with severe head injury. Moreover, the means to accomplish this maneuver must be clearly defined. Tracheal intubation and suctioning, unless preceded by adequate ventilation and paralysis of the patient, may cause large increases in ICP. Bucking must also be avoided. Although these abrupt, transient increases in ICP are usually not as dangerous as they might appear to be from examination of the pressure tracing, prolonged pressure waves can be initiated which can readily result in herniation.

Thus, intubation should be performed as atraumatically as possible after sedation with intravenous thiopental and lidocaine and the use of appropriate doses of intermediate-acting relaxants, such as atracurium or vecuronium. Cricoid pressure to reduce the risk of aspiration is indicated. Insertion of a nasotracheal tube is not indicated as the anesthesiologist is frequently less skilled in this maneuver, time to secure the airway is longer, nasal muscosal hemorrhage may occur, and suctioning and ventilation through a small diameter tube are more difficult. Moreover, if the base of the skull is disrupted, the tip of the endotracheal tube may be forced into the fracture site and increase cerebrospinal fluid rhinorrhea and the risk of infection.

Cardiovascular Assessment

Maintenance of adequate cerebral perfusion pressure (70–110mmHg) is essential to avoid brain ischemia.[20] Cerebral perfusion pressure is defined as follows:

$$CPP = MAP - ICP,$$

where CPP = cerebral perfusion pressure and MAP = mean arterial blood pressure.

Although transient hypotension is not infrequent after head injury, a prolonged decrease in arterial pressure in adults indicates, extracranial hemorrhage. A brain stem injury severe enough to destroy the vasomotor center is incompatible with life.[21]

Hypertension and tachycardia are the most frequently observed hemodynamic disorders following head injury. On admission to hospital, heart rates greater than 120 beats/min have been reported in over one third of patients, and systolic blood pressure greater than 160mmHg have been reported in one-fourth.[22] Cerebral vasomotor paralysis or impaired autoregulation occurs frequently after head injury.[23,24] Hypertension in the presence of these abnormalities increases cerebral edema and ICP, which further compromise the injured brain. Systemic arterial pressure greater than 30% above normal mean values should be treated. Intracranial pressure should be known to ascertain adequacy of CPP. Systemic vasodilators such as sodium nitroprusside and hydralazine, which increase cerebral blood flow and ICP, should be avoided.[25,26] As a hyperactive sympathetic nervous system exists in these patients, antihypertensive therapy requires adrenergic blocking agents.[27] One method is to infuse propranolol 1mg every 15 minutes until systolic pressure is less than 160mmHg, diastolic pressure is below 90mmHg, or the heart rate is less than 70 beats/min.

In most patients, both cardiac output and cardiac index are increased. The outcome in young patients with decreased cardiac output is poor.[27]

Electrocardiographic changes associated with subarachnoid hemorrhage include increased amplitude of P-waves, prolonged QT interval, large U waves, and ST and T wave changes.[28] The occurrence of peaked P-waves, long PR intervals, prolonged QT intervals and prominent U-waves indicates a poor prognosis.[29] Major ventricular extrasystoles, heart blocks and bradycardia are rare. However, fatal arrhythmias have been reported in young head injured patients without preexisting cardiac abnormalities.[30] Any abnormality of the ECG in a patient with subdural hematoma has been associated with an increased mortality rate.[31]

A combination of blood loss and diuresis often results in hypovolemia in the head injured patient. The hyperactive sympathetic system may mask this abnormality until thiopental, given for sedation, precipitates severe hypotension. Adequate fluid resuscitation is essential. Irrespective of heart rate, urine loss should be replaced with equal volumes of crystalloid solution. One study has shown that sugar infusion that causes insignificant changes in blood glucose can result in significant increases in cerebral injury in primates.[32] Thus, replacement should be with lactated Ringer's or saline solutions. Frequent estimations of serum electrolyte levels are required to ensure that hypokalemia does not develop.

Coagulopathies

Severe brain injury initiates the outpouring of tissue thromboplastin. Disseminated intravascular coagulopathy and fibrinolysis syndrome (DICF) results. The process occurs immediately after head injury and has a significant influence on outcome.[33] If the coagulation profile does not return to normal, this indicates continuing brain injury. Treatment consists of fresh frozen plasma, cryoprecipitate and, if necessary, fresh platelet packs.

Control of Intracranial Pressure

Normal ICP is 10–15mmHg. Although more than half of all deaths from head trauma are associated with increased ICP, any casual role or association of degree of elevation with outcome is unclear.[34] Nonetheless, significant intracranial hypertension can reduce intracranial perfusion pressure below the critical level and cause secondary damage. Therapy, for intracranial hypertension includes hyperventilation, dehydration with diuretics, and infusion of intravenous drugs (barbiturates, etomidate hydroxybutyrolactone, etomidate.) The use of corticosteroids in head injury remains controversial.

Neurologic Assessment

Observations of changes in level of consciousness, changes in respiratory pattern or cardiac rhythm indicate changing status. The Glasgow Coma Scale, which consists of eye opening, motor response, and verbal response, has been internationally accepted as a prognostic indicator of outcome after head injury and as a means of assessing deterioration in intracranial status or efficacy of treatment.[35] See Table 2. Hourly recording of coma scale affords some indication of improvement or deterioration in the disease process. Patients who score greater than 9 generally have a better outcome than those who score 8 or less.

Neuroradiologic Testing

Accurate assessment of head injury is generally best achieved by CT scanning. However, increased ICP, hypoxia, hypercapnia, pain, and intoxication cause patients to become restless, agitated, or belligerent, making studies difficult and the results equivocal.

Cooperation is especially difficult to obtain from young children. These patients should be sedated only after the cause of their restlessness has been established and appropriate therapy is initiated. Administration of opioids or barbiturates to a hypoxic patient breathing spontaneously may convert a life-threatening situation to one that is fatal. If there is any doubt of the adequacy of the airway in these restless patients, they must be managed with a general endotracheal anesthetic technique for the duration of the study. It has also been suggested that reduction of $PaCO_2$ levels will, by decreasing cerebral blood flow, allow better angiographic studies.

Anesthetic Plan

Preanesthetic medication should be avoided as effects are variable and accurate neurologic assessment is no longer possible. Appropriate monitoring includes continuous ECG, arterial cannulation (for blood pressure and gas analyses), temperature, serum electrolytes, and airway pressures. A pulmonary artery catheter affords valuable information on fluid status, but in an emergency situation (eg, arterial epidural hematoma), adequate time for placement is not available.

The anesthetic technique depends on the pathology of the injury and the elapsed time. Immediately following head trauma in children, and after missile injury in adults, hyperemic states tend to prevail. A regimen which decreases flow, ie, hyperventilation and barbiturate infusion, is appropriate. However, most head trauma in adults is characterized by hypoperfusion. A technique which maintains flow but decreases metabolic demand (ie, low-dose isoflurane) is perferable. Nitrous oxide should be avoided as it increases cerebral blood flow, increases metabolic rate and increases the risk of tension pneumocephalus in patients with fractured skulls.

References

1. Kalsbeek W.D., McLaurin R.L., Harris B.S.G. III, et al: The national head and spinal cord injury survey: major findings. *J Neurosurg* 53:S19–S31, 1980.
2. Caveness W.F.: Incidence of craniocerebral trauma in the United States with trends from 1970 to 1975, in Thompson R.A., Green J.R. (eds): *Complications of Nervous System Trauma*, New York, Raven Press, 1979.
3. Annegers J.F., Graybow J.D., Kurland L.T., et al: The incidence, causes and secular trends of head trauma in Olmsted County, Minnesota, 1935–1974. *Neurology* 30:912–9, 1980.
4. Cooper K.D., Tabaddor K., Hauser W.A., et al: The epidemiology of head injury in the Bronx. *Neuroepidemiology* 2:70–88, 1983.
5. Klauber M.R., Barrett-Conner E., Marshall L.F., et al: Epidemiology of head injury; a prospective study of an entire community, San Diego. California. *Amer J Epidemiol* 113:500–9, 1981.
6. Wassertheil-Smoller S., Tabaddor K., Feiner C., et al: Factors affecting short-term outcome of head trauma patients. *Neuroepidemiology* 1:154–66, 1982.
7. National Safety Council: *Accident Facts*. Chicago, 1978.
8. Galbraith S., Murray W.R., Patel A.R., et al: The relationship between alcohol and head injury and its effect on the conscious level. *Br J Surg* 63:228–30, 1976.
9. Honkanen R., Visuri T.: Blood alcohol levels in a series of injuried patients with special reference to accident and type of injury. *Ann Chirurg Gynaecol* 65:287–94, 1976.
10. Frankowki R.F., Klauber M.R., Tabaddor K., et al: Head injury mortality: a comparison of three metropolitan counties. *Am J Public Health*. In press.
11. Rose J., Valtonen S., Jennett B. Avoidable factors contributing to death after head injury. *Br Med J* 2:615–7, 1977.
12. Miller J.D., Jennett W.B. Complications of depressed skull fracture. *Lancet* 2:991–5, 1968.
13. Butler E.G., Pucket W.O., Harvey E.N., et al: Experiments on head wounding by high-velocity missiles. *J Neurosurg* 2:358–63, 1945.
14. Barnett J.C. Hematomas associated with penetrating wounds, in Coates J.B. Jr (ed): *Neurological Surgery of Trauma*. Washington, D.C., Office of the Surgeon General, Department of the Army, 1965, pp 131–4.
15. Crockard H.A. Early intracranial pressure studies in gunshot wounds of the brain. *J Trauma* 15:339–47, 1975.
16. Carey W., Young H.F., Rish B.L., et al: Follow-up study of 103 American soliders who sustained a brain wound in Vietnam. *J Neurosurg* 41:542–9, 1974.
17. Gildenberg P.L., Makela M.E.: The effect of early intubation and ventilation on outcome following head trauma. *Symposium of Neural Trauma*, Charlottesville, V.A., New York, Raven Press, 1982.
18. Frost E.A.M., Arancibia C.U., Shulman K.: Pulmonary shunt as a prognostic indicator in head injury. *J Neurosurg* 50:768–72, 1979.
19. Cruz J.: *Miner M.E. Modulating Cerebral Oxygen Delivery and extraction in Acute Traumatic Coma Neuroytauma*. Boston, Butterworths 1986, pp 55–72.
20. Lassen N.A.: Control of cerebral circulation in health and disease. *Circ Res* 34:749–59, 1974.
21. Clifton G.L., McCormick W.F., Grossman R.G.: Neuropathology of early and late deaths after head injury. *Neurosurgery* 8:309–14, 1981.

22. Brown R.S., Mohr P.A., Cavey J.S., et al: Cardiovascular changes after cranial cerebral injury and increased intracranial pressure. *Surg Gynecol Obstet* 125:1205–11, 1967.
23. LaBrosse E.H., Cowley R.A.: Tissue levels of catecholamines in patients with different types of trauma. *J Trauma* 13:61–4, 1973.
24. Langfitt T., Weinstein J., Kassell N.: Cerebral vasomotor paralysis produced by intracranial hypertension. *Neurology* 15:62–41, 1965.
25. Cottrell J., Patel K., Ransohoff J., et al: Intracranial pressure changes induced by sodium nitroprusside in patients with intracranial mass lesions. *J Neurosurg* 48:329–31, 1978.
26. Overgaard J., Skinhoj E.: A paradoxical cerebral hemodynamic effect of hydralazine. *Stroke* 6:402–4, 1975.
27. Clifton G., Ziegler M., Grossman R.: Circulating catecholamines and sympathetic activity after head injury. *Neurosurgery* 8:10–14, 1981.
28. Boddin M., Van Bogaert A., Dierick W.: Catecholamines in blood and myocardial tissue in experimental subarachnoidal hemorrhage. *Cardiology* 58:229–37, 1973.
29. Cruickshank J.M., Neil-Dwyer G., Brice J.: Electrocardiographic changes change the prognostic significance in subarachnoid hemorrhage. *J Neurol Neurosurg Psychiatry* 37:755–9, 1974.
30. Hersch C.: Electrocardiographic changes in head injuries. *Circulation* 23:853–60, 1961.
31. Vander Ark G.D.: Cardiovascular changes with acute subdural hematoma. *Surg Neurol* 3:305–8, 1975.
32. Lanier W.L., Stangland K.F., Scheithauer B.W., et al: Effects of IV dextrose and head position in neurologic outcome after complete cerebralsi chemia. *Anesthesiology* 63:A110, 1985.
33. Miner M.E., Kaufman H.H., Graham S.H., et al: Disseminated intravascular coagulation and fibrinolysis following head injury in children: frequency and prognostic implications. *J Pediatr* 100:687–91, 1982.
34. Langfitt T.W.: The incidence and importance of intracranial hypertension in head injured patients, in Becks J.W.F., Bosch D.A., Brock M. (eds): *Intracranial Pressure. III* New York, Springer–Verlag, 1976, pp 67–72.
35. Teasdale G., Jennett B.: Assessment of coma and impaired consciousness, a practical scale. *Lancet* 2:81–4, 1974.

CHAPTER 15

The Patient with Pregnancy-Induced Hypertension*

Richard B. Patt

Case History. *A 25-year-old parturient, para 2-0-1-2, at 36 weeks gestation, was admitted to the labor floor complaining of seeing spots before her eyes and sudden weight gain. Blood pressure was 180/120. There was a history of two previous cesarean sections under general anesthesia, indications and uterine scars unknown. Details of prenatal care during this pregnancy were unobtainable.*

Physical examination showed generalized edema and 3+ patellar reflexes. The cervix was closed, and the fetus was in vertex presentation. Examination of the urine showed 2+ protein. A 16-G intravenous catheter was placed, and blood was drawn for SMA 18, CBC, and a coagulation profile. External monitoring of the fetal heart revealed some variable decelerations. An infusion of magnesium sulfate was started. Diastolic blood pressure ranged from 100–120mmHg, and hydralazine was administered intravenously in 5mg increments.

It was decided to proceed with a C-section once blood pressure and hyper-reflexia were controlled, and an anesthesia consult was obtained. Prior to induction of lumbar epidural analgesia, a central venous catheter was inserted through the right internal jugular vein. The initial pressure was 12cmH$_2$O but review of the chest x-ray demonstrated extension of the catheter into the right ventricle. CVP was initially zero, but increased to 8cmH$_2$O following the slow infusion of 500cc 5% albumin and 500cc lactated Ringer's solution. Laboratory values were within the normal range, except for platelet count 143,000/min^3, sodium 133mEq/L, albumin 2.4mg/dl, total protein 4.8ml/dl, and uric acid 5.8mg/dl.

Following continued therapy with magnesium sulfate and hydralazine, the blood pressure was consistently measured at 130/80. After the administration of an antacid solution, the patient was transferred to the OR for C-section under epidural anesthesia.

---

*Reviewed by Dr. Gertie F. Marx, Professor and Director of Obstetric Anesthesiology, Albert Einstein College of Medicine of Yeshiva University, Bronx, New York.

Introduction

Preeclampsia is a pregnancy induced disorder, occurring in 5–7% of parturients. Early recognition and intervention are essential to prevent progression to eclampsia, and to limit maternal and fetal morbidity. Rational care of the preeclamptic patient requires that the anesthesiologist be consulted early and that the anesthetic and obstetric teams work in concert to implement a well-considered treatment plan.

Preeclampsia is defined clinically as a syndrome of hypertension, proteinuria, and generalized edema occurring after the twentieth week of gestation. Hypertension commencing before this time is termed chronic hypertension. The combination of pathologically elevated blood pressure and proteinuria of greater than 2 grams in 24 hours is considered adequate for diagnosis. Edema is common even in normal pregnancy, but the physician should be alerted by severe or rapidly accumulated edema. Accepted criteria for mild preeclampsia include either a blood pressure of 140/90, a systolic pressure increase of 30mm, or a 15mm elevation in diastolic pressure from prepregnancy values. Blood pressures exceeding 160/110 and urinary protein loss of greater than 5 grams per 24 hours signify severe preeclampsia, and impending eclampsia. Severe preeclampsia may be characterized further by headache, visual disturbances, epigastric pain, oliguria, azotemia, liver function abnormalities, or evidence of disseminated intravascular coagulation (DIC). Preeclampsia with superimposed convulsions, not related to coexistent neurologic disease, comprise eclampsia.

The term "toxemia of pregnancy" had been used to refer to preeclampsia and eclampsia, but has been abandoned along with the hypothesis that a circulating toxin was responsible for this condition. Recommendations have been made that the more precise terms "pregnancy induced hypertension" (PIH), or "EPH gestosis" (edema-proteinuria-hypertension) be used when referring to preeclampsia and eclampsia.[1]

PIH is a multisystem disease which places the parturient and the fetus at grave risk. Maternal morbidity exceeds that for hemorrhage. In 1971 in the United States, 107 pregnant women died from PIH, 127 from sepsis, and 94 from hemorrhage.[2] PIH accounts for 6–10% of maternal deaths in the peripartum period in the United States.[3] Causes of maternal death in PIH include intracranial hemorrhage (30–40%),[4] pulmonary edema with congestive heart failure (33%), renal failure, abruptio placentae, and pituitary necrosis. The fetus is at risk due to marginal placental function secondary to reduced uteroplacental blood flow. Newborns are frequently premature and small for gestational age. Forty-two percent of fetal deaths are due to large placental infarcts, 15% to fetal growth retardation, and 13% to abruptio placentae.[5] The patient with PIH should be managed in a center with adequate facilities for maternal and neonatal resuscitation.

The incidence of PIH is increased with inadequate prenatal care, and in young and elderly primigravidae. It is also more common in association with conditions causing rapid uterine enlargement, ie, multiple gestation, diabetes mellitus, polyhydramnios, and hydatiform mole.

Pathophysiology

The etiology of PIH is unclear. There is decreased uteroplacental blood flow secondary to placental vasculitis, which predisposes to uterine hypoperfusion and intrauterine growth retardation in the fetus. The causes of acute uteroplacental atherosclerotic changes are not understood; alternative explanations include hypertension,[6] decreased uterine prostaglandins,[7] and an antigen-antibody reaction between maternal and fetal tissues.[8] Placental changes are postulated to play a central role in other derangements.

Uterine ischemia may release uterine renin,[7] with activation of the renin-angiotensin-aldosterone axis, and contribute to sodium retention and generalized vasospasm. In PIH there is exquisite sensitivity to angiotensin, in contrast to normal pregnancy which is characterized by angiotensin insensitivity.[9] Placental hypoxia further decreases prostaglandins and may stimulate the release of thromboplastin-like substances, which leads to fibrin deposition.[7] The deposition of fibrin and the occurrence of vasopasm contribute to renal dysfunction and proteinuria. Normally, pregnancy is accompanied by a 30–50% elevation in glomerular filtration rate (GFR) and 40% reductions in serum BUN and creatinine levels. In mild PIH, GFR decreases 25% from nonpregnant values.[10] There are reductions in the clearance of urea (to 50–70% that of normal gravidae), and of uric acid. High uric acid levels correlate directly with the severity of PIH.

Derangements of fluid and electrolytes are of particular concern to the anesthesiologist. Due to vasopasm, there is reduced intravascular capacitance, with decreased plasma volume. Plasma volume in the mild preeclamptic is, on the average, 9% less than in the normal parturient.[11] This reduction is similar to that seen with essential hypertension,[12] and still represents an increase in plasma volume from the nonpregnant state. In severe PIH, plasma volume may be 30–40% less than in the normal parturient.[13] Despite a decrease in intravascular volume, there is abnormal retention of sodium and water, with an absolute increase in total body water. Salt and water retention are favored by increased tubular reabsorption of sodium, decreased GFR, and elevated levels of aldosterone. There is increased permeability of vessel walls which, together with hypoproteinemia, results in the accumulation of salt and water in the interstitium and generalized edema. Intravascular depletion of fluid and proteins leads to hemoconcentration and hyperviscosity, but serum electrolyte values are usually normal.

The most common clotting abnormalities are decreased platelet count and prolonged thrombin time. Although bleeding diathesis is rare, platelet counts below 150,000/mm³ have been observed in 15% of preeclamptic women,[14] and 29% of eclamptic women.[15] Thrombocytopenia is probably a result of increased platelet destruction from slow DIC and/or abnormal adherence to disrupted vascular endothelium. Abnormalities of platelet function frequently occur, with or without thrombocytopenia. In a recent prospective series,[16] 50% of thrombocytopenic and 25% of nonthrombocytopenic preeclamptic patients had prolonged bleeding times. Thromboxane B_2 was significantly reduced in 50% of patients, independent of platelet count, and in all patients with prolonged bleeding time. Determination of bleeding time is simple, inexpensive, and provides important information. In most centers, platelet count is still the most commonly used screening test for platelet defects.

There is central nervous system irritability, exaggerated deep tendon reflexes, and the potential for grand mal seizures. Liver injury is variable, and more common in severe PIH. Pulmonary function is not usually grossly abnormal, although an increased alveolar-arterial oxygen gradient has been observed. Pulmonary edema may result from acute myocardial failure or fluid overload. Varying degrees of pulmonary injury may occur when aspiration of gastric contents accompanies eclamptic seizures. Other associated disturbances include carpal tunnel syndrome, visual disturbances, and phlebitis.

Therapy

Specific therapy will depend on the condition of the mother and fetus, stage of pregnancy, severity of PIH, status of target organs, and the philosophy of the obstetric and anesthesiology teams. The general goals of therapy are outlined in Table 1. While most therapeutic maneuvers are undertaken by the obstetric staff, they have widespread effects on anesthetic care and must be understood.

Definitive therapy is delivery of the placenta. The condition of the mother and fetus must be evaluated, and if the fetus can benefit by remaining in the intrauterine environment without threatening maternal well-being, the pregnancy will be allowed to continue while efforts are made to improve maternal status. Delivery is indicated if intrauterine conditions jeopardize fetal viability, or if PIH is severe and the mother is not responding to treatment.

TABLE 1. General therapeutic goals in PIH

---

1. Regulate blood pressure
2. Reduce vasospasm
3. Enhance circulation (especially to uteroplacental unit and kidneys)
4. Improve intravascular volume
5. Diminish central nervous system irritability and peripheral reflexes
6. Correct acid-base and electrolyte disturbances
7. Assure fetal viability

TABLE 2. Clinical correlates to serum magnesium levels

Observation	Plasma Level*
Normal plasma level	1.5–2.0mEq/L
Therapeutic range	4.0–6.0mEq/L
Alteration in ECG (prolonged P-Q, widened QRS)	5.0–10.0mEq/L
Loss of deep tendon reflexes	10mEq/L
SA and AV block	15mEq/L
Respiratory arrest	15mEq/L
Cardiac arrest	25–30mEq/L

*These are average values. Findings may differ in some patients.

Preeclampsia

Bedrest in the lateral decubitus position to minimize aortocaval compression cannot be emphasized strongly enough.[17] Light sedation may be employed. Meticulous monitoring of blood pressure, fluid intake and output, weight change, reflex irritability, and fetal heart rate is essential. Although there is salt and water retention, cautious volume expansion is generally undertaken to promote diuresis and improve perfusion. Intravenous fluids should contain sodium, particularly when oxytocin is administered, to avoid water intoxication and convulsions.[7]

Magnesium sulfate is administered as an infusion in an attempt to prevent seizures (see Table 2) which may occur even in the absence of hyperreflexia. Other salutary effects of magnesium therapy include sedation, vasodilation, and a decrease in uterine tone, with attendant increases in uterine prefusion. Decreased uterine tone, however, may slow the progress of labor. Observation of deep tendon reflexes is the best clinical guide to the adequacy of magnesium therapy. Dosage should be reduced in the presence of renal compromise or oliguria. Calcium chloride should be available for the treatment of magnesium overdose.

Magnesium alone is usually inadequate to control blood pressure; if diastolic pressure still exceeds 100mmHg, an antihypertensive may be added. Hydralazine, administered in frequent intravenous boluses (5–10mg) or as a continuous infusion, is used commonly. Hydralazine relaxes arteriolar smooth muscle, and improves blood flow to the kidneys, uterus, brain, and heart. Other beneficial properties include rapid onset of action, short half-life, and reversibility of hypotension with volume infusion. Hydralazine frequently causes reflex tachycardia and consequently increased cardiac output. The raised cardiac output, together with decreased systemic vascular resistance, usually results in a greater reduction in diastolic than systolic pressure. Trimethaphan is an excellent choice for the treatment of hypertensive crisis. Despite theoretical risks of fetal cyanide toxicity, sodium nitroprusside is being utilized with increasing frequency. Once popular, diuretics are generally avoided unless oliguria persists despite volume expansion.

Eclampsia

In managing eclampsia, the priorities are to control grand mal seizures and to secure an adequate airway. Thiopental 50–100mg or diazepam 5mg is administered intravenously, and 100% oxygen is applied. Phenytoin (Dilantin®) is reserved for prevention of subsequent convulsions. It has a relatively slow onset and initially must be administered slowly to avoid hypotension. If ventilation is inadequate or there is a risk of aspiration, oral endotracheal intubation should be carried out. If necessary, intubation can be facilitated with succinylcholine. Muscle paralysis has the additional benefit of reducing oxygen debt. If there is postictal hypoventilation, assisted ventilation is instituted.

If arterial blood gas analyses demonstrates a significant metabolic acidosis, half of the calculated bicarbonate deficit is given as sodium bicarbonate. Acute left ventricular failure and pulmonary edema may occur in eclampsia. Treatment with furosemide is usually effective, but if it is not, digitalis should be considered. In the presence of heart failure, cardiac filling pressures should be monitored by a central venous or pulmonary artery catheter. Raised afterload usually selectively induces left heart failure, making a pulmonary artery catheter particularly useful. If cerebral edema is suspected, mannitol and dexamethasone can be given.

As PIH worsens, subclinical clotting defects may progress to frank DIC. In this setting, coagulation studies should be performed (PT, PTT, platelet count, fibrinogen). If DIC is diagnosed, preparation should be made for the administration of platelets, fresh frozen plasma, and whole blood. Heparin is rarely indicated. Definitive treatment for DIC, as well as for the underlying PIH, is delivery of the fetus, although many patients remain critically ill for the first 48 hours postpartum.

Based on the status of the mother and fetus, a decision is made when delivery should take place, and whether vaginal delivery is feasible. Since symptoms resolve with childbirth, delivery is favored unless gestational age is less than 34 weeks. No effect to stimulate labor or prepare for cesarean section is begun until the mother's condition has been stabilized. If vaginal delivery is anticipated, oxytocin is frequently administered to augment labor. In PIH the hyperactive uterus is very responsive to oxytocics, and induction is usually successful.[17]

Anesthesia for Labor and Delivery

Labor

Of the methods available for producing analgesia for labor in PIH, lumbar epidural analgesia (LEA) is the most advantageous.[7,17,18] Parenteral sedatives and opioids can depress the fetus and newborn.[19] Analgesia is incomplete, and elevations in heart rate, blood pressure, and oxygen debt can be expected during the second stage.[20] Paracervical block is not recommended. The high incidence of fetal bradycardia and acidosis associated with paracervical block are unacceptable risks,[21] since uteroplacental insufficiency is assumed in PIH. Bilateral lumbar sympathetic block is rarely used in modern obstetric anesthesia because it is difficult to perform, requires two needles, and provides only a finite duration of analgesia. In PIH, this technique carries increased risks of hemorrhage and increased uterine activity and tetany. Caudal analgesia is inferior because of early perineal anesthesia and relaxation, the need for large volumes of anesthetic, difficulty in passing a catheter, and inability to perform cesarean section without the risk of introducing potentially toxic doses of local anesthetics.[7] Inhalation analgesia with nitrous oxide (30–40%) in oxygen or low-dose volatile anesthetics can be used safely.

LEA is not regarded as therapy for PIH, although it reduces blood pressure and has other salutary effects on the mother and fetus. The use of LEA has been a subject of controversy. The main objection is that should maternal hypotension develop from sympathetic blockade, further compromise in uteroplacental circulation is likely to occur.[22,23] The preeclamptic patient is already volume contracted, and therefore at a greater risk for hypotension. Exquisite attention to the prophylaxis of hypotension by cautious volume infusion and the use of left uterine displacement should alleviate these concerns. Ephedrine should be available. The current concensus in obstetric anesthesia is that properly administered continuous LEA is, in most instances, the preferred method of analgesia for labor and vaginal delivery for preeclamptic patients under good medical control.[7,17,18] However, intravascular or intrathecal injection of local anesthetics intended for epidural placement portend disaster. Ordinary precautions are employed.

Besides providing excellent analgesia and reductions in blood pressure, LEA theoretically enhances uterine and renal perfusion by limiting endogenous catecholamine secretion. There is no ventilatory depression, and by eliminating maternal expulsive efforts, elevations in cerebrospinal fluid pressure (which often exceed 50mmHg[24]) are attenuated. In a series of 10 patients with severe PIH, LEA did not reduce cardiac output.[25]

Coagulation studies, particularly a platelet count, are required prior to epidural blockade in women with PIH. Epidural and spinal anesthesia are probably best avoided in patients with platelet counts less than 100,000/mm³ to guard against hematoma. A central venous pressure (CVP) catheter should be inserted prior to volume loading. A chest x-ray is required to verify location of the catheter tip and to exclude pneumothorax. Initial CVP readings are frequently zero. Volume expansion with a balanced salt solution or albumin is carried out cautiously, since venous capacitance is reduced and CVP may rise precipitously.

Once a right atrial pressure of 6–8cm H_2O or a wedged pulmonary artery pressure of 10–12mmHg is obtained, the epidural catheter may be inserted. A segmental block of T10–L1 can be obtained by utilizing small increments of a dilute concentration of local anesthetic (2% chloro-procaine, 0.25% bupivacaine, 0.75% lidocaine). Epinephrine should be omitted. Fetal heart rate should be monitored continuously, and blood pressure should be checked repeatedly following epidural blockade.

A fall in systolic blood pressure of 25% from preblock levels or to less than 100mmHg should be treated immediately. Hypotension and decelerations usually respond to the administration of 100% oxygen, further left uterine displacement, and the rapid infusion of intravenous fluids. If these measures are not effective, intravenous ephedrine is administered in repeated small increments (2.5–5.0mg). If LEA is conducted properly, hypotension will rarely occur, and ephedrine will almost never be required. In a study in England,[26] 2000 PIH patients received lumbar epidural analgesia for labor and delivery, with an average of 4–5 injections per patient. Systolic blood pressure fell more than 20% below preblock levels following only 6% of injections. Hypotension resolved rapidly with volume infusion and oxygen in all but one case in which the blood pressure responded to ephedrine.

Vaginal Delivery

For all the reasons mentioned, LEA is favored for vaginal delivery. It permits controlled delivery and facilitates the application of outlet forceps, if these prove necessary. Prematurity and intrauterine growth retardation are common in PIH, and delivery over a relaxed perineum minimizes trauma to a baby that may already be compromised.

A low level of spinal analgesia (saddle block) is a reasonable approach, provided hypotension is scrupulously avoided. Pudendal block, with or without nitrous oxide supplementation, is less effective than LEA or low spinal. General anesthesia is occasionally required. Endotracheal intubation is mandatory, and the considerations for general anesthesia for cesarean section (vide infra) are operative.

Cesarean Section

It must be emphasized that the anesthesiologist caring for the severe PIH patient is dealing with a critically ill individual. It is a multisystemic disease, "incurable" except by delivery. All the considerations involved in anesthetizing a pregnant patient and insuring fetal well-being exist, in addition to the special implications of preeclampsia. General or conduction anesthesia may be chosen, based on the case, and each technique has advantages and limitations. One caveat applies, regardless: for the best outcome, the manifestations of PIH should be well controlled prior to the induction of anesthesia.

Regional Anesthesia for Cesarean Section

Well-conducted LEA is preferable to spinal anesthesia. Both techniques avoid the hazards of general anesthesia (see below), but hypotension is less common and less precipitous with LEA. While the epidural block may be less dense, anesthetic level is controlled more readily, and anesthesia can be reinforced. Subarachnoid and epidural blockade are contraindicated in the presence of coagulopathy, hypovolemic shock, patient refusal, and local infection.

Most of the guidelines described for the conduct of LEA for labor and vaginal delivery apply equally during cesarean section. The incidence of maternal hypotension can be minimized by cautious volume preloading, left uterine displacement, and the anesthesiologist's vigilance. Continuous monitoring of the blood pressure via a radial artery catheter is helpful, but not mandatory.

If PIH is severe, cardiac filling pressures should be monitored to gauge volume status and myocardial reserve. If placement of a central venous or pulmonary arterial catheter is impractical or is deemed unjustified, volume is administered empirically on an individual basis. Usually 1000cc balanced salt solution or lesser amounts of colloid is given. Colloids are favored because of decreased extravasation. Fluids should be given cautiously. There have been case reports of cardiac failure and cerebral edema with and without pulmonary edema, attributed to injudicious volume infusion.[27] Urine output should be maintained at 1–2cc/kg/hr, but may not accurately reflect volume status in the presence of nephropathy or diuretics.

Magnesium sulfate should be discontinued before administering LEA for cesarean section.[18] Magnesium causes vasodilation, which predisposes to hypotension, and blunts compensatory vasoconstriction rostral to sympathetic blockade. A slowly advancing block is obtained by serial administration of 5ml boluses of local anesthetic. Any of the local anesthetic agents commonly used in obstetric anesthesia may be employed, eg, 2-chloroprocaine, lidocaine, bupivacaine. Chloroprocaine's rapid ester hydrolysis in the maternal and fetal bloodstream (seconds to minutes) may make it the preferred drug.[17] After placement of the epidural catheter, 100% oxygen is administered by facemask to maximize fetal oxygenation.

Local infiltration and field block are feasible when performed by experienced personnel, but are not recommended. Although hypotension and the hazards of general anesthesia are avoided, inadequate anesthesia may exacerbate hypertension, and there is a risk of local anesthetic toxicity.

General Anesthesia for Cesarean Section

General anesthesia is indicated in the presence of acute fetal distress. If general anesthesia is elected, it is conducted with the patient tilted 15–30 degrees to the left to minimize the effects of aortocaval compression. Electrocardiogram, blood pressure, temperature, neuromuscular blockade, and breath sounds are monitored. It is recommended that blood pressure be monitored either by an automated device or continuously via an indwelling radial catheter. Additional parameters (central venous pressure, wedged pulmonary artery pressure, end-expired gases) should be monitored in selected cases of severe PIH.

If magnesium sulfate has been administered, precurarization is omitted, and dosages of relaxants should be adjusted downwards, using the peripheral nerve stimulator as a guide. The effects of the nondepolarizing relaxants are more markedly potentiated than is the action of succinylcholine; regular intubating doses of the latter should be used. In the presence of hepatic or renal dysfunction, atracurium may be the agent of choice for maintenance of muscle paralysis. Reversal of relaxants should be attempted only after partial recovery has been documented.

If, upon evaluation of the patient's airway, a difficult intubation is anticipated, a regional technique should be reconsidered, or awake intubation contemplated. Conscious intubation amplifies considerations of reflex hypertension and its sequelae and should be undertaken only with ultimate caution and preparedness: with an experienced assistant, a ready selection of tubes and blades, vasodilators, and with continuous monitoring of blood pressure.

For general anesthesia, the patient is preoxygenated, and induction is with sodium thipental (4mg/kg) followed by succinylcholine in rapid sequence. Ketamine is not recommended in the presence of severe hypertension. Positive pressure ventilation is withheld and cricoid pressure is applied until the trachea has been intubated. Mucous membrane engorgement may be exaggerated in PIH, with increased likelihood of trauma and difficult intubation; hence, a small caliber endotracheal tube (6.0–7.0mm) should be utilized. Nasotracheal intubation should be avoided.

Reflex responses to tracheal intubation may raise plasma catecholamine levels,[20] pulmonary arterial pressures,[28] and blood pressure. Untoward sequelae may include stroke, pulmonary edema, and fetal distress. A rapidly acting, titratable vasodilator should be on hand, ie, trimethaphan, nitroglycerin, or sodium nitroprusside. Nitroprusside administration may be accompanied by fetal cyanide toxicity,[29] and it may be prudent to avoid its use pending further study. Trimethaphan may be preferable to nitroglycerin, because the latter increases intracranial pressure, and theoretically may cross the placental barrier more readily (molecular weight of trimethephan versus nitroglycerin is 597 versus 227).

Anesthesia is maintained with low concentrations of halothane (0.5–0.8%), enflurane (0.5–1.0%), or isoflurane (0.5–0.75%) in a 60:40 oxygen:nitrous oxide mixture. Oxygen 100% is recommended for the critically ill parturient or in the presence of acute fetal distress. Recent work suggests that enflurane nephrotoxicity is not of practical concern,[30] especially for a short anesthetic. Halothane may be the best choice if a rapid hypotensive response is desired.

Generally, once delivery has taken place, volatile anesthetics are discontinued, and the procedure is completed using an opioid-nitrous oxide technique. Low-dose inhalation anesthesia can usually be continued for blood pressure control if uterine tone is adequate. The obstetrician should be informed of this decision. Uterine massage and the administration of a dilute infusion of oxytocin (10–40 units/L) usually initiate contraction of the uterus and cessation of bleeding. Oxytocin should not be administered as a bolus because of transient vasodilation, hypotension, and reflex tachycardia. The administration of methylergonovine may be accompanied by exacerbation of hypertension, and it should be avoided. Intrauterine injection of prostaglandin 15- methyl $F_{2\alpha}$ by the obstetrician to promote uterine contraction may produce bronchospasm.

Intensive care should be extended for at least the first 48 hours after delivery. There is frequently a continued need for anticonvulsants, blood pressure reduction, and invasive cardiac monitoring. Up to 20% of patients may require postpartum ventilatory support, especially after eclampsia or cesarean section.

Conclusion

The patient with pregnancy induced hypertension is critically ill, and multiple organ systems are affected. Well-coordinated obstetric-anesthetic management based on a thorough knowledge of pertinent pathophysiology and pharmacology will effect substantial reductions in maternal and fetal morbidity and mortality.

References

1. Hughes E.C. (ed): *Obstetric-Gynecologic Terminology.* Philadelphia, F.A. Davis CO, 1972.
2. Thompson J.F.: The vital statistics of reproduction, in Danforth D.N. (ed): *Obstetrics and Gynecology,* 3rd ed, New York, Harper and Row, 1977.
3. Friedman E.A., Neff R.K.: *Pregnancy Hypertension.* Littleton, Mass, PSG Publishing Co, 1977.
4. McLean R., Mattison E.T., Cochrane N.E.: Maternal mortality study annual report 1970–1976. *NY State J Med* 55:39, 1979.
5. Naeye R.L., Friedman E.A.: Causes of perinatal death associated with gestational hypertension and proteinuria. *Am J Obstet Gynecol* 133:8, 1979.
6. Robertson W.B., Brosen S.I., Dixon H.G.: The pathological response of vessels of the placental bed to hypertensive pregnancy. *J Pathol Bacteriol* 93:581, 1967.
7. Gutsche B.B.: Anesthetic considerations for eclampsia-preeclampsia, in, Shnider S.M., Levinson G. (eds): *Anesthesia for Obstetrics.* Baltimore, Williams and Wilkins, 1979.

8. Redman C.W.G.: Immunological factors in the pathogenesis of preeclampsia. *Contrib Nephrol* 25:120, 1981.

9. Gant N.F., et al: A study of angiotensin II pressor response throughout primigravid pregnancy. *J Clin Invest* 52:2682, 1973.

10. Wright J.P.: Anesthetic considerations in preeclampsia-eclampsia. *Anesth Analg* 63:590, 1983.

11. Assali N.S., Vaughan D.L.: Blood volume in preeclampsia: Fantasy and reality. *Am J Obstet Gynecol* 129:355, 1975.

12. Tarazi R.C., et al: Relation of plasma to interstitial fluid volume in essential hypertension. *Circulation* 40:357, 1969.

13. Chesley L.C.: Disorders of the kidney, fluids and electrolytes, in, Assali N.S., Brinkman C.R. (eds): *Pathophysiology of Gestation, Vol. 1. Maternal Disorders*. New York, Academic Press, 1972.

14. Kleckner H.B., et al: The association of maternal and neonatal thrombocytopenia in high-risk pregnancies. *Am J Obstet Gynecol* 128:235, 1977.

15. Pritchard J.A., et al: Coagulation changes in eclampsia: their frequency and pathogenesis. *Am J Obstet Gynecol* 124:855, 1976.

16. Kelton J.G., et al: A platelet function defect in preeclampsia. *Obstet Gynecol* 65:107, 1985.

17. Marx G.F., Bassell G.M.: Anesthetic considerations in hypertensive disorders of pregnancy, in, Gallagher T.J. (ed): *Advances in Anesthesia*. Chicago, Year Book Medical Publishers, 1984.

18. James F.M.: Pregnancy induced hypertension, in, James F.M., Wheeler A.S. (eds): *Obstetric Anesthesia: The Complicated Patient*. Philadelphia, F.A. Davis Co., 1982.

19. Goodlin R.C.: Fetal medication in high-risk pregnancies. *Obstet Gynecol* 34:109, 1969.

20. Shnider S.M., Wright R.S., Levinson G. et al: Uterine blood flow and plasma norepinephrine changes during maternal stress in the pregnant ewe. *Anesthesiology* 50:525, 1979.

21. Shnider S.M., Gildea J.: Paracervical block in obstetrics. III. Choice of drug: Fetal bradycardia following administration of lidocaine, mepivacaine, and prilocaine. *Am J Obstet Gynecol* 116:320, 1973.

22. Gibbs C.P.: Anesthetic management of the high risk gravida, in, Spellacy W.N. (ed): *Management of the High-risk Pregnancy*. Baltimore, University Park Press, 1976.

23. Pritchard J.A., Pritchard S.A.: Standardized treatment of 154 consecutive cases of eclapsia. *Am J Obstet Gynecol* 123:543, 1975.

24. Donaldson J.O.: *Neurology of Pregnancy*. Philadelphia. W.B. Saunders, 1978.

25. Graham C., Goldstein A.: Epidural analgesia and cardiac output in severe preeclamptics. *Anaesthesia* 35:709, 1980.

26. Op cit ref 18, Crawford J.S., personal communication to James F.M., p 257.

27. Benedetti T.J., Quilligan E.J.: Cerebral edema in severe pregnancy induced hypertension. *Am J Obstet Gynecol* 137:860, 1980.

28. Hodgkinson R., Husain F.J., Hayashi R.H.: Systemic and pulmonary pressure during cesarean section in parturients with gestational hypertension. *Canad Anaesth Soc J* 27:389, 1980.

29. Lewis P.E.: Placental transfer and fetal toxicity of sodium nitroprusside. *Gynecol Invest* 8:46, 1977.

30. Crowhurst J.A., Rosen M.: General anesthesia for cesarean section in severe preeclampsia: Comparison of the renal and hepatic effects of enflurane and halothane. *Br J Anaesth* 56:587, 1984.

CHAPTER 16

The Patient with Neurofibromatosis*

David Amar

Case History. *A 17-year-old boy was admitted with severe neck pain and intermittent paresthesias of the arms and legs. Neurofibromatosis had been diagnosed at the age of 2 years. He had been operated upon on multiple occasions for excision of peripheral neuromata. Intellectual development was normal.*

Physical examination showed a well-developed male, weight 210lb. Gross deformity of the neck with diffuse swelling and some displacement of the head to the right was obvious. Severe pain was elicited by extension and lateral rotation of the neck. However, such movement did not provoke neurologic changes in the extremities.

X-ray of the neck showed marked distortion and instability of the cervical vertebrae by neurofibromatous growth. See Figure 1. Other aspects of the physical examination showed: BP right arm 140/80mmHg, left arm 165/95mmHg; pulse 80/min and regular. Arterial blood gas data on room air were: pH 7.36, $PaCO_2$ 45mmHg; PaO_2 78mmHg. CBC and SMA-6 were within normal limits. The patient was scheduled for neck exploration, excision of the tumor, and bony stabilization using an iliac bone graft.

Introduction

Neurofibromatosis is of importance to the anesthesiologist because multiple organ systems may be involved. It has been described in both a generalized or classical form (by von Recklinghausen in 1882) and in a central or acoustic form.[1] The disease is an autosomal dominant trait occurring with a frequency of 1 in 3000. The phenotypic expressivity is variable, but its genetic penetrance is complete.[2]

The pathogenesis of neurofibromatosis has been linked to neural crest disorders. Abnormal crest cells migrate to various parts of the body

---

*Reviewed by Dr. Thomas Kaye, Assistant Professor in Neurosurgery, State University of New York, Stony Brook, New York.

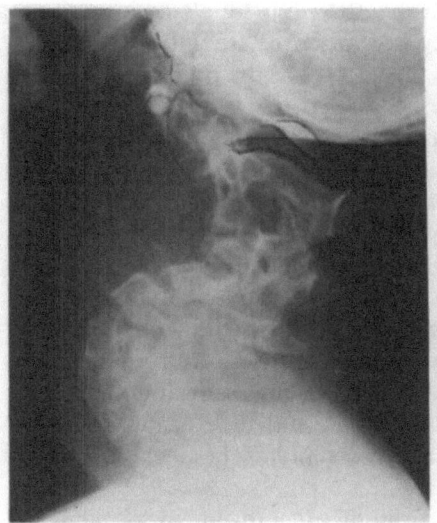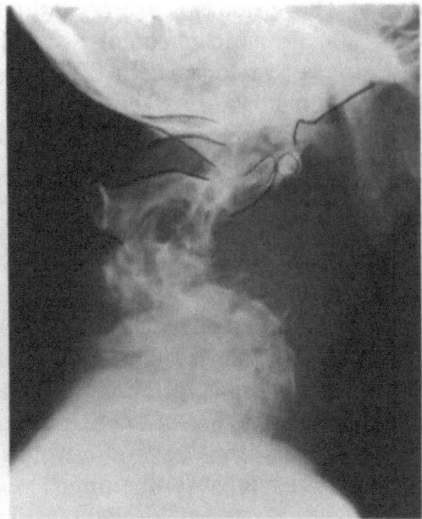

FIGURE 1.

to form, among other types, neuronal, neural-supportive (eg, glial or Schwann cells), pigmentary, and endocrine tissues. In light of the varied manifestations of this disease, other complex interactions with chemical or cellular elements may contribute to its progression. The natural history of the disease is of unrelenting increase in the number and/or size of the skin lesions and tumors. No single feature correlates with the severity of neurofibromatosis. The course is unpredictable. Malignant degeneration to neurofibrosarcoma or malignant schwannoma may occur, especially in tumors subject to constant irritation.[1]

Clinical Characteristics of Neurofibromatosis

The three defining features of neurofibromatosis are café-au-lait spots, Lisch nodules, and neurofibromas. Café-au-lait spots are areas of cutaneous hyperpigmentation present in over 99% of patients with neurofibromatosis. Occurrence of six or more café-au-lait spots larger than 1.5cm in diameter has been used as a criterion in establishing the diagnosis. Freckling in the axilla, groin and inframammary region is common. Of particular importance are the hyperpigmented areas (darker than the typical café-au-lait spots) whose borders overlap with underlying plexiform neurofibromas that extend to the midline. This association often indicates that the tumor involves the spinal cord, a condition that represents a relative contraindication to subarachnoid or epidural analgesia.

Lisch nodules are pigmented hamartomas of the iris and occur in 94% of patients afflicted with classic neurofibromatosis who are older than 6 years of age. These nodules are not found in healthy individuals or in patients with acoustic neurofibromatosis.[3] They do not correlate with other manifestations of the disease or the degree of severity of the affliction.

Neurofibromas (also called neurinomas or neurilemmomas) most commonly involve the skin but other structures such as deep nerves, nerve roots, viscera, blood vessels, the spinal cord, pharynx, larynx, as well as lung parenchyma may be affected. Histologically they are benign. However, they may cause functional compromise and cosmetic disfigurement (eg, elephant man). Plexiform neurofibromas may be extremely vascular. In the mediastinal or cervical areas, they may cause potentially life-threatening impairment of airway, pulmonary, and vascular functions.

Central nervous system tumors associated with neurofibromatosis include optic gliomas, meningiomas, astrocytomas, and schwannomas. The combined frequency of such tumors is 5–10%, and they account for the major portion of the severe morbidity and mortality of the disease.[5] Spinal tumors are usually meningiomas.

Varying extents of intellectual impairment are present in as many as 40% of patients with neurofibromatosis.[6] Macrocephaly associated with neurofibromatosis is usually an incidental finding, although it should prompt a search for hydrocephalus or a brain tumor. Major and minor motor seizures, severe headaches, and cerebrovascular compromise due to neurofibromatosis are well documented.[5] Rarely, hypertension (in less than 3% of neurofibromatosis patients) is secondary to renal artery obstruction (extra- or intramural neurofibromatous involvement of the artery), pheochromocytoma, or multiple cervical neurofibromas that are secreting excessive amounts of norepinephrine.[7]

Neurofibromas of bladder, bowel, liver, and other viscera may cause bleeding and mechanical obstruction. Obstructed labor from neurofibromas preventing vaginal descent has been reported.[8] Kyphoscoliosis occurs in at least 2% of patients. Typically, the deformity involves the lower cervical and upper thoracic spine with acute anterior angulation and S-shaped rotary scoliosis. Untreated kyphoscoliosis in these patients progresses to cardiorespiratory and neurologic compromise. Up to 20% of neurofibromatosis patients between 35 and 60 years of age develop interstitial fibrosing alveolitis that may progress to respiratory failure, cor pulmonale, and death.[9] Congenital heart defects, in particular pulmonary stenosis, are reported to occur frequently in patients with neurofibromatosis.[10] However, coincidence cannot be discounted.

At present, laboratory diagnosis of neurofibromatosis is not possible. Serum levels of nerve-growth factor, though reliable in distinguishing classical from central neurofibromatosis, have not been reliable in distinguishing patients with classical neurofibromatosis from healthy individuals. Nonetheless, all subjects with a strong family history for neurofibromatosis should undergo routine and extensive evaluation to establish the diagnosis, identify complications, and follow progression. The evaluation should include intelligence-quotient measurement and psychological testing, electroencephalography, audiography, slit-lamp ocular examination, radiologic survey of the skull, optic foramina, and spine, head CT scan with and without contrast to include the orbits and optic chiasm, and 24-hour urinary excretion levels of epinephrine and norepinephrine. Repeat visits should be scheduled at 6- to 9-month intervals.

Preanesthetic Assessment

Most patients with neurofibromatosis have a normal life span unless the disease is complicated by malignancy or cardiorespiratory failure. Early recognition of surgically amenable complications and correction are essential. In view of the multiple organ systems involved in patients with neurofibromatosis, the preanesthetic approach should include an assessment of several major systems.

Airway Evaluation and Respiratory Tests

Conditions that may lead to difficult airway management are: neurofibromas of the larynx and pharynx, vagus nerve involvement with vocal cord paralysis, and cervical spine deformity from kyphoscoliosis. Therefore, meticulous preoperative evaluation of the airway should be performed by an anesthesiologist and possibly by an otolaryngologist. Documented range of neck motion and results of extension and flexion x-rays should be available. Conditions should be available to perform an awake endotracheal intubation with or without the fiberoptic laryngoscope.[10, 11] Occasionally, as for example in the case history given, the integrity of the neck is so severely compromised (Figure 1) that a relatively pain-free state can only be maintained during muscle spasm. Administration of diazepam to this patient relaxed the cervical muscles to the extent that compression of the nerves caused severe pain.

Pulmonary function tests and arterial blood gas analyses are needed to determine the extent of damage caused by neurofibromatous interstitial alveolitis and/or kyphoscoliosis. Severe kyphoscoliosis leads to respiratory failure by lowering vital capacity and chest wall compliance, and increases areas of ventilation–perfusion mismatch and pulmonary vascular resistance. Some criteria useful in diagnosing actual or impending respiratory failure are listed in Table 1.

Neurologic Examination

Assessment of involvement of the central nervous system (tumors, hydrocephalus, seizures, headaches, cerebrovascular insufficiency), the peripheral nervous system, and spinal cord should be made. Spinal cord tumors that have caused transection at or above T7 may result in autonomic hyperreflexia under certain conditions, most commonly bladder and bowel stimulation or surgical stimulation under light anesthesia. Other

TABLE 1. Criteria in the diagnosis of actual or impending respiratory failure

If one or more of these conditions exist, a diagnosis of respiratory insufficiency is made.

Respiratory pattern	Irregular
Respiratory rate	< 10/min or > 40/min
Tidal volume	< 3.5ml/kg
Vital capacity	< 15ml/kg
$PaCO_2$	> 50mmHg
PaO_2	< 70mmHg on room air
Inspiratory force	> −25cmH$_2$O

structures that may be affected include the acoustic, that may be affected include the acoustic, optic, trigeminal, glossopharyngeal, and vagus cranial nerves. The corresponding manifestations may include deafness, blindness, trigeminal neuralgia, and vocal cord dysfunction. Preanesthetic documentation is essential.

Endocrine Evaluation

Several endocrine dysfunctions have been associated with major aspects of neurofibromatosis.[1] However, except for pheochromocytoma, medullary thyroid carcinoma, and hyperparathyroidism, such abnormalities are rare. There is no direct evidence that the disease represents a hypothalamic disorder mediated in hormonal terms. Tests for 24-hour urinary catecholamine levels in the hypertensive patient to rule out pheochromocytoma are indicated.

Radiologic and Laboratory Tests

Physical examination and review of the radiologic spine films in the presence of spinal cord tumors or severe kyphoscoliosis should be conducted to determine any anticipated difficulty in accessing the epidural or subarachnoid space. Laboratory tests to screen for obstructive uropathy, hepatobiliary and hematopoietic involvement are indicated as several types of leukemias are excessively represented among patients with neurofibromatosis.

Anesthetic Plan

There is no particular anesthetic technique or agent that is universally recommended for patients with neurofibromatosis. Anesthetic management must be tailored according to the presenting features and complications of the disease. There are considerations, however, that should be borne in mind that relate to the choice of general or regional anesthesia and managing the patient once the choice of anesthetic technique has been made.

General Anesthesia

If intracranial pressure is elevated, further increases must be prevented by careful attention to avoidance of hypercarbia, hypoxia, acidosis, and extreme blood pressure swings. Barbiturates, lidocaine, fentanyl, and isoflurane may be used. Ketamine is contraindicated.[13]

Prolonged neuromuscular block in patients with neurofibromatosis has been reported with the use of succinylcholine, d-tubocurarine, and pancuronium.[14] Both administration and reversal of muscle relaxants requires continued monitoring. Furthermore, in patients with neuromuscular involvement and muscle atrophy, succinylcholine can induce severe hyperkalemia.[15] In many instances, intracranial surgery can be successfully performed using little or no muscle relaxation after intubation has been accomplished. This latter maneuver is probably best performed after administration of one of the new nondepolarizing relaxants, atracurium or vecuronium.

In neurofibromatosis patients at risk of developing a hypertensive crisis secondary to a pheochromocytoma, sodium nitroprusside, trimethaphan, and phentolamine must be available in the operating room. Succinylcholine should be avoided under these circumstances as it stimulates autonomic ganglia and regularly evokes hypertensive episodes. Pancuronium is not recommended due to vagolytic properties. Vecuronium may provide the desired hemodynamic stability.[16]

In patients with interstitial alveolitis and severe kyphoscoliosis, intraoperative monitoring of pulmonary function, including inspiratory pressure and arterial blood gas analyses, is indicated. Before extubation, these patients must demonstrate return of adequate neuromuscular function and respiratory reserve. A classification system based on 0–3 to predict risk of pulmonary complications (lower number indicates less risk) is shown in Table 2.[17] This scheme, although initially devised for patients undergoing thoracic and abdominal procedures, integrates the evaluation of multiple organ systems and is thus applicable to patients with neurofibromatosis. Patients scoring 0 do not require oxygen therapy after discharge from the recovery room. Moderate-risk patients (score 1–2) have an increased incidence of atelectasis, pneumonia, and hypoxemia. Careful pulmonary hygiene, and administration of humidified oxygen is indicated for several days. High-risk patients (3 or more points) require observation in an intensive care facility postoperatively. Patients with pulmonary hypertension and cor pulmonale require monitoring after placement of a pulmonary artery catheter.

Regional Anesthesia

Regional anesthesia, whenever possible, may be the technique of choice in the patient with a spinal cord lesion above T7 due to the potential hazard of inducing autonomic hyperreflexia under light general anesthesia. How-

TABLE 2. Classification system for risk of pulmonary complications

Expiratory Spirogram	
Normal (% FVC + % FEV_1/FVC > 150)	0
% FVC + % FEV_1/FVC = 100–150	1
% FVC + % FEV_1/FVC < 100	2
Preoperative FVC < 25ml/kg	3
Postbronchodilator FEV_1/FVC < 50%	3
Cardiovascular System	
Normal	0
Controlled hypertension, MI without sequelae > two years ago	0
Dyspnea on exertion, orthopnea, paroxysmal nocturnal dyspnea, dependent edema, congestive heart failure, angina, recent MI	1
Nervous System	
Normal	0
Confusion, obtundation, agitation, spasticity, discoordination, bulbar malfunction	1
Significant muscular weakness	1
Arterial Blood Gas Measurement	
Acceptable	0
$PaCO_2$ > 50mmHg or PaO_2 < 60mmHg on room air	1
Metabolic pH abnormality > 7.50 or < 7.30	1
Ambulatory Status	
Expected ambulation (at minimum, sitting at bedside) within 36 hours	0
Expected complete bed confinement for at least 36 hours	1

0 = Low risk
1–2 = Moderate risk
> 3 = High risk

Adapted from Shapiro B.A., Harrison R.A., Kacmarek R.M., and Cane R.D. (eds): *Clinical Application of Respiratory Care*, ed 3. Chicago, Year Book Medical Publishers, 1985. Reproduced with permission of author and publisher.

ever, if major conduction anesthesia appears to be the technique of choice, radiologic spine films, especially in the presence of spinal cord tumors or kyphoscoliosis, must be carefully examined to rule out possible difficulty in locating the epidural or subarachnoid space.

Summary

In the patient with neurofibromatosis, whether the surgical problem requires emergent or elective care, it would be wise to assume that some or all of the above complications are present and to apply the appropriate precautions to provide a safe anesthetic.

References

1. Riccardi V.M.: von Recklinghausen neurofibromatosis. *N Engl Med* 305:1617–1627, 1981.

2. Riccardi V.N., Kleiner B., Lubs M.L.: Neurofibromatosis: Variable expressivity is not intrinsic to the mutant gene. *Birth Defects* 15(5B):283–9, 1979.

3. Lewis R.A., Riccardi V.M.: von Recklinghausen neurofibromatosis incidence of iris hamartomata. *Ophthalmology* 88:348–54, 1981.

4. Riccardi V.M.: Pathophysiology of neurofibromatosis IV. Dermatologic insights into heterogeneity and pathogenesis. *J Am Acad Dermatol* 3:157–66, 1980.

5. Rubenstein A.E., Mytilineau C., Yahr M.D., et al: Neurological aspects of neurofibromatosis. *Ad Neurol* 29:11–21, 1981.

6. Rosman N.P., Pearce J.: The brain in multiple neurofibromatosis (von Recklinghausen's disease): A suggested neuropathological basis for the associated mental defect. *Brain* 90:829–37, 1967.

7. Schuch W., Messerli F.H., Genest J., et al: Arterial hypertension and neurofibromatosis: Renal artery stenosis and coarctation of abdominal aorta. *Can Med Assoc J* 113:879–85, 1975.

8. Katz J., Benumof J., Kadis L.B. (eds): *Anesthesia and Uncommon Diseases*. Philadelphia, W.B. Saunders Company, 1981, pp 571–572.

9. Sagel S.S., Forrest I.V., Askin F.B.: Interstitial lung disease in neurofibromatosis. *South Med J* 68:642, 1985.

10. Neiman H.L., Mena E., Holt J.F., et al: Neurofibromatosis and congenital heart disease. *Am J Roentgenol Radium Ther Nucl Med* 122:146–9, 1974.

11. Fisher M.M.: Anesthetic difficulties in neurofibromatosis. *Anesthesia* 30:648–650, 1975.

12. Holt G.T.: ENT manifestations of von Recklinghausen's disease. *Laryngoscope* 88:1617–32, 1978.

13. Frost E.A.M.: *Clinical Anesthesia in Neurosurgery*. Boston, Butterworth, 1984, pp 43–63.

14. Yamashita M.: Anesthetic considerations in von Recklinghausen's disease. Abnormal response to muscle relaxants. *Der Anaesthetist* 26:317, 1977.

15. Cooperman L.H.: Succinylcholine induced hyperkalemia in neuromuscular disease. *JAMA* 21:1967, 1970.

16. Verner J.: Management of theochromocytoma. ASA 1984 Annual Refresher Course Lectures, 216.

17. Shapiro B.A., Harrison R.A., Trout C.A.: *Clinical Application of Respiratory Care*, ed. 3. Year Book Medical Publishers, Inc., Chicago, 1985, pp 523–525.

CHAPTER 17

The Patient with Trigeminal Neuralgia*

Zenaida Aurellano-Hoh

Case History. *A 33-year-old white female was admitted for a posterior fossa craniectomy for microvascular decompression of the trigeminal nerve. The patient had been suffering for eight years from brief, extremely intense paroxysms of pain, which she described as lightning-like stabbing sensations on her right cheek and around her lips, precipitated by chewing, brushing her teeth, talking, washing her face, and applying make-up. The pain would last seconds to minutes and rarely occurred at night. For the past year, she had been experiencing attacks several times daily, despite carbamazepine 1200mg by mouth daily in four divided doses.*

Past medical history was unremarkable. Physical examination showed a slim, mildly anxious female; height 152cm; weight 48kg. Vital signs were within limits. HEENT (head, eyes, ears, nose, throat) heart, lungs, and neurologic examinations were normal.

Preoperative evaluation included routine blood work (CBC, SMA-16), ECG, chest x-ray, skull x-ray, and CAT scan with contrast. All were normal.

Historical Description of Trigeminal Neuralgia

Although cephalgia is one of the oldest painful syndromes mentioned in medical literature, specific entities such as trigeminal neuralgia were not identified until the eighteenth century. Sixteenth century carvings in the Wells Cathedral are said to depict sufferers of this syndrome. The first clearly recognizable description of the condition is contained in a eulogy of Johannes Laurentius Bausch written in 1672.

The term "tic douloureux" was introduced in 1756 by Nicolaus André. Fothergill, in 1773, gave a classic account of the disease and stressed that it should be distinguished from toothache and rheumatism of the face. Medi-

---

*Reviewed by Dr. Ronald Apfelbaum, Associate Professor of Neurosurgery, University of Utah, Salt Lake City, Utah.

cinal, physical, balmeal, electric, and herbal therapies were tried with little success. Lotions, vesicants, and cautery were applied to the painful points. Drugs used included quinine sulfate, ferrous carbonate, and hemlock. Facial numbness resulting from exposure to trichloroethylene suggested that this gas might be a satisfactory remedy. Sectioning of facial nerves was advocated, but it was not until the sensory function of the trigeminal and the motor action of the facial nerve were demonstrated in 1822 by Magendi and Bell that the cause of the pain was understood.[1]

Pathology of Tic Douloureux

Trigeminal neuralgia (tic douloureux) is a clinical syndrome characterized by short paroxysms of high-intensity facial pain. It is a sensory disorder of the peripheral distribution of the fifth cranial nerve, affecting the second, third, and first division, in order of frequency of involvement. It has an estimated incidence of 15 per 100,000 population. Its onset is typically after age 40, it affects women more often than men, and occurs more frequently on the right than left side.[2]

The history is diagnostic. The pain seldom lasts more than a few seconds or a minute or two but may be so intense that the patient winces, hence, the term, tic. It is a shooting, stabbing sensation, frequently precipitated by touching a trigger zone around the lips or the buccal cavity. Attacks may occur spontaneously or be precipitated by light touch, temperature change, facial movement, emotional disturbance, or trauma. Spontaneous remissions and exacerbations are common; the exacerbations tend to occur in the spring and fall. Between paroxysms of pain, the patient is asymptomatic. Tic pain rarely occurs at night.

No neurologic abnormality can be identified clinically. However, hyperesthesia of the affected side of the face may accompany an attack.[3]

Numerous pathophysiologic mechanisms have been proposed to explain the occurrence of trigeminal neuralgia. Infection, trauma, inflammation, neoplastic and vascular lesions, mechanical compression, and degenerative demyelination may precipitate the disorder by causing development of an abnormal sensory response to minimal stimuli. Cross-circuiting of autonomic pathways and reverberations of peripheral impulses produce a repetitive, independent, multineuronal discharge within sensory channels.[4] Pain results.

Therapy

Pharmacologic Management

Carbamazepine (Tegretol®, Geigy Pharmaceuticals, Ardsley, NY) is the drug of choice for the treatment of trigeminal neuralgia. Anticonvulsant agents are believed to depress the response of the mechanoreceptive neurons in the spinal trigeminal nucleus and antagonize synaptic transmission.[5] The drug is given in doses varying from 400–800mg a day. Because of its sedative properties, the initial dose is 100mg twice daily, gradually increased to the required maintenance dose. No more than 1200mg should be taken daily. The drug is reported to be effective initially in 80% of patients. However, one fourth become refractory. More important, serious idiosyncratic side effects such as rash, leukopenia, thrombocytopenia, gastrointestinal upset, lack of coordination, mental obtundation, renal and liver abnormalities and, rarely, aplastic anemia may necessitate withdrawal of the drug.[6]

Approximately 50% of those afflicted with trigeminal neuralgia will respond to phenytoin (Dilantin®, Parke-Davis, Morris Plains, NJ) in doses of 400mg a day. Toxicity may be manifested by ataxia, nystagmus, slurred speech, mental confusion, cutaneous eruptions, gastrointestinal upset, and hematopoietic complications.[7]

When one of the aforementioned drugs has not proven efficacious, the two combined may provide pain relief at nontoxic levels. Several other medications have been used as ancillary drugs. Chlorphenesin carbamate (Maolate®, Upjohn, Kalamazoo, MI) 400mg four times a day and baclofen (Lioresal®, Geigy) 20–80mg per day, have, on occasion, been of benefit.[4]

Surgery

Surgery is reserved for those patients in whom medical treatment has failed to relieve the pain, or those in whom side effects force discontinuation of drug treatment. There are several surgical approaches in the treatment of tic douloureux. A specific procedure can best be recommended after considering the patient's age, associated conditions, general health, state of facial sensation, the acceptance of associated risks, and response to prior surgical intervention.

For a patient whose age is less than 65 years and who is in good general health, the Janetta microsurgical decompression of the trigeminal root is the procedure of choice.[8] The procedure is based on the observation that many patients with trigeminal neuralgia have a tortuous vessel, usually arterial, looped against the trigeminal root near the brain stem. The operation consists of a craniectomy, using the operating microscope to expose the trigeminal root at the brain stem, and interposing a piece of sponge between the nerve and any vascular structure impinging on it. Microvascular decompression spares the nerve and treats the apparent cause of the pain.[9] This therapy does not cause numbness, dysesthesia, or corneal anesthesia. Drawbacks include the need for a formal craniectomy requiring general anesthesia and exposing the patient to increased risk of serious, even lethal, complications. Although the Janetta procedure is usually performed in the sitting position, it may be done in a lateral or park-bench position.[10]

Trigeminal neuralgia will occur in 1–3% of patients afflicted with multiple sclerosis, and 1–3% of patients with trigeminal neuralgia will be found to suffer from multiple sclerosis.[11] For patients who are elderly or debilitated, or those with tic associated with unresectable intracranial masses or with multiple sclerosis, a percutaneous procedure such as radiofrequency lesioning or glycerol chemoneurolysis is the recommended procedure.

Radiofrequency lesioning involves selective destruction of the postganglionic retrogasserian trigeminal nerve by graded radiofrequency ablation.[12] It has also been called radiofrequency trigeminal neurolysis, radiofrequency gangliolysis, or thermocoagulation stereotaxic rhizotomy. Successful performance of this procedure requires patient cooperation because of the need for assessment of the response to physiologic stimulation. After ascertaining correct needle placement through the foramen ovale under radiographic control, radiofrequency current is incrementally applied to the needle until selective destruction of pain fibers is achieved as ascertained by repetitive testing of the patient.

Percutaneous retrogasserian glycerol rhizotomy uses chemical rather than thermal injury to the nerve. Glycerol in 99% anhydrous form is a weak neurolytic alcohol which is injected into the trigeminal cistern of Meckel's cave. Precise placement of a small volume (0.15–0.35ml) of sterile glycerol is ensured by demonstrating the anatomy of the trigeminal cistern using a water-soluble contrast agent, metrizamide (Amipaque®, Winthrop-Breon, New York, NY). The most likely explanation of pain relief after glycerol neurolysis lies in selective destruction of the previously damaged large-fiber population that can be implicated in the etiology of trigeminal neuralgia.[13] Results with glycerol neurolysis are as good as those after radiofrequency lesioning. The procedure is more easily tolerated because repeated testing is not required and it tends to produce less numbness and a decreased incidence of dysesthesia.

Percutaneous trigeminal neurolysis is safe and well tolerated despite an advanced age or poor medical condition; it requires only brief hospitalization and is easily repeated if needed. Its disadvantages are that symptoms, rather than underlying pathology, are treated. The procedure is destructive, permanently altering facial sensation. Risk of corneal anesthesia is present as are dysesthetic sequelae and an increased recurrence rate with the passage of time.

The ultimate choice of surgical procedure depends on patient preference after thorough discussion of the alternatives, risks, and benefits of each approach.

Preanesthetic Assessment

Several factors peculiar to patients with trigeminal neuralgia must be considered in the preanesthetic evaluation.

Evaluation of Drug Therapy

The majority of patients with tic douloureux are on high-dose carbamazepine and/or phenytoin. Patients on the latter agent might present with swollen, bleeding gums which may complicate airway management. Interactions between drugs may occur under anesthesia. Carbamazepine is capable of inducing the synthesis of drug-metabolizing enzymes, particularly those of the hepatic endoplasmic reticulum.[14] Such induction can enhance the metabolism not only of the inducing agent but also of a variety of drugs administered during anesthesia. These patients usually require higher than normal doses of barbiturates and opioids to maintain an adequate anesthetic state.

A complete blood count immediately prior to surgery is important in all patients maintained on carbamazepine because of the risk of idiosyncratic hematopoietic effects. Renal and hepatic function must also be evaluated and any abnormalities noted prior to the administration of anesthetic drugs.

One of the ancillary drugs for the pharmacologic management of trigeminal neuralgia, baclofen, is an analog of the inhibitory neurotransmitter, gamma aminobutyric acid (GABA). It is inevitable that some patients taking baclofen will require surgical management of their tic pain, necessitating general anesthesia. Case reports have recently been published that severe bradycardia and hypotension have occurred under general anesthesia in patients who received baclofen.[15] The mechanism to explain this dangerous hemodynamic complication is unknown. When anesthetizing such patients, the possibility of severe bradycardia and hypotension should be anticipated and drugs appropriate for treating this emergency (atropine, neosynephrine) should be readily available. It may be prudent to discontinue baclofen therapy prior to anesthesia and surgery, although it should not be suddenly discontinued after long-term administration. Hallucinations, seizures, or both can occur following abrupt withdrawal after more than two months of therapy. It is recommended that dosage be gradually reduced by 5–10mg per day at weekly intervals.

As in all cases of patients who have suffered painful syndromes for years, the potential for drug abuse exists in patients with trigeminal neuralgia. If the patient has been receiving large doses of anxiolytic or opioid preparations, abrupt discontinuation should not be attempted immediately preoperatively. Rather, tapering of dosage with psychologic counseling and other support mechanisms should be commenced immediately after surgery. Although immediate pain relief is obtained in most cases, in some instances, attacks of lesser intensity may continue for a few days to a few weeks. The patient should be cautioned about this possiblity.

Neurologic Assessment

As noted previously, trigeminal neuralgia may be associated with multiple sclerosis. A careful neurologic assessment is important prior to anesthesia, particularly if microvascular decompression is undertaken. Any diminution in protective airway reflexes should be assessed and the possible need for prolonged postoperative intubation evaluated. Other neuropathies such as foot drop or any areas of diminished sensation (eyes, face, etc) should be documented.

Anesthetic Plan

Neurolysis

Percutaneous trigeminal neurolysis is usually performed in the x-ray department. A properly functioning anesthesia machine and suction apparatus must be available. Monitors used in this procedure are an electrocardiogram, blood pressure cuff, and a precordial stethoscope. Review of anesthetic records of patients who had trigeminal themocoagulation have consistently noted a marked increase in blood pressure during percutaneous trigeminal rhizotomy.[16] Blood pressure should be monitored closely during these procedures and treatment should be readily available to control excessive rises (hydralazine, furosemide, propranolol).

In attempting to analyze the requirements of the anesthetic technique for percutaneous trigeminal neurolysis, four factors are necessary: the ability to produce sedation and anesthesia with rapid reversal; the avoidance of nausea; formulation of a technique acceptable to patients, some of whom may require further treatment; and maintenance of the patient in a stable physiological state.[17]

The patient is usually fasted after midnight. After premedication with an anticholinergic drug (atropine or glycopyrrolate) and an anxiolytic (hydroxyzine, diazepam, or droperiodol), the patient is anesthetized with a short-acting barbiturate and an opioid such as fentanyl for the most painful part of the procedure (the penetration of the foramen ovale).[18]

Decompression

Although patients undergoing microvascular decompression of the trigeminal nerve are usually relatively young and in good general health, anesthetic management is more complicated because this approach involves a formal craniectomy usually done with the patient in the sitting position. The obvious dangers to the patient in this position include air embolism, hypotension, cranial nerve palsies, airway obstruction, and vital sign changes during brain stem manipulation.[19] Anesthetic management should be directed at the prevention, early detection, and treatment of these problems.

Monitoring should include an electrocardiogram, intra-arterial blood pressure measurement, temperature probe, esophageal stethoscope, and measurement of urinary output, arterial blood gases, and end-tidal carbon dioxide tension. Monitoring for venous air embolism is with a precordial

Doppler ultrasound unit, which is presently the most sensitive readily available method for detection.[19] Routine use of a right atrial catheter, especially for posterior fossa craniectomy for nerve decompression, has been questioned for it was found to offer no advantage while subjecting the patients to considerable risk.[20]

Premedication should be minimal to avoid depression of the respiratory center and the possibility of postural hypotension as the patient is moved into the sitting position. Anxiolytics such as diazepam are preferable to opioids. For induction of anesthesia, thiopental 2–4 mg/kg, lidocaine 1–1.5mg/kg, and succinylcholine 1mg/kg may be used, keeping in mind that these patients might require more barbiturates especially if they are receiving carbamazepine. Anesthesia can be maintained with isoflurane (0.5–1%) in a 50:50 mixture of oxygen and air with incremental doses of fentanyl.

Prior to position change from supine to sitting, rapid infusion of about 100ml of fluid to acutely increase the intravascular volume is recommended. The position change should be achieved gradually. An adjunct to the sitting position includes wrapping the legs with elastic bandages. All pressure points should be adequately padded and the eyes protected.

At the end of the procedure, prevention of excess movement, particularly while the patient is still secured by the pin headholder, can be accomplished by administration of lidocaine 1mg/kg intravenously as a bolus during skin closure.[21] Rapid emergence from anesthesia is desired to allow immediate postoperative neurologic evaluation. In the rare event that a hematoma impinges on the brain stem, this complication may be rapidly diagnosed by the patient's decreasing consciousness, hypertension, tachycardia, and disorders of respiration.

References

1. Walker A.E.: *A History of Neurological Surgery*. New York, Hafner Pub Co., 1967, pp 309–313.
2. Victor M., Adams R.D.: Diseases of cranial nerves, in Harrison T.R. (ed): *Principles of Internal Medicine*. New York, McGraw-Hill Book Co, 1980, p 2023.
3. Voorhies R., Patterson R.H.: Management of trigeminal neuralgia (tic douloureux). *JAMA* 245:2521–2523, 1981.
4. Greenberg C., Papper E.M.: The indications for Gasserian ganglion block for trigeminal neuralgia. *Anesthesiology* 31:566–573, 1969.
5. Fromm G.H., Terrence D.F., Chattha A.S.: Baclofen in the treatment of trigeminal neuralgia: Double-blind study and long-term follow-up. *Ann Neurol* 15:240–244, 1984.
6. Killian J.M., Fromm G.H.: Carbamazepine in the treatment of neuralgia. *Arch Neurol* 19:129–136, 1968.
7. Loeser J.D.: The management of tic douloureux. *Pain* 3:155–161, 1977.
8. Apfelbaum R.I.: Surgery for tic douloureux. *Clin Neurosurg* 31:667–683, 1984.

9. Lundsford L.D., Apfelbaum R.I.: Choice of surgical therapeutic modalities for treatment of trigeminal neuralgia: microvascular decompression, percutaneous retrogasserian thermal, or glycerol rhizotomy. *Clin Neurosurg* 31:319–333, 1984.

10. Janetta P.J.: Treatment of trigeminal neuralgia by suboccipital and transtentorial cranial operations. *Clin Neurosurg* 23:538–549, 1976.

11. Penman J.: Trigeminal neuralgia, in Vinken P.K., Bruyn G.W. (eds): *Handbook of Clinical Neurology*, New York, Elsevier Publishing Co, 1968, p 296.

12. Apfelbaum R.I.: Surgical management of disorders of the lower cranial nerve, in Schmidek H.H., Sweet W.H. (eds): *Operative Neurosurgical Techniques, vol 2*. New York, Grune & Strutton, 1982, pp 1063–1082.

13. Lundsford L.D.: Treatment of tic douloureux by percutaneous retrogasserian glycerol injection. *JAMA* 248:449–453, 1982.

14. Melmon K.L., Gilman A.G.: Drug interactions, in Goodman L.S., Gilman A.G. (eds): *The Pharmacological Basis of Therapeutics*. New York, Macmillan, 1980, pp 1739–1740.

15. Sill J.C., Schumacher K., Southorn P.A., et al: Bradycardia and hypotension associated with baclofen used during general anesthesia. *Anesthesiology* 64:255–258, 1986.

16. Brodsky J.B., Samuels S.I., Britt R.H., et al: Anesthesia for trigeminal nerve thermocoagulation, correspondance. *Anaesthesia* 38:912–913, 1983.

17. Lowe S.S., Meurer M., Ingram O., et al: Anesthesia for trigeminal nerve thermocoagulation. *Anaesthesia* 38:152–154, 1983.

18. Apfelbaum R.I.: Technical considerations for facilitation of selective percutaneous radiofrequency neurolysis of the trigeminal nerve. *Neurosurgery* 3:396–399, 1978.

19. Cucchiara R.F.: Positioning the neurosurgical patient: Special considerations. ASA Annual Refresher Course Lectures, 116, 1984.

20. Mogos B., Phillips P.L., Apfelbaum R.I., et al: Is right artrial catheterization always indicated for anesthesia in the sitting position? *Anesth Analg* 61:205, 1982.

21. Frost E.A.M., Rubin R.C.: Posterior Cranial Fossa Surgery, in Frost E.A.M. (ed): *Clinical Anesthesia in Neurosurgery*. Boston, Butterworth, 1984, pp 155–185.

CHAPTER 18

The Patient with Acquired Immune Deficiency Syndrome*

Elizabeth A.M. Frost

Case History. *A 42-year-old, unmarried, white male, native to New York, was admitted to the hospital complaining of severe intermittent headache of 4 weeks duration, stiff neck, dizziness, and intermittent lethargy. He reported an approximate 30lb weight loss over the previous year associated with almost constant diarrhea.*

Past history included herniorrhaphy without complications 5 years previously. The patient admitted to heroin abuse but at present attended a methadone clinic. His family suspected him of bisexual preference.

Physical examination showed a thin, slightly disoriented male who coughed frequently. Height was 170cm and weight, 55kg. Vital signs included oral temperature 38.1°C, pulse 107/min; blood pressure 110/90, and respiratory rate 22/min. Chest examination revealed bilateral basal crepitations. There were white plaques on the oral mucosa. Diffuse lymphadenopathy of the axillae, submandibular, and inguinal areas was present.

Neurologic examination showed lack of finger-to-eye coordination, right-grip weakness, foot drop, and positive Kernig's and Brudzinski's signs. Computerized tomography (CT) scan visualized several intracranial masses, including a cerebellar mass with ring enhancement and obstructive hydrocephalus.

Laboratory studies showed: white blood cell count 4,300/mm³; Hgb 9.8gm/dl; platelet count 180,000/min³; SMA-6 normal. Analysis of cerebrospinal fluid obtained via lumbar puncture gave the following results: mononuclear pleocytosis, white blood cell count 175/ml³; protein 98mg/dl. Chest x-ray showed diffuse bilateral fibrotic changes. ECG was normal.

The ELISA serum test for HIV antibody was positive as was the Western blot test, confirming the presence of antibody to the virus of acquired immune deficiency syndrome (AIDS). Immunoglobulin (Ig) M toxoplasma titers were elevated.

---

*Reviewed by Dr. R. Klein, Associate Professor of Medicine, Albert Einstein College of Medicine of Yeshiva University, Bronx, New York.

Medications included pyrimethamine, sulfadiazine, dexamethasone, nystatin, and phenytoin. The patient was scheduled for stereotaxic brain biopsy.

Definition and Incidence of AIDS

The Centers for Disease Control (CDC) have defined AIDS as a "reliably diagnosed disease that is at least moderately indicative of an underlying cellular immunodeficiency in a person who has no underlying cause of cellular immunodeficiency nor any other cause of reduced resistance reported to be associated with that disease."[1] AIDS patients characteristically present with malignant tumors such as Kaposi's sarcoma and non-Hodgkin's lymphoma and/or infections that are rare in immunocompetent persons. These opportunistic infections most frequently include *Pneumocystis carinii* pneumonia, cryptococcal meningitis, atypical *Mycobacterium* infections and toxoplasmosis. AIDS-related complex (ARC) has been diagnosed in a larger number of patients who present with lymphadenopathy syndromes and/or abnormal laboratory findings (low T-helper/T-suppressor cell ratio or decreased number of T-helper cells), suggesting a milder or prodromal form of AIDS.

As of June, 1987, over 36,000 cases of AIDS have been reported to the CDC of which more than 20,000 have already died. A large majority of cases have occurred in just a few states: New York, 42%; California, 20%; Florida, 7%; and New Jersey, 6%. Although there are monthly fluctuations, the number of cases reported to the CDC has been doubling approximately everly 12–14 months. It has been estimated that a million people in the United States have been infected with the virus that causes AIDS,[2] which has been called human T-cell lymphotropic virus type III (HTLV-III) lymphadenopathy-associated virus (LAV), or, more recently, human immunodeficiency virus (HIV). The brief history of AIDS is shown in Table 1.

A recent study has shown that AIDS victims live an average of 224 days

TABLE 1. The brief history of AIDS

The number of cases of AIDS reported to the Centers for Disease Control continues to double every 12–14 months.

1978 Retrospective recognition
1981 Association with Kaposi's sarcoma and *Pneumocystis carinii* recognized; identification of high-risk groups—homosexuals and intravenous drug abusers
1982 Opportunistic infections reported in 4 homosexual males
1983 Isolation of a T-lymphotropic retrovirus
1984 Identification of HTLV-III
1985 Identification of pathways toward developing a vaccine
1986 18,000 cases reported to CDC
1987 1 million infected persons in US

after their first hospitalization. The direct lifetime hospital cost of the care of such patients is calculated to be $42,000. If only 8000 new cases are diagnosed in 1987, the estimated cost of inpatient care for these cases will approximate $336 million. If one adds to this the cost of outpatient services, social considerations (lost employment, reduced productivity, shortened life expectancy, welfare services), and antibody testing of the 12 million units of blood collected annually, it has been estimated that AIDS cost society more than half a billion dollars in 1985,[3] and by 1991 it will cost New York City alone over 1 billion dollars.

Etiology

It has been speculated that the HIV virus was transferred to man from monkeys in Central Africa during the 1970s.[4] A cultural preference existing in Africa for medications delivered by injection, based on traditional beliefs about disease causation and neutralization, may have helped spread AIDS. The colonial medical services introduced needles and syringes, which were also used for scarification linked to cupping. The authorities reinforced the preference for injectables to achieve compliance, as pills were often sold or given away. Widespread reuse of unsterilized needles resulted.

Spread of the disease throughout other parts of Africa has been linked tc heterosexual activity.[5] Moreover, HIV disease in Africa is characterized mainly by lymphadenopathy and has a female:male incidence of 1:1. (In the U.S. the ratio is 1:16.) Although Kaposi's sarcoma does occur in Africa, it is less commonly associated with the AIDS virus. Mortality rates are lower than those in the U.S.

AIDS was first reported in the United States in 1981.[6] Evaluation of the overall distribution of AIDS in this country indicates that 71% of patients are homosexual or bisexual males, 17% are heterosexual intravenous drug abusers of either sex, 3% have received blood donations, and 1% are female sexual partners of AIDS patients.[6] Approximately 3% of cases occur in infants who are presumably infected in utero or perinatally. The patient category breakdown for New York City in the early part of 1987 is shown in Table 2. Ethnic breakdown shows a preponderance of white males afflicted. (See Figure 1.)

Diagnosis

AIDS is a disease of the immune system caused by a horizontally transmitted retrovirus. Retroviruses contain the enzyme reverse transcriptase that allows the conversion of RNA to DNA which is then incorporated into the cell's genome. The virus preferentially infects lymphocytes of the T-helper subset and destroys them, leaving the cell unable to cope with infection and neoplastic diseases.[7] The incubation period ranges from 6 months to at least 5 years.

TABLE 2. New York City AIDS cases: patient profiles*

Patient Category	Males Cases (%)	Females Cases (%)	Total Cases (%)
Homosexual/bisexual, not intravenous drug user	5,101(55.5)	0 (0.0)	5,101(55.5)
Homosexual/bisexual, I.V. drug use unknown	138 (1.5)	0 (0.0)	138 (1.5)
Homosexual/bisexual, I.V. drug user	451 (4.9)	18 (0.2)	469 (5.1)
I.V. drug user, heterosexual	2,086(22.7)	544 (5.9)	2,630(28.6)
I.V. drug user, sexual orientation unknown	93 (1.0)	11 (0.1)	104 (1.1)
Born in country where heterosexual transmission is believed common	159 (1.7)	39 (0.4)	198 (2.2)
Transfusion-associated	38 (0.4)	35 (0.4)	73 (0.8)
Hemophiliac, or other blood-factor deficiency	17 (0.2)	2 (0.0)	19 (0.2)
Sex partner of person from known risk-group	4 (0.0)	209 (2.3)	213 (2.3)
Interviewed, no risk factor determined	44 (0.5)	23 (0.3)	67 (0.7)
Unable to interview adequately	51 (0.6)	24 (0.3)	75 (0.8)
Under investigation	74 (0.8)	27 (0.3)	101 (1.1)
TOTAL	8,256(89.8)	932(10.2)	9,188(100)

*Number of cases of acquired immune deficiency syndrome as of Feb. 25 1987, by patient group and percentage of total cases.
Source: New York City Department of Health

The Western blot test is the most extensively used diagnostic assay for HIV antibody. The test identifies antibodies within a range of molecular weights that have been associated with the HIV virus. An enzyme-linked immunosorbent assay (ELISA) has also been developed that detects the specific antibodies to HIV.[8] This test permits widespread screening of donated blood. Approximately 3.2 million patients receive blood annually in the U.S., and about 3% of AIDS cases have been associated with transfusions. ELISA also identifies asymptomatic persons who have been infected with the HIV virus. The Western blot test is less sensitive than ELISA, but it is more specific if positive.

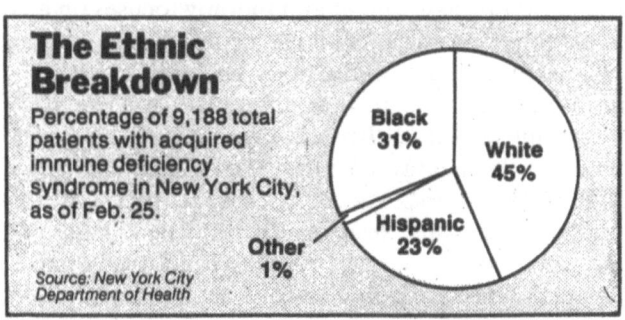

FIGURE 1.

Serologic surveys have yielded variable seropositive rates in the high-risk groups: 22–65% of homosexual men, 87% of intravenous drug abusers in a detoxification program, 56–72% of hemophiliacs, and 35% of women who were sexual partners of men with AIDS. HIV antibody has been detected in less than 1% of persons with no known risk factors.[9]

The time to development of a positive antibody test is unknown. One case of seroconversion has been reported between 4 and 7 weeks after a needle stick.[10] The CDC has recently (May 1987) reported that three health care workers, contaminated with blood from AIDS patients, have become infected. In each case direct exposure was through cuts or abrasions on the hands or through the mouth.

For research purposes, peripheral blood mononuclear cells can be cultured and assayed for the presence of HIV virus activity. HIV virus can be cultured from 68–100% of seropositive individuals, and from greater than 85% of seropositive symptomatic patients, that is, individuals with AIDS or ARC. Virus can also be cultured from 84–100% of persons with AIDS-related conditions, such as generalized lymphadenopathy.[8,11,12]

That the virus has also been recovered from 95% of high-risk seropositive blood donors 2 or more years after initial donation indicates that viremia may persist for years in asymptomatic individuals. If there is a reactive test for antibody to HIV in blood donors, the Public Health Service recommends that additional serologic testing be done.

During a follow up period of 2–5 years, AIDS developed in 4–19% of HIV seropositive persons. Nonspecific symptoms suggesting early states of AIDS-related illnesses developed in an additional 25%.[13] However, with time, the percentage of symptomatic patients increases.

Pathophysiology

The pathologic pathway of the AIDS virus is outlined in Figure 2. The virus itself is described as a poor pathogen but subject to frequent subtype variations, which makes development of a vaccine difficult.[14]

In adults, preanesthetic assessment and therapy focuses on an evaluation of the effects of opportunistic infections, chemotherapeutic agents, and (often) intravenous drug abuse on the body systems.

The picture in children is somewhat different. Children are often born infected with cytomegalovirus, Epstein-Barr, herpes, or rubella virus. Craniofacial dysmorphism may coexist. The incubation period of HIV in children is about 6 months, and the children usually present with recurrent bouts of pneumonitis, oral thrush, diarrhea, lymphadenopathy, parotid disease, and failure to thrive. As they cannot generate an immune response to antigens, they are prone to contract all the childhood diseases despite immunization attempts.

In the preanesthetic assessment of the patient presented in this lesson, several body systems require particular attention.

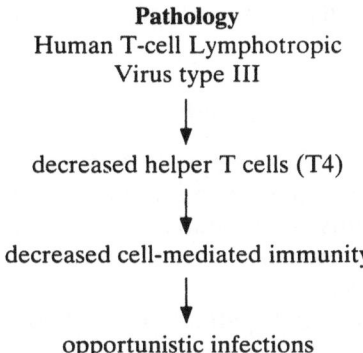

Pathology
Human T-cell Lymphotropic
Virus type III

↓

decreased helper T cells (T4)

↓

decreased cell-mediated immunity

↓

opportunistic infections

FIGURE 2. Pathway taken by the HIV virus as it is incorporated into the cell.

Respiratory System

The respiratory system is vulnerable to attack by several opportunistic infections. Complications include *Pneumocystis carinii* pneumonia, aspergillosis, herpetic infections, oral and pharyngeal candidiasis, and cytomegaloviral pneumonia, which may be the terminal event for the AIDS victim.[15] Other pulmonary infections are caused by *Mycobacterium* and, rarely, coccidioidomycosis. Inert substances used to dilute street opioids frequently cause pulmonary fibrosis in the intravenous drug abuser.

Thus, both acute and chronic lung disease occur. Establishment of a diagnosis is helpful, and some of the infections may respond to therapy. For example, aspergillosis may respond to amphotericin B; herpes simplex, to acyclovir; tuberculosis, to isoniazid (INH); and cytomegalovirus, to dihydroxypropoxymethyl guanine (DHPG).[16]

Appropriate preanesthetic assessment requires careful evaluation of pulmonary function, including arterial blood gas analyses and evaluation of tidal volume, vital capacity, and timed expiratory volumes. If a general anesthetic technique is planned, provision may be necessary for postoperative ventilatory care.

Cardiovascular System

Although perhaps less of a target system than the lungs, many cardiac abnormalities may be caused by opportunistic bacterial infections, ranging from endocarditis to congestive cardiac failure. Of particular importance are vegetations which may form on heart valves in association with intravenous drug abuse. Embolic phenomena may require replacement of heart valves. Central nervous system pathology causing brain stem lesions and intracranial hypotension may cause almost any type of cardiac dysrhythmia. Electrocardiography and echocardiography may be indicated to differentiate between cardiac and cerebral disease and initiate appropriate therapy.

Gastrointestinal System

Diarrhea, vomiting, and loss of appetite commonly occur in the AIDS patient. Oral candidiasis makes eating and swallowing difficult and painful. Cytomegaloviral colitis and proctitis cause debilitating diarrhea. Other intestinal infections are caused by cryptosporidium and *Mycobacterium avium* and *M. intracellulare*.

Thus, the majority of AIDS patients are dehydrated, in negative nitrogen balance, and have electrolyte abnormalities. Preanesthetic correction is essential whenever time permits.

Hematologic abnormalities

Anemia, thrombocytopenia, and leukopenia are common in AIDS patients. Treatment of opportunistic infections with DHPG, vinblastine, doxorubicin, and other chemotherapeutic agents increases immunosuppression and causes neutropenia, eosinophilia, and thrombocytopenia. Radiation therapy for lymphoma may cause further hematologic abnormalities. Clearly, these patients are already infected, and the caveats pertaining to withholding of blood and blood product transfusions are unimportant.

Although bone marrow transplantation was suggested as potentially curative for the AIDS victim,[17] early results were discouraging.

Central Nervous System

The HIV virus appears to be harbored within the central nervous system.[18] Table 3 outlines some of the neurologic manifestations.

TABLE 3. Neurologic Manifestations of AIDS

Cranial or Peripheral Neuropathies	CNS Complications
Bell's palsy	Subacute encephalitis
Polyneuropathies	Aseptic meningitis
Guillain-Barré syndrome	Herpes simplex encephalitis
Herpes zoster	Multifocal leukoencephalopathy
Myalgias	Viral myelitis
Polymyositis	Varicella-zoster encephalitis
	Nonviral infections (toxoplasmosis, *Cryptococcus, Candida, Mycobacterium, E. coli, Treponema, Aspergillus*)
	Tumors (lymphoma, Kaposi's sarcoma)

The HIV virus preferentially attacks the CNS. It may manifest in many different forms.

Approximately 30% of AIDS patients develop neurologic complications, usually secondary to opportunistic infection. Both central and peripheral involvement has been described. Subacute encephalopathy characterized by general malaise and altered consciousness is not uncommon. Neoplasms such as primary lymphoma of the brain and spinal cord or, rarely, epidural plasmacytoma may also occur. Vascular complications arise from nonbacterial thrombotic endocarditis, cerebral hemorrhage and parainfectious cerebral arteritis. Autoimmune phenomena may cause peripheral neuropathies as seen in Guillain-Barré syndrome, thrombocytopenic purpura, and polymyositis.

Protozoal infection may cause toxoplasmosis, which has been shown to respond to pyrimethamine and sulfadiazine. Many of the patients have intracranial hypertension, dementias, paresis or paralysis, seizures or other neurologic changes. All of these factors must be carefully considered in planning a rational anesthetic technique. If possible, intracranial hypertension should be decreased prior to surgery by administration of steroids and diuretics and cerebrospinal drainage.

Anesthetic Management

A plan for a general anesthetic should include adequate premedication and induction with thiopental and lidocaine (intravenously and topically) to avoid bucking during endotracheal intubation. Depolarizing muscle relaxants should not be used in the patient with hemiparesis because these agents may cause a sudden increase in serum potassium. Mental status and neurologic manifestations of disease should be documented preoperatively to ensure accurate comparison at postoperative examination. Drugs such as droperidol and trimethaphan, which cause extrapyramidal signs, should be avoided. Seizures are not uncommon. Enflurane and high-dose fentanyl should be avoided. Patients receiving bleomycin should not be given high oxygen concentrations because of the risk of pulmonary failure. Silent aspiration is a possible hazard. Antiseizure medication, such as phenytoin and phenobarbital, can cause hepatic microsomal enzyme induction and increase drug tolerance. A similar effect is often found in the intravenous drug abuser, a situation that may co-exist.

Because of the rapid and changing profile of AIDS, subarachnoid and epidural block analgesia should be performed only after careful evaluation and documentation of neurologic deficits.

For the patient presented in this case report, the best type of anesthesia probably includes infiltration of the scalp with a local anesthetic solution (bupivacaine), and I.V. administration of small doses of a potent opioid, such as fentanyl, to provide sedation and analgesia during drilling of the bone. Careful monitoring of vital signs is essential.

Further problems in the anesthetic management of the AIDS patient may include considerations pertaining to anesthetizing the drug abuse patient: lack of venous access, and hepatic, neurologic, cardiac, and renal involvement. For a discussion of these considerations, see Chapter 3. Also, AIDS patients may be receiving multipharmacologic agents, such as broad-spectrum nephrotoxic antibiotics, phenytoin, barbiturates, and immuno-suppressive drugs, and the possibility of drug interaction must be considered.

Precautions During Care of AIDS Patients

An important issue in the care of the patient with AIDS concerns the possible transmission of a lethal disease to health care workers and the exposure of the patient to opportunistic pathogens.

No occurrence of AIDS has been reported in physicians or nurses who are not already members of a high-risk group although seropositivity has been obtained.[19] A recent study of heterosexual household contacts of AIDS patients indicated minimal or no risk of infection with the HIV virus.[20]

A report of the cases of 25 hospital employees exposed to the blood of patients with AIDS by accidental needle puncture showed that none of the individuals had any evidence of defects in cell-mediated immunity over the study period (up to 12 months); however, the authors advise monitoring for several years.[21] Two thirds of the exposures occurred during needle disposal, 37% during recapping and 30% during disposition of the used needle. The more recent report, referred to at the beginning of this chapter, would indicate that careful precautions in handling of body fluids of AIDS victims is essential. Precautions should be directed at reducing hospital personnel exposure to blood and body fluids, and reducing the possibility of transmission of opportunistic pathogens to the patient. The patients are at far greater risk than the physicians.

Suggested precautions for hospital personnel include wearing gowns and gloves while handling blood and secretions, and frequent hand washing. Masks are probably indicated for physicians or patients who are actively coughing. Instruments can be sterilized with ethylene oxide or glutaraldehyde. Needles should be placed in puncture-resistant containers and not reinserted in their original sheaths. There is absolutely no justification for using substandard monitoring or therapy in the care of these seriously ill individuals.

References

1. Center for Disease Control: Prevention of acquired immune deficiency syndrome (AIDS): report of interagency recommendations. *MMWR* 32:101–3, 1983.

2. Curran J.W., Morgan W.M., Hardy A.M., et al: The epidemiology of AIDS: current status and future prospects. *Science* 229:1352–7, 1985.
3. Landerman S.H., Ginzburg H.M., Weiss S.M.: The AIDS epidemic. *N Engl J Med* 312:521–5, 1985.
4. Saxinger W.C., Levine C.M., Dean A.G., et al: Evidence for exposure to HTLV-III in Uganda before 1973. *Science* 227:1036–8, 1985.
5. Kreiss J.K., Koech D., Plummer F.A., et al: AIDS virus infection in Nairobi prostitutes. *N Engl J Med* 314:414–8, 1986.
6. Center for Disease Control: Acquired immunodeficiency syndrome (AIDS) update—United States. *MMWR* 32:309–11, 1983.
7. Ma P., Armstrong D., eds: *The Acquired Immune Deficiency Syndrome and Infections of Homosexual Men*. New York, York Publishing, 1984.
8. Sarngadhavan M.G., Popovic M., Bruch L., et al: Antibodies reactive with human T-lymphotropic retroviruses (HTLV-III) in the serum of patients with AIDS. *Science* 224:506–8, 1984.
9. Center for Disease Control: *MMWR* 34:5–7, 1985.
10. Anonymous: Needlestick transmission of HTLV-III from a patient infected in Africa. *Lancet* 2:1376–7, 1984.
11. Safai B., Sarngadhavan M.G., Groopman J.E., et al: Seroepidemiological studies of human T-lymphotropic retrovirus type III in acquired immunodeficiency syndrome. *Lancet* 1:1438–40, 1984.
12. Laurence J., Brun-Vezenet F., Schutzer S.E., et al: Lymphadenopathy-associated viral antibody in AIDS. *N Engl J Med* 311:1269–73, 1984.
13. Darrow W.W., Joffe H.W., Braff E.: AIDS in a cohort of homosexual men. 24th Intensive Conference on Antimicrobial Agents and Chemotherapy. Washington, DC, 1984.
14. Osborn J.E. The AIDS epidemic: multidisciplinary trouble. *N Engl J Med* 314:779–82, 1986.
15. Macher A.M., Reichert C.M., Straus S.E., et al: Death in the AIDS patient: role of cytomegalovirus. *N Engl J Med* 309:1454, 1983.
16. Collaborative DHPG Treatment Study Group: Treatment of serious cytomegalovirus infections with 9-(1,3 dihydroxy-2-propoxymethyl) guanine in patients with AIDS and other immunodeficiencies. *N Engl J Med*. 314:801–5, 1986.
17. Amimann A.J., Dritz S.K., Volberding P., et al: The acquired immune deficiency syndrome—a multidisciplinary engima. *West J Med* 140:66–81, 1984.
18. Levy R.M., Bredesen D.E., Rosenbaum M.L.: Neurological manifestations of the acquired immunodeficiency syndrome (AIDS). Experience at UCSF and review of the literature. *J Neurosurg* 62:475–95, 1985.
19. Conte J.E.: Guidelines for the care of hospitalized patients with AIDS. *Infect Surg* 3:265–9, 1984.
20. Friedland G.M., Saltzman B.R., Rogers M.F., et al: Lack of transmission of HTLV-III/AV infection to household contacts of patients with AIDS or AIDS-related complex with oral candidiasis. *N Engl J Med* 314:344–9, 1986.
21. Wormser G.P., Joline C., Duncanson F., et al: Needle-stick injuries during the care of patients with AIDS. Correspondence, *N Engl J Med* 310:1461, 1984.

CHAPTER 19

The Patient with Porphyria*

Gary Hartstein

Case History. *A 26-year-old woman was scheduled for elective cholecystectomy. The patient complained of intermittent right upper quadrant pain, nausea, and vomiting for two weeks. A low grade fever (101.2°F) was documented. Initial therapy included ampicillin and gentamicin. Past history was unremarkable. Notably, she had no previous complaint of abdominal pain, no neuropsychiatric symptoms, and no cutaneous lesions. She has no allergies and took no medications.*

Acute intermittent porphyria (AIP) was documented in her sister in 1980 during investigation of abdominal and neurologic symptoms. At that time, the sister was referred to the National Institutes of Health where screening showed mildly elevated urinary levels of δ-aminolevulinic acid and porphobilinogen and reduced red blood cell levels of uroporphyrinogen synthase (50% of normal). These tests confirmed the presence of latent-phase AIP.

Vital signs showed: temperature 101.2°F, pulse 110/min, blood pressure 140/90mmHg, and respiratory rate 20/min. The patient was in no acute distress. Physical examination was negative for cutaneous lesions, muscle weakness, or sensory deficit. The right upper quadrant was mildly tender with minimal peritoneal signs. No difficulty was anticipated in establishing or maintaining an airway.

Laboratory examinations, including CBC and SMA-18 were within normal limits. A gallbladder scan confirmed the diagnosis of acute cholecystitis.

Introduction

The porphyrias are a group of diseases with the common denominator of a partial defect in the metabolic chain leading to heme synthesis. The biochemical hallmark is the overproduction of heme precursors. Clinical man-

---

*Reviewed by Dr. Maria Santorineou, Professor of Pediatrics, Albert Einstein College of Medicine of Yeshiva University, Bronx, New York.

Succinate

```
          1        2        3                         5
  +        →  ALA  →  PBG  →  Uroporphyrinogen III  →  Coproporphyrinogen III
                             4                                    ↓  6
Glycine                          8                    7
                    Heme  ←  Protoporphyrin IX  ←  Protoporphyrinogen IX
```

Abbreviations: ALA = δ-aminolevulinic acid, PBG = porphobilinogen. The enzymes are as follows: (1) δ-aminolevulinate synthase (ALA-S), (2) PBG synthase (or δ-aminolevulinic dehydratase), (3) uroporphyrinogen I synthase, (4) uroporphyrinogen III cosynthase, (5) uroporphyrinogen decarboxylase, (6) coproporphyrinogen oxidase, (7) protoporphyrinogen oxidase, (8) ferrochelatase.

FIGURE 1. The Heme biosynthetic pathway.

ifestations include a combination of photosensitivity, cutaneous lesions, abdominal symptoms, and neuropsychiatric problems.

The significance of porphyria for the anesthesiologist is twofold. First, three of the porphyrias, acute intermittent porphyria (AIP), variegate porphyria (VP), and hereditary coproporphyria (HC), have a course marked by clinical crises which can be induced by anesthetic drugs. These porphyrias are termed the inducible porphyrias.[1] Second, the neurologic manifestations of the inducible porphyrias include several problems of potential concern to the anesthesiologist, including variable muscle weakness, unpredictable motor neuropathy, and autonomic neuropathy. Other types of porphyria of lesser concern during anesthesia include protoporphyria and congenital erythropoietic porphyria.

Pathophysiology

The porphyrias are genetic diseases resulting from the partial deficiency of enzymes along the synthetic pathway to heme. See Figure 1 and Table 1. Heme, a planar tetrapyrrole compound, forms the prosthetic group of several proteins involved in oxygen and electron transport. These proteins include hemoglobin, myoglobin, catalase, and the cytochromes, including those involved in the mitrochondrial electron transport chain, and

TABLE 1. The deficient enzymes in the various porphyrias

	Abbreviations in text
AIP	Uroporphyrinogen I synthase
HC	Coproporphyrinogen oxidase
VP	Protoporphyrinogen oxidase
Protoporphyria	Ferrochelatase
Congenital Erythropoietic Porphyria	Uroporphyrinogen III cosynthase

TABLE 2. Heme precursor excretion patterns in the inducible hepatic porphyrias

Disease		Urine				Feces	
		ALA	PBG	Uro	Copro	Copro	Proto
AIP	Acute	↑↑	↑↑	↑↑	↑↑	↑	↑
	Latent	↑	↑↑↑	↑↑	↑↑	N	N
VP	Acute	↑↑	↑↑	↑↑↑	↑↑↑	↑↑	↑↑
	Latent	N	N	N	N	↑↑↑	↑↑↑
HC	Acute	↑↑	↑↑	↑↑	↑↑↑	↑↑↑	↑
	Latent	↑	↑	N	N or ↑	↑↑	N

Abbreviations in text, and, uro = uroporphyrins, copro = coproporphyrins, proto = protoporphins, N = normal.

cytochrome P450, a microsomal enzyme intimately involved in the metabolism of exogenous lipid-soluble compounds.

The heme pathway starts with succinylcoenzyme A, derived from the tricarboxylic acid (Krebs) cycle, and with glycine, derived from the intracellular pool of amino acids. These compounds are joined to form δ-aminolevulinic acid (ALA) by the enzyme δ-aminolevulinate synthase (ALA-S) with vitamin B_6 as a co-factor. The reaction takes place in the mitochondria and is the rate-limiting step of the entire metabolic pathway. Biologic control of the rate of heme biosynthesis is exerted via control of ALA-S, both quantatively and qualitatively (see below). All other reactions along the pathway are strongly favored thermodynamically.[2]

The ALA thus formed passes into the cytosol, where several steps occur leading to the formation of coproporphyrinogen III. The first of these involves the fusion of two molecules of ALA to form porphobilinogen (PBG). This compound enters the mitochondria where three more reactions culminate in the formation of heme.

The body synthesizes approximately 250mg of heme each day, 80% of which is used for hemoglobin. Normally, only small quantities of excess precursors are excreted (4mg ALA, 15mg PBG, 0.1mg uroporphyrinogen, 0.3mg coproporphyrinogen, 0.1mg protoporphyrinogen).[3] Since the organism's requirement for heme is relatively constant, partial blockages due to enzymatic deficiencies cause large increases in the amounts of precursors. The pattern of increased precursor production is easily predictable once the deficient enzyme is known. The total loss of an enzyme along this path would be incompatible with life.

The excretion pattern of the excess precursors in the porphyrias is predictable on the basis of water solubility. ALA, PBG, and uroporphyrinogen are water soluble, and are thus found in the urine. Protoporphyrins are insoluble in water and are excreted in the feces. Coproporphyrins are intermediately soluble, and appear in both urine and feces. Table 2 shows the characteristic excretion pattern of the various inducible porphyrias in acute crisis and in the latent phase.

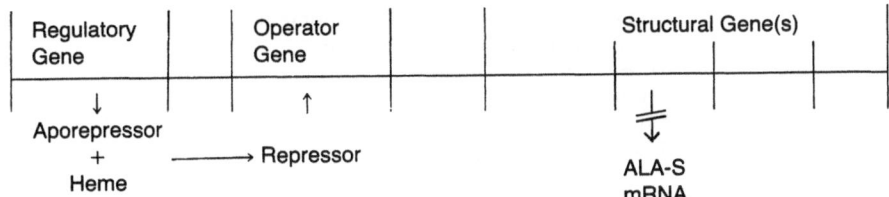

FIGURE 2. The ALA-S operon (see text for details).

The synthetic pathway to heme is controlled tightly at the ALA-S step, ie, flux through the reactions is regulated to fill the organism's requirement for heme. ALA-S is regulated via two feedback mechanisms. The major regulatory mechanism involves induction and repression of ALA-S synthesis. ALA-S synthesis is under the control of an operation, a set of genes that includes a regulator gene.[4] The regulator gene directs the synthesis of an aporepressor protein; heme combines with this protein to form a repressor, which in turn binds to an operator gene, blocking the synthesis of ALA-S messenger RNA at the structural gene(s). See Figure 2. The less important mechanism involves inhibition of enzyme activity by the end-product of the pathway, heme. Heme binds to a site on the ALA-S molecule and decreases its activity.[5]

Although all cells can (and must) synthesize heme, the erythropoietic system and the liver are the most active. The clinical syndromes of porphyria are expressed primarily in these organs. Porphyrias are classified as hepatic or erythropoietic. AIP, VP, and HC constitute the hepatic porphyrias.

Various factors are important in the induction and repression of ALA-S synthesis, the most relevant of which occurs in the liver, where most of the heme synthesized is incorporated into cytochrome P450.[1] This enzyme system is involved in the metabolism of nonpolar lipid-soluble compounds, including many anesthetic drugs. Cytochrome P450, located on the smooth endoplasmic reticulum of the hepatocyte, is itself inducible. Thus, in the presence of inducing compounds (some of which can exert a profound and prolonged induction after a single dose), cytochrome P450 is synthesized. Increased demand for heme results, lowering intracellular levels, and de-repressing ALA-S synthesis. If porphyria exists, the partial enzymatic blockade leads to accumulation of the heme precursors located "upstream" of the block; this is the end event that provokes the clinical crisis of porphyria.

Most drugs and compounds capable of inducing cytochrome P450 (and thus indirectly ALA-S) are capable of provoking prophyric crises. Starvation (via increased catabolism of heme), and steroids (both endogenous and exogenous) also induce ALA-S and have been reported to cause clinical crises. Table 3 lists the drugs that have been implicated in causing

TABLE 3. Drugs implicated in inducing attacks of the inducible prophyrias

Steroids
Althesin*
Hydroxydione
Estrogens
Progesterone
Metapyrone*

Antibiotics
Chloramphenicol*
Griseofulvin
Sulfonamides

Anticonvulsants
Phenytoin
Primidone
Methsuximide

Local Anesthetics
Lidocaine*

Sedatives
Barbiturates
Chlordiazepoxide
Glutethimide
Meprobamate

Analgesics
Pentazocine*
Amidopyrine
Antipyrine

Oral Antidiabetics
Chlorpropamide
Tolbutamide

Inhalation Anesthetics
Enflurane*
Methoxyflurane*

Miscellaneous
Amphetamine
Ferric chloride
Imipramine

*Shown to induce ALA-S synthesis in vivo, but not definitely associated with acute attacks in man.

porphyric crises. Glucose in large amounts administered intravenously represses ALA-S synthesis, and is therapeutic in acute crisis.

Incidence

The inducible porphyrias are all transmitted as an autosomal dominant trait.[2] The degree of clinical expression varies markedly among family members, with some who carry the gene remaining asymptomatic throughout life. This variability, coupled with the clinical course of crisis and remission, makes estimation of prevalence extremely difficult.

In one series, the reported incidence of porphyria was 1 in 7000 hospital admissions.[6] In Lapland, however, the prevalence may be greater than 1 in 1000 of the general population.[7] Estimates in the U.S. run to 1 in 100,000. Females with this disease outnumber males 3 to 2.[2]

AIP constitutes 75% of cases of inducible porphyria.[1] VP (20% of inducible porphyrias) is most common in South Africa (more than 3 cases per 1000 population) where it was introduced by a Dutch settler in 1688.[8] Five percent of inducible porphyrias are HC, most of which remain asymptomatic.

Clinical Presentation

Many patients may present a perfectly normal clinical picture. This disease is characterized by a sequence of crises and remissions.

Crisis

Acute crises of all three of the hepatic porphyrias are similar; the type of porphyria cannot be distinguished on the basis of the clinical presentation. VP and HC also are associated with skin lesions which are absent in AIP (see below).

A crisis consists of abdominal pain and neuropsychiatric symptoms, and can appear hours to weeks after a triggering agent. Attacks may be precipitated by four major groups of factors:

- drugs,
- hormonal levels (steroids),
- infection,
- starvation.

Abdominal Pain

The abdominal pain experienced by 90–95% of porphyria patients during crisis is described as colicky in nature and can radiate to the back. The pain is often (50–80%) accompanied by nausea, vomiting, and constipation, or, more rarely, by diarrhea.[2] On examination, there is less abdominal guarding and rigidity than symptoms might suggest. Abdominal x-ray usually shows dilated loops of bowel adjacent to areas of spasm. Fever and leukocytosis may or may not be present. However, in their presence, a source of infection must be aggressively sought. The pathogenesis of the abdominal pain is not known but is presumed to result from autonomic neuropathy. This may explain the effectiveness of ganglionic blockade in relieving pain. Phenothiazine derivatives, which are also very effective analgesics in porphyric crisis, may act by a similar mechanism.[3]

Neurologic Problems

Neurologic signs and symptoms result from variable involvement of the autonomic, peripheral, and central nervous systems. Theories of the pathogenesis of neurologic lesions include toxicity of porphyric precursors, pyridoxine deficiency, and intraneuronal heme deficiency. The pathologic neural lesion is primarily an axonopathy, with secondary demyelination.

Central nervous system involvement shows a clinical spectrum ranging from mild changes in mental status (emotional instability, irritability, confusion) to psychosis, seizures, and coma. Seizures occur in 10% of patients[3] and are usually, but not always, related to hyponatremia. When the cranial nerves are affected, the optic nerve can atrophy, and oculomotor function can be lost. Vocal cord pareses are also common, as are facial palsies. Of most concern to the anesthesiologist are the neuropathies affecting the respiratory muscles; respiratory failure is the major cause of death in porphyric crisis. Weakness of the muscles of deglutition may result in aspiration.

Peripheral nervous system manifestations consist primarily of motor neuropathy, which is greater proximally and is usually asymmetric. Sensory loss can sometimes also be demonstrated. Motor loss can range from mild weakness to mono-, para-, or quadriplegia. Some paralysis is seen in 40–50% of patients in crisis.[1] Pain can precede the motor symptoms, and deep tendon reflexes are frequently diminished or absent.

The autonomic nervous system is also affected in porphyric crisis. Sinus tachycardia is the most frequent sign and is related to vagal neuropathy. Labile hypertension with or without orthostatic hypotension is common.

Fluid Balance

Fluid and electrolyte derangements may accompany an acute attack. Hypovolemia and hypokalemia occur secondary to diarrhea and vomiting, and can lead to prerenal azotemia and oliguria or anuria. Hyponatremia is frequent, and is usually the result of inappropriate secretion of antidiuretic hormone.[3] Liver function is normal, except for slight bromsulphthalein retention during crisis.[5]

Skin Lesions

Cutaneous lesions of VP and HC presumably result from photoactivation by ultraviolet light of excess porphyrins, which are stored in lysosomes, releasing proteolytic enzymes into the skin. The skin is very sensitive to mechanical trauma and is prone to infection. Scarring often occurs resulting in hyperpigmentation and hypertrichosis.

Diagnosis

All the inducible porphyrias are associated with clinical crises. In VP and HC there are associated skin lesions. However, several factors make diagnosis difficult.

Although the porphyrias are genetic diseases, the variable clinical expression among family members makes a family history necessary but insufficient for diagnosis. The pattern of symptoms differs from patient to patient but tends to show individual uniformity. Another factor creating diagnostic difficulty is the variable delay (hours to weeks) between a triggering agent (eg, drug administration) and the onset of a crisis. Symptoms of disease rarely occur before puberty.

As mentioned above, on clinical grounds alone, one cannot distinguish the clinical crisis of AIP from that of VP or HC. Skin lesions narrow the diagnosis to HC or VP, but the presence of such lesions is not consistent.

Diagnosis is confirmed by measuring the pattern of precursor excretion in urine and feces.[9] Table 2 shows the various patterns seen in both acute attacks and in the latent phase. It can be seen that acute crises of all the inducible porphyrias are associated with increased urinary ALA and PBG levels. A crisis can be easily revealed with the Watson–Schwartz test, performed on fresh urine. In the presence of dimethylaminoparabenzaldehyde, PBG polymerizes, and an immediate red color indicates high levels of PBG. Further testing is necessary to distinguish the inducible porphyrias.

During acute crisis, VP patients show, in addition to elevated urinary levels of ALA and PBG, increased urinary coproporphyrins and fecal protoporphyrins. In HC, fecal and urinary coporporphyrins are elevated, with normal amounts of protoporphyrins. Both during crisis and remission, positive qualitative tests should be confirmed with quantitative tests, usually by chromatography. These quantitative tests are also most useful to detect increased precursor excretion during latent phases.

Screening of family members involves careful quantitative analyses of fecal and urinary precursors. Determination of levels of the enzymes suspected to be involved (usually in red blood cells) is also very useful, especially in prepubescent family members, whose symptoms may not yet be manifest. Laboratories equipped to perform thin-layer or high-pressure liquid chromatography can perform the diagnostic tests relatively quickly. However, such testing is not routinely available, and individual hospitals may have to send specimens to reference laboratories. Under these circumstances, results may not be available for several days, and delay of an emergent or semiemergent case is not justified. Provocative drugs should be avoided and the patient advised to undergo appropriate screening postoperatively.

Preanesthetic Care

Latent Phase

Preoperative evaluation should include a careful neurologic examination and documentation of the patient's status. Since the clinical situation can change rapidly, a repeat neurologic check should be completed immediately prior to administration of anesthesia.[5]

Respiratory capacity should be assessed by history, physical examination, and pulmonary function tests, when appropriate. Blood pressure, orthostatic changes, and pulse must be evaluated. Intravascular volume status and electrolytes (especially sodium and potassium) should be measured and corrected as necessary. Invasive monitors of volume status can be used as dictated by the patient's clinical condition and the proposed surgery. Glucose should be infused when the patient is fasted, since starvation can precipitate an acute attack. These supportive measures are especially important because an acute porphyric attack occurring under anesthesia is extremely difficult to diagnose.

Crisis

Treatment for the patient in crisis who presents for surgery includes both general supportive and more specific therapy. Correction of fluid and electrolyte disturbances is a primary concern prior to anesthesia. Ventilation must be supported if neurologic involvement includes respiratory embarrassment. Pain can be managed with opioids such as morphine; chlorpromazine has proven to be very effective for analgesia. Severe hypertension and tachycardia can be treated with titrated doses of propranolol.

More specific measures include intravenous glucose administration 10–20gm/hour for 24–48 hours to suppress ALA-S induction. Further therapy requires intravenous hematin, the purified heme fraction isolated from lysed red blood cells. Acutely increasing plasma (and presumably intracellular) levels of heme theoretically would suppress ALA-S induction.[11] Four mg/kg hematin is dissolved in 50ml 0.1M sodium bicarbonate at pH 8 and given over 10–15 minutes every 12 hours. Clinical remission usually occurs within 48 hours. Hospital pharmacies generally require 24 hours to obtain hematin.[12]

Anesthetic Plan

The inducible porphyrias are unpredictable diseases. Data regarding caveats involving anesthesia are conflicting. Some general guidelines, however, can be suggested.

Ultrashort-acting barbiturates should be avoided in all known or suspected porphyria patients. Evidence indicates that barbiturates may not induce symptoms if administered to a patient in remission, but are likely to aggravate symptoms if administered in crisis.[13] Prudence, however, suggests complete avoidance.

Although local anesthetic drugs do not induce crisis, the variable nature of neurologic involvement probably precludes regional anesthesia and major conduction block for medicolegal reasons. Inhalation agents have proven to be safe. Intravenous anesthesia, including opioids and muscle relaxants, is an alternative satisfactory technique. There are conflicting data between clinical and laboratory studies regarding the use of ketamine. The bulk of evidence indicates that ketamine may be safely used.[14,15]

Awake intubation in the well-prepared, topically anesthetized patient eliminates the need for an intravenous induction agent. Inhalation induction is an alternative.

Special care of the skin must be taken in patients with VP or HC. Blood pressure cuffs and tourniquets should be padded. Antibiotic ointment should be applied to all puncture sites. When a mask induction is used, undue pressure on the face should be avoided.

Acute porphyric crisis is part of the differential diagnosis of any patient with prolonged paralysis or coma, residual peripheral neurologic lesion, and/or severe abdominal pain following anesthesia. Follow-up for two to four weeks postoperatively is suggested, as acute attacks may be delayed after a triggering agent has been administered.

References

1. Orkin F.K.: Exacerbation of inducible porphyria, in Orkin F.K., Cooperman L.H. (eds): *Complications of Anesthesiology*. Philadelphia, JB Lippincott, 1982, pp 505–22.
2. Schmit R.: Porphyria, in Beeson P.B., McDermott W., Wynegaarden J.G. (eds): *A Textbook of Medicine*. Philadelphia, WB Saunders, 1979, pp 2044–9.
3. Samuels M.A., Shahani B.T.: Clinicopathological conference cases 39-1984. *N Engl J Med* 311:839, 1984.
4. Jacob F., Monod J.: Genetic regulatory mechanisms in the synthesis of proteins. *J Mol Biol* 3:318, 1961.
5. Katz J.: Hereditary hepatic porphyrias, in Katz J., Kadis L. (eds): *Anesthesia and Unusual Disease*. Philadelphia, WB Saunders, 1981, pp 23–31.
6. Ward R.J.: Porphyria and its relation to anesthesia. *Anesthesiology* 26:212, 1965.

7. Waldenstrom J.: The porphyrias as inborn errors of metabolism. *Am J Med* 22:758, 1957.
8. Dean G.: *The Porphyrias*. Philadelphia, JB Lippincott, 1963, p 10.
9. Elder G.H.: The porphyrias, in Conn H.F., Conn R.B. (eds): *Current Diagnosis*, ed 5. Philadelphia, WB Saunders, 1977, pp 713–23.
10. Vavra J.D., Avioli L.V.: Intermittent acute porphyrias. *Arch Intern Med* 142: 152, 1982.
11. Watson C.J., Pierach A., Bossenmaier I., et al: Use of hematin in the acute attack of the "inducible" hepatic porphyrias. *Adv Intern Med* 23:265, 1978.
12. Tishler P.V.: The porphyrias, in Conn H.F. (ed): *Current Therapy*. Philadelphia, WB Saunders, 1982, p 329.
13. Mustajoki P., Heinonen J.: Ceneral anesthesia in "inducible" porphyrias. *Anesthesiology* 53:15, 1980.
14. Rizk S.F., Jacobsen J.H., Silvay G: Ketamine as an induction agent for acute intermittent porphyria. *Anesthesiology* 46:305, 1977.
15. Kostrzewska E., Gregor A.: Ketamine in AIP—dangerous or safe? *Anesthesiology* 49:376, 1978.

CHAPTER 20

The Patient with Snakebite*

Robert Hirsh

Introduction

From antiquity, the snake has filled man with a special mix of fascination and loathing. As "The Beguiler of Eve," the Serpent plays a pivotal role in Genesis as antagonist to the Creator, luring "man to disobedience by the promise of increased conscious knowledge."[1] Apart from the Judeo-Christian tradition, the serpent is a recurring figure in the mythology of other peoples, "always as a central symbol for the life of the universe, and the continuity of creation."[2] For instance, a snake is wound around the Staff of Aesculapius as a magical symbol of the healing power of medicine. To the ancients, the power of the snake to wreak pathophysiologic mischief and morbidity to death, completely out of proportion to the size of the wound it inflicted (compared for example to that of a sabertoothed tiger), was magical.

Incidence

Snakebite is a significant world health problem: An estimated 300,000 episodes result in about 30,000 deaths annually. Approximately 45,000 snakebites are recorded each year in the United States. Of this number, some 8000 are caused by venomous snakes, which result in 10–15 deaths.[3] Over 85% of bites by venomous snakes result in symptomatic poisoning.[4]

Herpetology

Taxonomically, there are five families of venomous snakes, only two of which are indigenous to the United States.

---

*Reviewed by Dr. Warren Wetzel, Assistant Professor of Surgery, Albert Einstein College of Medicine of Yeshiva University, Bronx, New York.

Family Elapidae

The best-known example of Elapidae is the cobra but the only members of this family native to the U.S. are the coral snakes. The bites of Elapidae are generally neurotoxic. Elapidae are characterized by short, fixed, front fangs and are believed to account for much of the worldwide snakebite mortality. The cobra (*Naja naja*) is particularly feared in India. One subspecies, known as the spitting cobra, can actually project its venom, usually at the victim's eyes, with considerable accuracy over short distances.

The Western and Eastern coral snakes, native to the U.S., are found along the Gulf Coast in southern Florida, and in the southwestern United States. They are characterized by beautiful colored bands of alternating red, yellow (or white), and black encircling the snake from head to tail.

Family Hydrophidea

Hydrophidae, or sea snakes (eg, banded krait), have fangs similar to Elapidae and are adapted to their aquatic environment by virtue of a flattened tail for swimming. The venom is predominantly myotoxic. Sea snakes are indigenous to Asian and Western Pacific coastal areas, and fishermen of these seas are most often bitten.

Family Crotalidea

The pit vipers, or Crotalidae (from the Greek "krotalus," meaning rattle), are common in the American West and account for 95% of all snakebite injuries in the U.S.[5] See Figure 1. Pit vipers, such as the Western diamondback rattlesnake, can retract their front fangs to the roof of their mouths and have a pair of infrared heat-sensitive pits lateral to each nostril to locate warm-blooded prey. The venom is cytotoxic. The rattlesnake (*Crotalus*) typically assumes an S-shaped posture before striking which it can accomplish almost instantaneously. Having stunned its prey with a penetrating venomous bite, it opens its unhinged mandible much wider than itself and, moving its retractable fangs one after the other in a walking fashion, forces its prey inside. Humans are typically bitten on the extremities. Twenty to thirty percent of these bites are "dry," in the sense that no envenomation occurs. For elapid bites, 40–50% are dry.[3]

Other Families

The other two families of snakes include the Viperidae, or Old World vipers (eg, Cleopatra's asp), and the Colubridae. This last group, represented by the boomslang, are tree-climbing snakes with fixed rear fangs and are indigenous to Africa. (There is not a single specimen of boomslang in the Bronx Zoo).

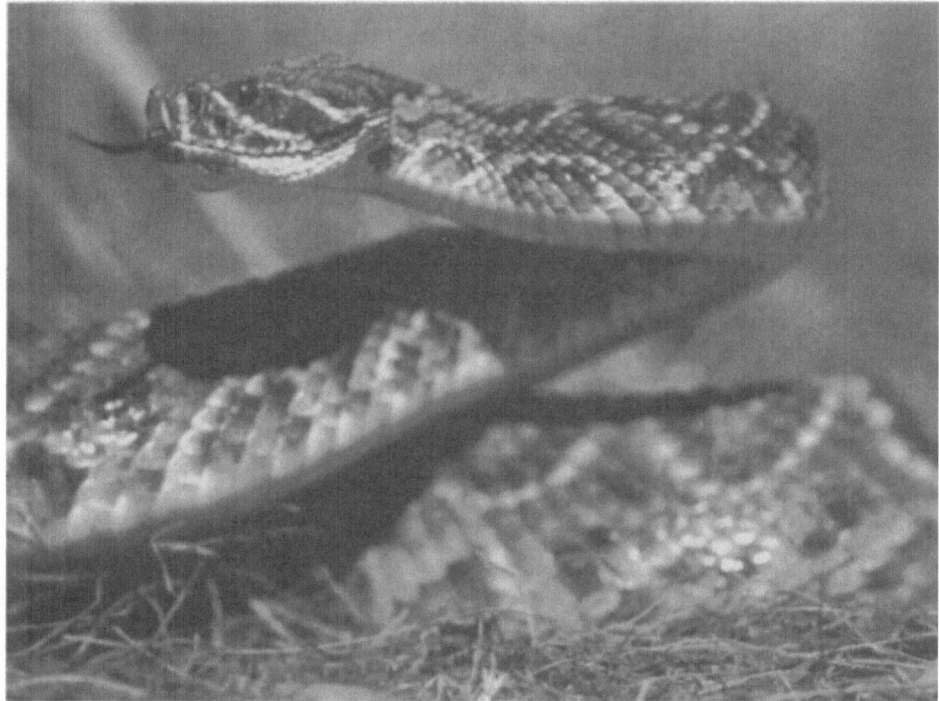

FIGURE 1. Eastern diamondback rattlesnake.

The Venom

By evolution, the snake's venom gland is a modified digestive gland. Thus, snake venom is a complicated mixture of proteins and hydrolytic enzymes. Included are a fibrinogenase, prothrombinase, hyaluronidase, collagenase, proteinases, as well as less-clearly characterized neurotoxins, cardiotoxins, hemorrhagin, anticoagulants, and cytotoxins.[6] As the venom is pH- and temperature-activated,[7] first aid including application of ice packs is advocated by some. However, immersion of the envenomed extremity in ice water over many hours may result in frostbite, gangrene, and loss of limb. Application of a constricting band, tight enough to block lymphatic channels through which the poison is spread systemically but not tight enough to block deep venous return, has been proven effective in decreasing morbidity.[6] Ethyl alcohol is a vasodilator that serves to hasten the uptake of venom and is definitely contraindicated (unless by Hollywood license).

Apart from local necrosis, the venom acts hematologically, causing red cell lysis, thrombocytopenia, fibrinogenolysis, and capillary fragility. The hemorrhagin component of venom causes spontaneous oozing of blood (rhexis) from capillaries. This action does not depend upon the depletion of serum fibrinogen, since complete defibrinogenation can persist for days without spontaneous bleeding. The fibrinogenase acts to split fibrinopeptide-A from fibrinogen, resulting in hypofibrinogenemia. This enzyme activity is not inhibited by heparin.[8]

In small mammals, such as rodents, the unnatural species of fibrin that is produced overwhelms the natural fibrinolytic enzymes, causing the blood to coagulate within seconds. From the snake's point of view, this causes the blood of its small mammalian prey to curdle and the fluid to exit the vascular space, resulting in rapid death. Where the snake to mammalian-mass ratio is lower, the process is prolonged. In humans, the fibrinolytic capacity is not overwhelmed, and because much of the fibinogen is consumed, the blood is noncoagulable.

Three cases of snake bite are presented, the first two of which illustrate the most common clinical situations that may be encountered by the anesthesiologist.

Case One: Systemic Pit Viper Envenomation

A 15-year-old boy was bitten by a rattlesnake in the left calf and was seen by the referring physician approximately 45 minutes following the accident. Initial treatment consisted of 5 vials of Antivenin (Crotalidae) Polyvalent (Wyeth Laboratories, Philadelphia), intravenous corticosteroids, tetanus toxoid, and excision of hemorrhagic tissue around the bitten area. He was referred to a tertiary center approximately three hours following the accident because of facial swelling, hematemesis, and hematuria.

Upon examination, the patient was dyspneic and had marked angioneurotic edema involving the face and neck. There was minimal swelling of the left calf. Bleeding from the upper gastrointestinal tract was confirmed by aspiration of blood through a nasogastric tube. Laboratory studies revealed less than 10mg% serum fibrinogen, a prolonged prothrombin time, and a platelet count of 80,000/mm³. Arterial blood gas analyses showed PaO_2 60mmHg, $PaCO_2$ 52mmHg, and pH 7.32.

The anesthesiologist was consulted regarding airway and fluid management. Blind awake nasotracheal intubation was achieved after application of local anesthetic and vasoconstricting (cocaine) solutions. Muscle relaxants were avoided. After administration of four units of fresh blood obtained from family members, the serum fibrinogen level rose to 145mg%. The clinical status of the patient continued to improve over the next two to three days. The swelling around the face resolved after 48 hours and his trachea was extubated. He was scheduled for closure of the now necrotic calf wound by partial thickness graft.

Discussion

The severity of a snakebite depends upon a number of factors, including the size of the victim and the amount of venom that is injected. Because humans are relatively large prey for a snake, systemic envenomation can result in a comparatively prolonged reaction. The enzymes in the venom, acting over a period of time, react with fibrinogen to produce a species of fibrin that is more easily lysed by the natural fibrinolytic pathways. In this pathologic state, the fibrinolytic pathways can lyse clots as quickly as they are formed. This results in low serum fibrinogen, a low platelet count, and noncoagulable blood. Increased clotting time is a reliable bedside test of systemic envenomation[8] which typically presents with vomiting, headache, diarrhea, and cardiovascular collapse. Intravascular hemolysis may lead to hematemesis and hematuria (as in this case) and oliguric renal failure. Increased capillary permeability, especially pulmonary capillary permeability, causes pulmonary edema and hypoxia leading to dyspnea. Death may result in hours to days from intracerebral hemorrhage, intestinal infarction, or renal or pulmonary failure.[9] Hemorrhagic complications may be delayed for up to one week.

In the event that symptoms develop rapidly, the accident must be considered serious, and the prognosis is bad. This is always grave when the patient is small or young, when the amount of venom injected is large, or when the snake fang pierces a vein and venom directly enters the circulation.

Therapy

The patient was given polyvalent crotalid antivenin. Antivenin is a concentrated preparation of serum globulin derived from horses immunized with venom from four different rattlesnake species. It is supplied as a lyophilized powder with 10ml of diluent. Because many patients have been exposed to horse serum protein from tetanus toxoid, anaphylaxis is a serious risk. Skin testing with 0.03–0.1ml of a 1:10 dilution of reconstituted antivenin is routine prior to intravenous administration. Should a wheal or flare develop, epinephrine or diphenhydramine should be administered prior to injection of the full dose. Serum sickness is delayed for 7–21 days and is characterized by fever, malaise, urticaria, and arthralgia.

Antivenin should only be given if there is clear evidence of systemic envenomation. Dosage depends on the severity of symptoms: mild, 20–40ml; moderate, 50–100ml; severe, 100–150ml. Administration should be within four hours of the bite to be effective; it is of questionable value after 12 hours. Thus, although time is important, there is usually no cause for panic.

Considerable controversy has arisen over the use of antivenin. A case report in 1983 by Buntain[10] described a 3½-year-old girl given 750ml (75 vials) of polyvalent antivenin over 14 hours for treatment of an Eastern diamondback rattlesnake bite. The author concluded, "The successful therapeutic result reinforces the credibility of antivenin neutralization as the primary mode of therapy in venomous snake bite." Lindsey,[11] however, has noted there are no controlled studies that demonstrate that antivenin, in the range of doses presently used, has any therapeutic effect.

Lindsey has also argued that commercially available antivenin is "woefully weak in potency." Crotalid antivenin is standardized by mixing it with a measured amount of venom and injecting the mixture into the tail vein of a population of 18-gram mice. One vial of antivenin will protect 540, 18-gram mice from death, a total weight of less than 10kg. By comparison, a usual 1500-unit dose of tetanus antitoxin, which is also manufactured from horse serum, will protect 1.5 million 350-gram guinea pigs, weighing a total of 525 metric tons.

Steroids have been administered after snakebite to decrease swelling. Again, therapeutic effectiveness has not been established. Similarly, tetanus toxoid is administered more as reassurance against infection developing from the puncture wound than for any specific therapeutic effect. Antibiotics are also administered prophylactically.

Case Two: Local Pit Viper Envenomation

A 14-year-old boy was bitten by a pygmy rattlesnake on the proximal phalanx of the right thumb. He was brought to the emergency room three hours later, where it was noted that his hand was extremely swollen, especially in the thenar compartment. Although the radial artery pulse was palpable and the circulation to the fingers seemed adequate, the thumb was cyanotic with no capillary filling of the nailbed. Motion was painful and limited by the extent of edema. The forearm was also tense and the patient complained of parasthesias in the thumb and median nerve distribution.

Intracompartmental pressures were measured in the thenar, volar, and dorsal forearm compartments by the Whiteside technique. The thenar compartment pressure was 60mmHg; the volar and dorsal compartment pressures were both 30mmHg. The patient received 7 vials of antivenin and intravenous fluid support. No steroid therapy, cryotherapy, or local wound suction were employed. He was scheduled for fasciotomies of the thenar and volar forearm compartments as well as carpal tunnel release.

Discussion

Short of systemic envenomation, local manifestations of rattlesnake bite may be sufficiently severe to require the services of an anesthesiologist.

After envenomation of an extremity, the venom hydrolyzes small blood vessels, lymphatics, and muscle tissue. Intracompartmental hemorrhage occurs, and cell debris raises the interstitial osmotic pressure, causing further loss of intravascular fluid into the wound.[9] The limb appears dusky, ecchymotic, and edematous. It is extremely tender. Dysesthesias, as well as spotty areas of anesthesia, occur with diminished motor function. The clinical picture is almost identical to that of compartment syndrome.

The rationale for performing fasciotomy is to prevent the fascial compartment pressures from becoming sufficiently high for the time required to cause a compartment syndrome, the consequences of which may be ischemic necrosis and Volkmann's contracture. The critical compartment pressure that must be exceeded for this to occur is 30mmHg.[6] Normal resting (supine) intracompartmental pressure for the forearm and leg is 4mmHg.[12]

Intracompartmental pressure is measured with a wick catheter, which is similar to the Whiteside technique. An epidural catheter containing a braided "wick" is placed into the fascial compartment through a needle. The fibrils that protrude from the tip prevent tissue blockage of the catheter, allow free exchange of fluid between the interstitium and the fluid-filled catheter, and carry the pressure signal which is electronically transduced.

Controversy has arisen over the efficacy of fasciotomy. A study by Garfin et al[13] using the wick catheter measured the pressure in the anterolateral compartment of dog hindlimbs after 3mg desiccated crotalid venom was injected at various depths. With direct muscular envenomation, the mean pressure in 10 limbs was 83.75 ± 9.98mmHg. If the venom was injected into limbs that had previously undergone fasciectomy and skin closure, the mean pressure was 19.60 ± 1.75mmHg. This demonstrated that fasciectomy prevented a compartment syndrome; however, histologically, no difference could be seen between the treated and untreated limbs.

The authors maintained that the clinical picture of crotalid limb envenomation is explained by the tissue-destroying action of the enzymes contained in the venom rather than by the mechanism of compartment syndrome, and therefore muscle destruction was not prevented by fasciotomy.

Later studies have suggested that whereas routine fasciotomy is not indicated, patients in whom intracompartmental pressures are higher than 30mmHg are deserving of such therapy.

Anesthetic Care

Anesthetic management begins with evaluation of the patient's coagulation system. Typed and crossmatched blood should be available. Complete blood count, platelet count, prothrombin time, partial thromboplastin time, fibrinogen level, fibrin split products, SMA-6 and calcium levels should be obtained. The patient may already have received 4–5 vials of antivenin over 30 to 60 minutes. The anesthesiologist should be alert to signs of allergic reaction.

Whole blood and blood component therapy is directed to controlling the bleeding diathesis; fresh whole blood or commercial fibrinogen is preferable.[9] The coagulation profile should be checked intraoperatively, as venom may continue to be absorbed systemically.

Adequate volume replacement is essential. Invasive monitoring may be indicated for appropriate fluid therapy, especially if renal or cardiac failure is suspected or if pulmonary edema has developed.

Respiratory assessment may indicate the need for immediate intubation and may warn against early postoperative extubation. Cautious extubation is warranted especially if only a few hours have elapsed since the injury. It is important to remember that the severity of response to snakebite is unpredictable, and all victims should be observed carefully in an intensive care setting for at least 24 hours.

Regional anesthesia is contraindicated because of the unpredictability of the development of bleeding diathesis. There is no particular advantage to an opioid anesthetic over an inhalational technique. However, these patients are often in severe pain from the injury and may require large doses of opioids pre- and postoperatively. Thus, continued administration of opioids during surgery may be warranted.

Depolarizing muscle relaxants should be avoided or used with caution, since synergism with any neurotoxic fraction of the venom may occur. Although neurotoxicity is rare with crotalid envenomation, the venom of at least one species, the Mojave rattlesnake, has been shown to produce this effect. Extubation should be delayed if there are any neuromuscular symptoms, such as ptosis or drooling.

Case Three: Elapid Envenomation

A 10-year-old child was aamitted to the emergency room with marked cyanosis and no respiratory activity. Ventilation was assisted manually. Immediate endotracheal intubation was performed, and oxygen-enriched air was administered with the help of an AMBU resuscitator. Within a few minutes, the child's color improved. However, respiration remained inadequate, and continued ventilatory support was required.

The child, who had been in good health, was bitten on the dorsum of the left foot by a pet snake 3–4 hours earlier. His father immediately applied a tourniquet and made an incision on the dorsum of the foot. The child was then taken to a local hospital where he was given tetanus toxoid and antibiotics and transferred to a tertiary care center some 30 miles away.

On clinical examination, the heart rate was 160beats/min. The pupils were dilated and reacted sluggishly to light, and the patient was in a state of cardiovascular collapse. Dextrose in saline, hydrocortisone acetate, mephentermine, and sodium bicarbonate were administered intravenously. Type specific anti-snake venom was given intravenously. However, there was no improvement in the child's respiration, and assisted ventilation was continued with an AMBU bag.

Respiratory failure associated with neurotoxin was considered, and it was thought that neostigmine might be effective. Initially, neostigmine 0.5mg diluted to 5ml with distilled water was given slowly intravenously. After a few minutes, the heart rate was 120beats/min and there was respiratory improvement. The dose was repeated 10 minutes later and again after 20 minutes. The heart rate decreased to 90beats/min and respiratory effort was adequate. The endotracheal tube remained in position for a further period of two hours. Over the next two days, ventilation was maintained spontaneously, but cellulitis and sloughing of the dorsum of the foot necessitated excision and grafting.

Discussion

Elapid envenomation, due to cobra bite, presents a different clinical picture from rattlesnake bite. Local effects are more moderate and usually consist of swelling, pain and ecchymosis, with blisters containing dark-brown fluid. After several days, skin necrosis with sloughing and pyogenic infections occur.[14] The venom contains among its constituents an ophioxidase, which promotes autolysis and putrefaction. Like crotalid venom, it contains proteases and hyaluronidase, which facilitate the spread of toxin.[15]

Cobra venom forms fine needle-like crystals on drying. It contains three active ingredients: a hemolysin, a cardiotoxin, and a neurotoxin. The hemolysin is similar to that of crotalid venom, and when given separately, causes red cell lysis, hemorrhage, and acute hemolytic anemia, though this is not part of the usual clinical picture of systemic cobra envenomation. The cardiotoxin is poorly characterized. Rarely, patients present with cardiovascular collapse with myocardial depression and asystole.[16]

By far, the most common effect of cobra envenomation is neurotoxicity. The effect is similar to nondepolarizing neuromuscular blockade. Onset is relatively slow and lasts many hours. Death is usually caused by respiratory arrest.

Systemic envenomation usually begins with drowsiness and ptosis, with frothy saliva and slurred speech, progressing to generalized skeletal, and finally, respiratory, muscle weakness.[14] Apnea can occur as soon as 1.5 hours after a bite.

Therapy

Questions have arisen regarding the relative value of cobra antivenom versus anticholinesterases in reversing apnea and dyspnea. In vitro, anticholinesterases do not antagonize neuromuscular blockade.[14] That this effect sometimes occurs in vivo suggests that the neuromuscular blockade, which is caused by binding of neurotoxin to the acetylcholine receptor, is only partial. The function of unoccupied receptors can be augmented by anticholinesterases.

A pediatric study showed that children apneic after cobra bites who received an average of 189ml type specific cobra antivenom required 13 hours for resolution of neurologic symptoms.[14] Patients with dyspnea required only 127ml antivenom and recovered in 9 hours. The periods of 13 and 9 hours may have sufficed for the synthesis of new neuromuscular end-plate acetylcholine receptor molecules. Again, the efficacy of antivenom has not been established.

Edrophonium chloride was given to two patients who received large doses of antivenom, and whose dyspnea had already resolved, but whose ptosis had persisted. The ptosis dramatically disappeared after edrophonium was administered.[14] Current therapy suggests the use of both anticholinesterase agents and antivenom.

Anesthetic Plan

Because of the neurotoxic complications of elapid bites, regional anesthesia is probably best avoided. Intubation is usually indicated early in treatment. Extubation should be delayed until spontaneous ventilation is adequate. Neuromuscular blocking agents should be avoided.

References

1. Thomas L.: *The Lives of a Cell*. New York, Bantam Books, 1974, p 144.
2. Jung C.G.: *Memories, Dreams, Reflections*. New York, Vintage Books, 1955, p 327.
3. Kunkel, D.B., Curry S.C.: Reptile envenomations. *J Toxicol Clin Toxicol* 21:505, 1983.
4. Parrish H.: Incidence of treated snakebites, U.S.A. Public Health Rep 81: 269, 1966.
5. Podgorny G.: Snakebites in U.S. *Ann Emerg Med* 12 651, 1983.
6. Garfin S.R., Mubarak S.J.: Rattlesnake bites, current concepts. *clin Orthop* 140:51–57, 1979.
7. Henderson B.M., Edgardo B.J.: Snakebite in children. *J Pediatr Surg* 5: 730, 1973.
8. Reid H.A., Theakston R.D.G.: The management of snakebite. *Bull WHO* 61:885–95, 1983.
9. Glass T.G.: Early debridement in pit viper bites. *JAMA* 235:2513–6, 1976.
10. Buntain W.L.: Successful venomous snakebite neutralization with massive antivenin infusion in a child. *J Trauma* 23:1012, 1983.
11. Lindsey D.: Controversey in snake bite—time for a controlled appraisal. *J Trauma* 25:462, 1985.
12. Mubarak S.J., Hargens A.R.: The wick catheter for measurement of intramuscular pressure. *J Bone Joint Surg* 58A:1019, 1976.
13. Garfin S.R., Castilonia R.R., Murabak S.J.: Rattlesnake bites and surgical decompression: Results using a laboratory model. *Toxico* 22:177–82, 1984.
14. Mitrakul C., Dharmkrong-At A: Clinical features of neurotoxic snake bite, and response to antivenom in 47 children. *Am J Trop Med Hyg* 33:1258–9, 1984.
15. Naphade R.W., Shette R.N.: Use of neostigmine after snake bite. *Br J Anaesth* 49:1066, 1977.
16. Stueven H.: Cobra envenomation, an uncommon emergency. *Ann Emerg Med* 12:638, 1983.

CHAPTER 21

The Patient with Sleep Apnea*

Ingrid Hollinger

Case History. *An 8-year-old boy came to the emergency room complaining of coughing, shortness of breath, and stomachache for 2 days. He had a history of dyspnea, snoring, and restless sleep for several years and had been admitted elsewhere 1 year previously for evaluation. His mother was told that he had large tonsils and a large heart and that tonsillectomy was indicated. The child was known to be markedly overweight for at least 3 years and had behavioral and learning problems. He attended a special school for the learning disabled. There was no history of other medical or surgical problems.*

Physical examination revealed an obese (53kg, 132cm) youngster in marked respiratory distress with inspiratory stridor. Large tonsils were easily visualized. Auscultation of the chest revealed poor air entry, bilateral râles, and a loud S_2 murmur.

Chest x-ray taken in the emergency room indicated pulmonary edema. The electrocardiogram was interpreted as showing sinus tachycardia with right ventricular hypertrophy, and right axis deviation. Arterial blood gases on room air were pH 7.33, $PaCO_2$, 42mmHg, PaO_2, 56mmHg. Pulse was 130/min, respiratory rate, 36/min. Laboratory values included: Hct 44%, white blood cell count 40,000/mmm^3 with marked left shift, SGOT 46 units/ml, SGPT 94 units/ml, alkaline phosphatase 237U/L, lactic dehydrogenase 380U/ml.

The child was transferred to the intensive care unit with a diagnosis of obstructive sleep apnea, cor pulmonale, and acute cardiac decompensation due to airway obstruction secondary to upper airway infection. He was treated with I.V. antibiotics and IM morphine sulfate 8mg for sedation. Bilateral nasopharyngeal tubes were placed to relieve the upper airway obstruction. Oxygen 60% by mask and furosemide 1mg/kg were given to treat the pulmonary edema.

---

*Reviewed by Dr. Michael J. Thorpy, Director of the Sleep Wake Disorder Center, Montefiore Medical Center, and Associate Professor of Neurology, Albert Einstein College of Medicine of Yeshiva University, Bronx, New York.

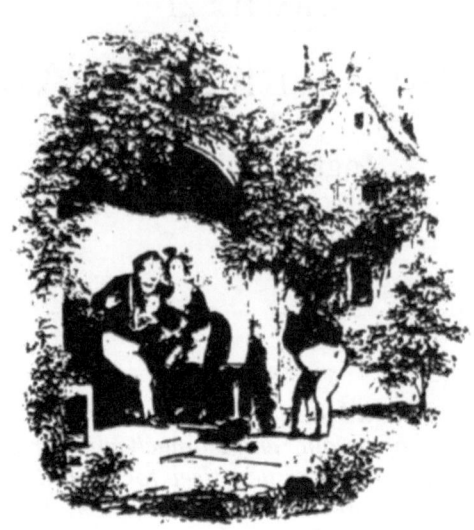

FIGURE 1. "The Fat Boy Awake." Drawing by Halbot Browne, "Phiz."

The child remained somnolent and partially obstructed. Twenty-four hours later, hypercarbia developed despite a vigorous stir-up regimen. His trachea was intubated. Thereafter arterial blood gas values normalized, and the child was able to sleep without evidence of hypoventilation. Occasional short periods of apnea (5 seconds or less) persisted. Chest x-ray was reported clear. Intubation was continued for 4 days.

Following extubation a polysomnogram was performed. It demonstrated obstructive and central sleep apnea. The child was scheduled for endoscopy of the nose, hypopharynx, and larynx; tonsillectomy; and adenoidectomy. All preoperative laboratory values were within normal limits.

Introduction

The combination of obesity and hypersomnolence in a young boy was first described in 1837 by Charles Dickens[1] in *The Posthumous Papers of the Pickwick Club.* See Figure 1. Nearly 50 years elapsed before further studies showed that these patients suffered periodic states of airway obstruction and suffocation during sleep.[2] Not until 1936 was the association of these clinical symptoms with significant cardiocirculatory problems, cor pulmonale, and congestive heart failure recognized.[3] Only recently has systematic research been undertaken to elucidate the underlying physiologic and anatomic features of this and other syndromes associated with apnea during sleep.

Apnea or an apneic period is defined as cessation of airflow for more than 10 seconds, and a sleep apnea syndrome is characterized by 30 or more such episodes during a 7-hour sleep period.[4] The incidence and prevalence of sleep apnea syndromes have not been well determined, but studies examining excessive daytime sleepiness have found an incidence of approximately 1% in the general adult population.[5] Sleep apnea occurs more commonly in males than in females, at a ratio of 2:1. Sleep apnea is also found more frequently in children less than 6 years of age, due to the lymphoid tissue hyperplasia common in this age group.

Excessive daytime sleepiness, although easily appreciated in adults and teenagers with sleep apnea, is often not recognized in small children. Principal clinical features in this group are restless sleep; sleep walking; enuresis; and abnormal, particularly aggressive, behavior patterns. Withdrawal and even bizarre behavior may be observed. Delayed language acquisition and poor school performance may be present. Small children may show failure to thrive, while older children tend to be obese. Children with obstructive sleep apnea frequently suffer recurrent otitis media.[6] The diagnosis is established objectively by polysomnography monitoring during sleep in a controlled environment. Physiologic parameters monitored during sleep include EEG, ECG, respiratory effort (by chest and/or abdominal strain gauges or esophageal pressure transducer), airflow at the nostrils, extraocular muscle movement, chin muscle tone, and arterial oxygen saturation.[7]

Normal sleep consists of cyclic alterations between rapid eye movement (REM) and non-REM sleep stages. Non-REM sleep is the predominant sleep pattern during the first half of night sleep after the first year of life. During non-REM sleep, heart and respiratory rates are slow and regular, and muscles are relaxed but muscle tone is preserved.

REM sleep, in contrast, is associated with profound physiologic changes. Muscle tone reaches its lowest level during REM sleep and is most pronounced in the neck muscles. Extraocular muscles, however, are not paralyzed and rapid conjugated eye movements together with muscle twitching occur. Phasic episodes of autonomic variability occur, including elevated and irregular heart rate, respiratory rate and blood pressure. Cerebral blood flow is increased, as is cerebral oxygen consumption. Temperature regulation is suspended.

Because of the profound muscle relaxation during REM sleep, airway obstruction tends to occur more readily, and since arousal thresholds are increased, severe levels of oxygen desaturation may develop before the patient awakens.

Sleep Apnea Syndromes

Sleep apnea syndromes are commonly classified into central sleep apnea, obstructive sleep apnea, and mixed apnea. Each of the three syndromes presents a different clinical picture, each has a characteristic polysomno-

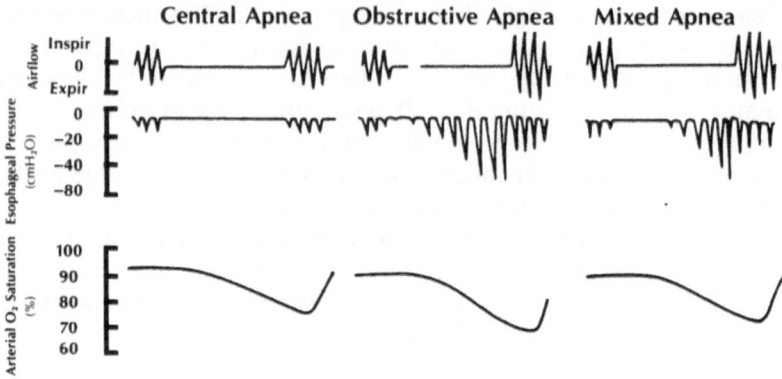

FIGURE 2. Schematic representation of polysomnograms of various types of sleep apnea.

gram, and effective treatment depends on the differential diagnosis. (See Figure 2.)

Central Sleep Apnea

Central sleep apnea is characterized by repeated apneic periods without respiratory effort, caused by a lack of neuronal output to the respiratory muscles. The underlying cause appears to be reduced or absent chemoreceptor sensitivity, particularly to carbon dioxide. Central sleep apnea is relatively uncommon and constitutes 10% or less of all sleep apneas. Patients usually have normal body habitus and complain of depression and insomnia rather than hypersomnolence. Periods of apnea tend to be brief causing little arterial desaturation.

Central sleep apnea is associated with various neurologic disorders, in particular familial dysautonomia, Shy-Drager syndrome and central alveolar hypoventilation (Ondine's curse), diabetic neuropathy, brain stem lesions, and encephalitis; it is also associated with bilateral cervical cordotomies and bilateral carotid body resection. Congestive heart failure and nasal obstruction due to various causes, including the common cold, may be associated with central apnea.[9, 10]

Obstructive Sleep Apnea

More than 85% of patients with sleep apnea have the obstructive type, and over two thirds of these patients are overweight.[11] The syndrome is more common in males and in the elderly.[11] Fatigue and daytime sleepiness are common complaints. Deterioration of memory and judgment with attacks of morning confusion occur. Patients snore loudly at night and exhibit periods of snorting or silence during an apneic episode. This is followed by gasping and choking as respiration resumes. Sleep is restless with frequent movements. Sleepwalking and, particularly in children, enuresis are common.[6, 12]

The immediate cause of obstructive sleep apnea is obstruction of the upper airway during sleep resulting in cessation of airflow despite continuing respiratory efforts. Asphyxia develops progressively, which leads to arousal from sleep and restoration of upper airway patency. The primary site of obstruction appears to be the pharynx. Normally, the pressure in the pharynx during inspiration is slightly below atmospheric pressure. Collapse of the airway is prevented by the activity of the dilator and abductor muscles of the upper airway, which generally results in an actual dilatation of the upper airway.

During REM sleep, muscle activity in the upper airway is reduced. In the patient with obstructive sleep apnea, negative airway pressure is generated with the onset of diaphragmatic contraction that leads to collapse of the hypotonic pharyngeal walls and, in a small pharyngeal cavity, causes complete airway obstruction. Continuing diaphragmatic activity increases negative airway pressure and increases the obstruction. Progressive asphyxia with hypoxemia and respiratory acidosis develop resulting in arousal from sleep which is accompanied by activation of the upper airway muscles. Stimulation by these muscles is greater than diaphragmatic activity resulting in dilatation of the upper airway and resumption of airflow.[13]

Patients are usually unaware of the sleep fragmentation that ensues. Frequent arousal results in reduction of deep non-REM sleep and some REM sleep. Persistent sleepiness causes the common clinical features of obstructive sleep apnea, ie, drowsiness and intellectual, personal, and behavioral deterioration.

Obstructive sleep apnea is associated with a variety of anatomic abnormalities of the upper airway, particularly in children. These include facial dysmorphism with micrognathia or retrognathia, and relative or absolute macroglossia. Obstructive sleep apnea is found in Pierre Robin and Treacher Collins syndromes, hemifacial microsomia, craniosynostosis (Apert's syndrome, Apert-Crouzon syndrome), metaphyseal dysplasia, and Down's syndrome (trisomy 21) and may occur following the repair of a cleft palate particularly after a pharyngeal flap reconstruction. Achondroplasia, Prader-Willi syndrome, and congenital myxedema in addition to various hemoglobinopathies are associated with obstructive sleep apnea. Several neuromuscular disorders may also present with obstructive sleep apnea. These include various forms of Arnold-Chiari malformation with or without Klippel-Feil syndrome, syringobulbia, cerebral palsy, and myotonic dystrophy,[9, 14–16]

The majority of children who present with signs of obstructive sleep apnea have adenotonsillar hypertrophy that results in narrowing of the airway and increased airway resistance. As the negative intraluminal pressure during inspiration increases, the velocity of airflow rises. The decrease in

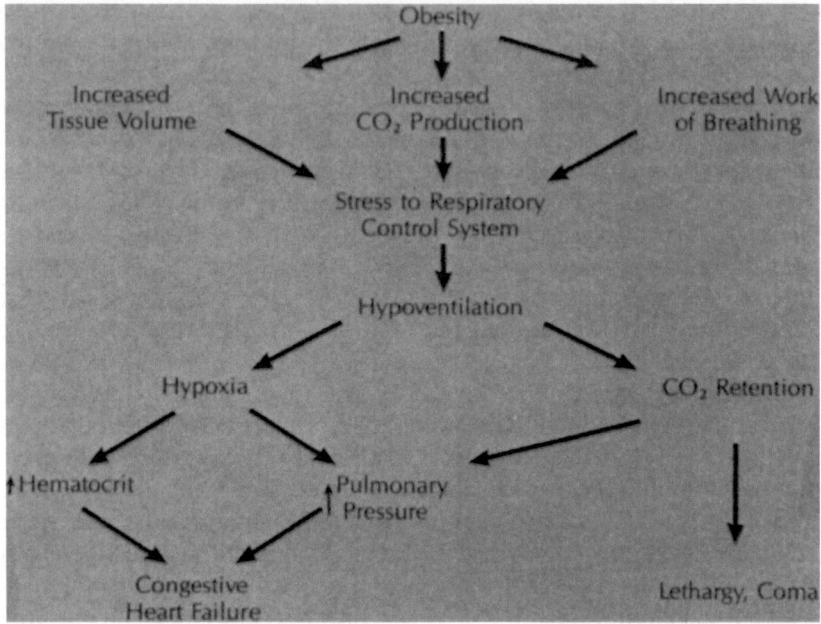

FIGURE 3. The schematic representation of the pathogenesis of pulmonary hypertension in the Pickwickian syndrome.

muscle tone during sleep facilitates the development of pharyngeal wall collapse and airway obstruction.[13]

The repeated episodes of nocturnal asphyxiation have several cardiovascular consequences. Arterial hypoxemia increases systemic and pulmonary arterial pressures. Negative intrathoracic pressure exerted against an upper airway obstruction increases left ventricular transmural pressure and left ventricular and left atrial volumes and pressures. The increase in left atrial pressure may precipitate pulmonary edema.

Although systemic blood pressure tends to normalize with resumption of ventilation, systemic hypertension may persist during wakefulness even in the absence of daytime hypoventilation. Patients with obstructive sleep apnea have a high incidence of systemic hypertension.

Pulmonary pressures, in contrast, tend to remain elevated. Persistent pulmonary hypertension and cor pulmonale, however, usually develop only in the presence of either lung disease or persistent hypoventilation during the daytime as well as during sleep. The degree of pulmonary hypertension is proportional to the degree of arterial hypoxemia. See Figure 3. The amount of arterial desaturation is determined in part by preapnea oxygen saturation and lung volumes. If lung volumes are reduced, as in obesity, significant desaturation occurs more rapidly.

The cardiovascular aberrations of greatest clinical significance are the changes in heart rate and rhythm. All forms of sleep apnea causing arterial hypoxemia result in vagally mediated bradycardia. Sinus arrhythmia, with variability exceeding 30 beats/min, is present in nearly all patients. Severe sinus bradycardia (less than 30 beats/min) or sinus arrest with pauses in excess of 10 seconds may be present in more than 10% of patients. Arterial oxygen desaturation below 60% commonly results in second degree heart block and ventricular ectopy. Malignant ventricular arrhythmias (multifocal, bigeminy, ventricular tachycardia) are observed. Increased sympathetic neural activity may play an important role in generating these arrhythmias. Sudden death during sleep in patients with obstructive sleep apnea is probably due to fatal cardiac arrhythmias (ventricular fibrillation or complete heart block without ventricular escape).[11,17,18]

Mixed Sleep Apnea

Both central and obstructive sleep apnea may be observed, and this is termed mixed sleep apnea. Central apnea usually precedes an obstructive episode.

Dickens' fat boy Joe exhibited this syndrome. It is characterized by marked obesity, somnolence, periodic breathing, hypoventilation, hypercarbia, hypoxia, polycythemia, and cor pulmonale. The syndrome is rare and present in only about 5% of patients with sleep apnea. Degree of obesity, magnitude of hypoventilation, and severity of apnea do not necessarily correlate.

Obesity imposes an increased load on the respiratory muscles. Ventilation–perfusion relationships are abnormal, and lung volumes are diminished. Closing capacity increases, resulting in small airway closure and intrapulmonary shunting. Central blood volume is increased resulting in a decrease in lung compliance. Chest wall compliance is markedly diminished in obesity. Central control of ventilation is abnormal and, in conjunction with the increased work of breathing, leads to chronic hypercarbia and loss of hypoxic drive. Excess fat tissue leads to narrowing of the pharyngeal dimension and predisposes to the development of obstruction during sleep. Hypoxemia and sleep fragmentation result in somnolence. The abnormal control of ventilation results in more severe hypoxia before arousal and slowly increasing hypercarbia even during waking hours.[19]

Therapy

Therapy for central sleep apnea is difficult. Acetazolamide has been used successfully in some cases. Inspired low-flow oxygen during sleep has reduced the frequency of apnea in various studies. Severe cases of central sleep apnea require mechanical ventilation during sleep.[10]

Obstructive and mixed sleep apneas usually respond dramatically to therapy aimed at preventing upper airway closure during sleep. Positive nasal airway pressure via a mask or prongs acting as a pneumatic splint to hold the upper airway open may be sufficient.[20] Uvulopalatopharyngoplasty, which involves resection of the tonsils, uvula, non-muscular portion of the soft palate, and redundant pharyngeal mucosa, enlarges pharyngeal dimensions and is frequently curative. With skeletal abnormalities, mandibular osteotomy with or without maxillary advancement and hyoid suspension may be necessary to enlarge the upper airway and prevent obstruction. If obstruction cannot be relieved, tracheoplasty is performed which bypasses the obstruction during sleep and allows the patient to function normally during the day with the tracheoplasty occluded.[21]

Preanesthetic Evaluation

An assessment of the frequency and severity of apneic periods during sleep must be made. Patients may have a history of frequent upper respiratory infections and pneumonia, irregular heart beat, or even cardiac arrest. Family history may be significant for sudden infant death in a sibling or sleep apnea in another family member. The extent of psychomotor delay should be noted.

Physical Examination

Nutritional status should be assessed. Although the majority of adolescent and adult patients with obstructive sleep apnea are overweight, malnutrition may be present in infants and children with chronic upper airway obstruction. The physical stigmata of Down's syndrome or achondroplasia may be present. Presence of Arnold-Chiari deformity may be associated with hydrocephalus or laryngeal muscle paralysis.

Airway Assessment

The patency of the airway should be assessed, including patency of the nasal airways, the extent of tonsillar enlargement, and the presence of mouth breathing. Difficulties with intubation may be anticipated in patients with craniofacial anomalies. Use of topical anesthesia of the mouth and pharynx prior to induction will allow insertion of an oral airway that, together with positive pressure, will maintain airway patency.

Intravenous induction agents and muscle relaxants are relatively contraindicated in patients with anatomic airway abnormalities.

Cardiovascular Assessment

Sleep apnea patients have a high incidence of systemic hypertension. Heart beat may be irregular, and the heart sounds may indicate cor pulmonale.

The electrocardiogram may show evidence of right ventricular hypertrophy and pulmonary hypertension with right ventricular strain. Ventricular arrhythmias and various degrees of first and second degree heart block may also be present.

The bradycardia commonly observed during apneic episodes can be prevented or ameliorated by the prior administration of an anticholinergic agent. Generous atropinization prior to induction of anesthesia is therefore advisable. Blood pressure should be controlled medically prior to surgery. Also, any serious arrhythmias or congestive failure should be under control with medication.

Severe cases of sleep apnea may exhibit left ventricular hypertrophy and strain. Echocardiography will confirm the presence of right-sided hypertrophy and pulmonary hypertension and left ventricular dysfunction. The chest x-ray may show cardiomegaly and evidence of pulmonary congestion.

Laboratory Testing

The hematocrit may be elevated due to chronic hypoxemia with reactive polycythemia. This is, however, an unusual feature of pure obstructive sleep apnea. A metabolic alkalosis may be present with an elevated serum bicarbonate that compensates for respiratory acidosis. Intraoperative hyperventilation may result in prolonged postoperative apnea.

Anesthetic Management

Because of the unpredictability of the occurrence of prolonged apnea or the development of airway obstruction, no preoperative sedation or long-acting intravenous agents are used. Adult and adolescent patients with anticipated intubation problems should have their airways secured while awake under topical anesthesia, and pediatric patients may be intubated under deep halothane anesthesia with spontaneous ventilation. Otherwise, a short-acting barbiturate may be used and intubation facilitated with the use of a muscle relaxant. Topical anesthesia of the mouth prior to induction allows insertion of an oropharyngeal airway under light planes of anesthesia without triggering pharyngeal reflexes.

Patients with sleep apnea may be quite sensitive to all anesthetic agents, and they require very carefully titrated induction. Agents causing minimal cardiovascular depression with little arrhythmogenic propensity, such as low-dose isoflurane, are useful anesthetic choices.

Use of long-acting hypnotics and analgesics may result in prolonged apnea in the postoperative period even with relief of the obstructive component. Patients who exhibited preoperative hypoxemia may develop postoperative apnea in the presence of uncontrolled inspired oxygen concentrations since ventilatory control remains abnormal for many weeks. Ventilation should be controlled.

At the conclusion of the procedure the residual effect of any neuromuscular blocking agent should be reversed, and the patient completely awakened before removing the endotracheal tube. Nasopharyngeal airways inserted by the surgeon should be maintained for 24 hours following nasopharyngeal surgery in the absence of a tracheostomy. All patients require intensive monitoring for apnea for the first 48 hours postoperatively. Only if apnea or obstruction do not develop during observed sleep postoperatively may patients be transferred to the ward or discharged home after tonsillectomy. Monitoring during and after surgery should include, besides blood pressure and electrocardiogram, direct arterial blood gas measurements, and, if possible, continuous oxygen saturation monitoring. No patient with sleep apnea is a suitable candidate for outpatient or day care surgery.

References

1. Dickens C.: *The Posthumous Papers of the Pickwick Club*. London, Chapman and Hall, 1837.
2. Caton R.: A case of narcolepsy. *Br Med J* 358, 1880.
3. Kerr W.J., Lagen J.B.: The postural syndrome of obesity leading to postural emphysema and cardiorespiratory failure. *Ann intern Med* 10:569, 1936.
4. Guilleminault C., Lugaresi E.: *Sleep/Wake Disorders: Natural History, Epidemiology and Long Term Evolution*. New York, Raven Press, 1983.
5. Guilleminault C., Tilkian A., Dement W.C.: The sleep apnea syndromes. *Annu Rev Med* 27:465, 1976.
6. Mandel E.M., Reynolds C.F.: Sleep disorders associated with upper airway obstruction in children. *Med Clin North Am*. Philadelphia, W.B. Saunders, 1981; 28:897.
7. Orr W.C.: Utilization of polysomnography in the assessment of sleep disorders. *Med Clin North Am*. Philadelphia, W.B. Saunders, 1985· 69:1153.
8. Baker T.L.: Introduction to sleep and sleep disorders. *Med Clin North Am*. Philadelphia, W.B. Saunders, 1985; 69:1123.
9. Chung F., Crago R.R.: Sleep apnea syndrome and anesthesia. *Can Anaesth Soc J* 29:439, 1982.
10. White D.P.: Central sleep apnea. *Med Clin North Am*. Philadelphia, W.B. Saunders, 1985; 69:1205.
11. Guilleminault C.: Obstructive sleep apnea. The clinical syndrome and historical perspective. *Med Clin North Am*. Philadelphia, W.B. Saunders, 1985; 69:1187.
12. Brouillette R.T., Fernback S.K., Hunt C.E.: Obstructive sleep apnea in infants and children. *J Pediatr* 100:31, 1982.
13. Bradley T.D., Phillipson E.A.: Pathogenesis and pathophysiology of the obstructive sleep apnea syndrome. *Med Clin North Am*. Philadelphia, W.B. Saunders, 1985; 69:1169.
14. Kuna S.T., Remmers J.E.: Neural and anatomic factors related to upper airway occlusion during sleep. *Med Clin North Am*. Philadelphia, W.B. Saunders, 1985; 69:1221.

15. Schaefer M.: Upper airway obstruction and sleep disorders in children with craniofacial anomalies. *Clin Plast Surg* 9:555, 1982.
16. Roa N.L., Moss K.S.: Treacher Collins' syndrome with sleep apnea, anesthetic considerations. *Anesthesiology* 60:71, 1984.
17. Shepard J.W.: Gas exchange and hemodynamics during sleep. *Med Clin North Am*. Philadelphia, W.B. Saunders, 1985; 69:1243.
18. Weinberg S., Kravath R., Phillips L., et al: Episodic complete airway obstruction in children with undiagnosed obstructive sleep apnea. *Anesthesiology* 60:356, 1984.
19. Wittels E.H.: Obesity and hormonal factors in sleep and sleep apnea. *Med Clin North Am*. Philadelphia, W.B. Saunders, 1985; 69:1265.
20. Lombard R.M., Zwillich C.N.: Medical therapy of obstructive sleep apnea. *Med Clin North Am*. Philadelphia, W.B. Saunders, 1985; 69:1317.
21. Thawley S.E.: Surgical treatment of obstructive sleep apnea. *Med Clin North Am*. Philadelphia, W.B. Saunders, 1985; 69:1337.

CHAPTER 22

The Patient with Mitral Valve Prolapse*

Lydia Alcantara

Case History. *A 23-year-old woman was admitted with signs and symptoms of acute cholecystitis. Her past medical problems included a history of dizziness and difficulty in breathing associated with exercise, which had occurred once or twice per year since childhood. Six months previously, she had been admitted to another hospital for investigation of weakness, weight loss, and substernal pain. She thought that the results of her tests indicated that she had a "floppy" valve in her heart that was "normal" and certainly not harmful.*

Physical examination showed a tall, thin female in no distress. Her fingers were noted to be particularly long. Cardiac auscultation revealed a midsystolic click. No murmur was appreciated.

Laboratory data were within normal limits except for slight elevation of liver function tests. ECG showed sinus tachycardia with an occasional premature ventricular contraction and slight prolongation of the QT interval. Vital signs were: pulse 132/min, blood pressure 160/80mmHg, respiration 32/min, temperature 39.6°C. Diagnosis of acute cholecystitis was confirmed by HIDA scan. Her referring physician was contacted and he reported that echocardiography had confirmed the diagnosis of mitral valve prolapse.

Incidence of Mitral Valve Prolapse

Mitral valve prolapse (MVP) has been reported in up to 10–15% of the U.S. population. It occurs predominately among women in the younger age groups but without sex discrimination in older ages.[1,2] Familial transmission is common (primary MVP). Secondary or acquired MVP is associated with coronary heart disease, cardiomyopathy, left ventricular aneurysm, atrial septal defect, or idiopathic hypertrophic subaortic stenosis.[3–5]

---

*Reviewed by Dr. Martin N. Cohen, Professor of Medicine, Albert Einstein College of Medicine of Yeshiva University, Bronx, New York.

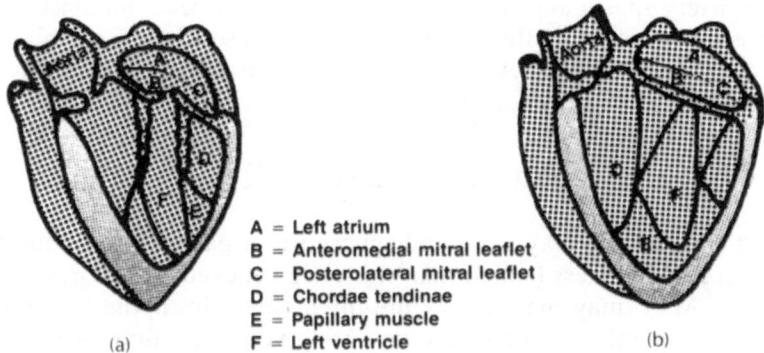

A = Left atrium
B = Anteromedial mitral leaflet
C = Posterolateral mitral leaflet
D = Chordae tendinae
E = Papillary muscle
F = Left ventricle

(a)   (b)

FIGURE 1. (a) Reduction of left ventricular volume increases the amount of prolapse of the mitral leaflets. (b) Increase in left ventricular volume decreases the degree of prolapse.

Pathophysiology

In mitral valve prolapse, the mitral valve is structurally abnormal with elongated chordae tendinae and redundant mitral leaflets. On histological examination, myxomatous degeneration is seen. Association with Marfan's syndrome (4%) and connective tissue disorders is well recognized.

The pathophysiology of MVP involves the prolapse of the redundant mitral leaflets into the left atrium during mid- to late systole as the ventricle empties. With reduction in ventricular volume, the degree of prolapse of the mitral leaflets is accentuated. See Figure 1a. Prolapse is also increased by factors that effectively reduce ventricular volume. Such a condition occurs during increased myocardial contractility, decreased afterload, decreased preload, and tachycardia. Factors that can contribute to MVP include various drugs, the Valsalva maneuver, or a stress response. Conversely, increased left ventricular volume, decreased contractility, increased peripheral resistance, and bradycardia reduce the degree of prolapse.[6] See Figure 1b.

Patients with MVP are often asymptomatic, or they may have vague complaints such as chest pain (30%), palpitations (50%), faintness, dyspnea, or decreased exercise tolerance.[7] Often patients are tall and thin with thoracic skeletal abnormalities such as scoliosis, pectus excavatum, or "straight back" deformity.

The mechanism that causes chest pain and arrhythmias in MVP is not known. A postulated cause is ischemia due to compression of the circumflex artery by the dilated posterior leaflet, but this obstruction has not been demonstrated.[8] An ischemic focus in the papillary muscle produced by billowing scallops of mitral valve leaflets may result in papillary muscle stress leading to dysrhythmias and pain.[9] Recently, an association between coronary artery spasm and mitral valve prolapse has been demonstrated, and it has been suggested that the spasm is the cause of the ischemia and its associated symptoms.[10] Another suggested cause of arrhythmia is increased sensitivity to catecholamines.

Preanesthetic Evaluation

Although this disease may exist undiagnosed in a patient presenting for elective surge y, it is less benign than was once believed. In the postsurgical patient, MVP may manifest as life-threatening dysrhythmias, mitral regurgitation, or infective endocarditis during hospitalization. A high index of suspicion based on the characteristically vague cardiac history and the patient's habitus should alert the anesthesiologist to careful evaluation and should prompt ordering of screening tests to establish or rule out the presence of MVP.

Cardiovascular Assessment

Cardiac assessment of the patient with suspected MVP is particularly important. A common auscultatory finding is a mid- to late systolic click due to the abrupt deceleration of blood contained within the undersurface of the prolapsing valve. Electrocardiographic changes may include T-wave inversion, flattening in leads II, III, and aVF, and prolonged QT- or ST-segment changes. Approximately 70% of patients show arrhythmias, including premature atrial or ventricular contractions.[11, 12]

Mitral regurgitation can occur if there is nonapposition of the mitral valve due to redundancy of the mitral leaflets. A late systolic or pansystolic murmur may be appreciated. Diagnosis is made by echocardiography, which shows "hammocking" of the posterior mitral leaflet into the left atrium. A midsystolic click is heard in approximately 50% of patients with echocardiographic evidence of MVP. A poor prognosis is associated with prolongation of the QT interval and a late systolic murmur.

Arrhythmias are a common complication of MVP. The most frequent arrhythmia is premature ventricular contractions. Atrial premature contractions, sinus bradycardia leading to sinus arrest, Wolff-Parkinson-White syndrome, A-V block, and right and left bundle branch blocks are also seen. Patients with MVP of congenital origin have an associated bradycardia.[13] Although the dysrhythmias are usually well tolerated, they may be symptomatic. Response to drug therapy is usually good, but sudden deaths due to ventricular fibrillation, profound bradycardia, acute rupture of chordae, or coronary spasm have been reported in 1.2–13% of cases.[14] Endocarditis is rare but has been reported.[15] Mitral regurgitation of either sudden or gradual onset leading to cardiac decompensation may also occur. Other coexisting cardiac problems, although extremely rare, may include aortic insufficiency, coarctation of the aorta, and tendency to dissecting aneurysm.

Pulmonary Assessment

Respiratory function in patients with mitral valve prolapse may be impaired due to pectus excavatum, kyphoscoliosis, emphysema, or pneumothorax. As dictated by the patient's physical examination, pulmonary function tests should be performed. The possibility of unstable joints and/or temporomandibular abnormalities should be evaluated as they may make intubation difficult.

Central Nervous System Assessment

Central nervous system symptoms related to MVP may include transient cerebral ischemic attacks or partial non-progressive strokes. These are related to emboli originating from the mitral valve when it is diseased by endocarditis or due to dysrhythmias associated with MVP.[16]

Documentation of any paresis or other neurologic symptoms should be made prior to any procedure but especially before performing a regional anesthetic technique.

Preanesthetic Medical Therapy

Propranolol may be used successfully for the treatment of pain and for dysrhythmias although treatment is empirical. The slower heart rate produced by propranolol increases the ventricular end-diastolic and systolic volumes and thus reduces the degree of prolapse and stretching of the mitral valve leaflets, which may decrease the ectopic input originating at these sites. Occasionally, drug resistance develops and cardiac pacing may be indicated. Surgical replacement of the valve is necessary if mitral regurgitation is severe. More than 10% of valve replacements for mitral regurgitation are performed for correction of redundant mitral leaflets.[17]

Patients with MVP are often taking many drugs, including corticosteroids for polyarteritis nodosa. Dosages should be maintained and even increased to compensate for the stress of surgery.

Once the diagnosis of mitral valve prolapse has been established, prophylactic antibiotic therapy should be initiated to decrease the risk of endocarditis, certainly in patients undergoing dental extractions or other procedures that are associated with bacteremia. Subacute bacterial endocarditis prophylaxis is probably not needed for patients with echocardiographic MVP but unthickened or unrolled leaflets without clicks or murmurs.

Anesthetic Plan

Based on the pathophysiology, our anesthetic goal for patients with MVP is directed toward decreasing myocardial contractility, providing volume loading, and avoiding decreases in systemic vascular resistance. Adequate premedication to avoid tachycardia associated with anxiety is essential. Drugs causing tachycardia or having an α-adrenergic blocking effect (droperidol) should be avoided. Hyoscine and glycopyrrolate are preferable to atropine because they cause less tachycardia. Scopolamine, because of its negative chronotropic effect, is preferable to atropine. Potentially dysrhythmic agents such as epinephrine are best avoided to prevent diagnostic confusion. Any antiarrhythmic agents the patient may be taking should be continued on the day of surgery. Prevention of hypovolemia, acidosis, hypoxemia, hypercarbia, hypokalemia, and overdose is also essential.

When selecting anesthetic agents, the pathophysiology of mitral valve prolapse should be kept in mind even though most patients have minimal hemodynamic consequences. Agents that reduce end-diastolic volume by decreasing both preload and afterload as well as agents that increase myocardial contractility or heart rate have been shown to exacerbate the degree of prolpase and the incidence of dysrhythmias and should be avoided.[14]

Blood volume should be maintained and an extreme head-up position avoided. In order to reduce the effects of positive intrathoracic pressure on cardiac output, the ventilatory pattern should be one of slow inspiratory flow.

Halothane causes myocardial depression and consequently decreases cardiac output; it also increases the diastolic filling time by both slowing the heart rate and increasing the end-diastolic volume. Halothane might thus seem a good anesthetic choice in patients with MVP; however, excessive end-diastolic pressure could predispose to subendocardial ischemia. The myocardium is usually healthy in patients with MVP, but if there is any evidence of potential decompensation, anesthetic agents with minimal myocardial depressant effect should be selected. Isoflurane causes little myocardial depression, but the tachycardia it causes may be hazardous for these patients.

Similarly ketamine, gallamine, atropine, and sympathomimetic drugs with predominant beta effect are known to cause tachycardia and are better avoided. Gallamine and pancuronium cause tachycardia by blocking vagal activity. In selecting a muscle relaxant, a neuromuscular blocking dose of atracurium, 0.3mg/kg, is a suitable choice. Light anesthesia should be avoided because of a potentially dysrhythmogenic effect.

Epidural and spinal anesthetic techniques are usually avoided because of possible increases in venous capacitance and lowered peripheral resistance that may accentuate the prolapse and regurgitation. However, the contraindications are relative, and regional techniques may be safely employed if they are performed slowly with adequate prehydration and maintenance of intravascular volume. Sensory blockade should be limited to T8. If vasopressor therapy is needed, an α-agonist such as phenylephrine or metaraminol is preferable.

For all patients, intraoperative monitoring of cardiac activity including rate and rhythm, blood pressure, temperature, and blood loss is mandatory. Continuous cardiac monitoring in the immediate postoperative period is advisable until cardiovascular stability and complete elimination of anesthetic effects are achieved.

References

1. Brown O.R., Kloster F.E., DeMots H.: Incidence of mitral valve prolapse in the asymptomatic normal. *Circulation* 52(suppl 2):77, 1975.
2. Markiewicz W., Stoner J., London E., et al: Mitral valve prolapse in one hundred presumably healthy young females. *Circulation* 53:464–73, 1976.
3. Scampardonis G., Yang S.S., Maranhao V., et al: Left ventricular abnormalities in prolapsed mitral leaflet syndrome. *Circulation* 48:287–97, 1973.
4. Aranda J.M., Befeler B., Lazzara R., et al Mitral valve prolapse and coronary artery disease. Clinical hemodynamic and angiographic correlations. *Circulation* 52:245–53, 1975.
5. Victoria B.E., Elliot L.P., Gessner I.H.: Ostium secundum atrial septal defect associated with balloon mitral valve children. *Am J of Cardiol* 3:668–73, 1974.
6. Nutter D.O., Wickliffe C., Gilbert C.A., et al The pathophysiology of idiopathic mitral valve prolapse. *Circulation* 52:297–305, 1975.
7. Fontana M.E., Pence H.L., Leighton R., et al The varying clinical spectrum of the systolic click-late systolic murmur syndrome. *Circulation* 41:807–16, 1970.
8. Barlow J.B., Bosman C.K.: Aneurysmal protrusion of the posterior leaflet of the mitral valve. *Am Heart J* 71:166–78, 1966.
9. Pocock W.A., Barlow J.B.: Etiology and electrocardiography features of the billowing posterior mitral leaflet syndrome. *Am Med* 51:731–9, 1971.
10. Buda A.J., Levene J.L., Myers M.G., et al: Coronary artery spasm and mitral valve prolapse. *Am Heart J* 96:457–62, 1978.
11. Jeresaty R.M.: Mitral valve prolapse—click syndrome. *Prog Cardiovasc Dis* 15:623–52, 1973.
12. Winkle R.A., Lopes M.G., Fitzgerald J.W., et al: Arrhythmias in patients with mitral valve prolapse. *Circulation* 52:73–81, 1975.
13. Koch F.H., Hancock E.W.: Ten-year follow up of forty patients with the mid-systolic click–late systolic murmur syndrome *Am J Cardiol* 37:149, 1976.
14. Thiagarajah S., Frost E.A.M.: Anesthetic considerations in patients with mitral valve prolapse. *Anaesthesia* 38:560–6, 1983.
15. Lachman A.S., Bramwell-Jones D.M., Lakie J.B., et al: Infective endocarditis in the billowing mitral leaflet syndrome. *Br Heart J* 37:326–30, 1975.
16. Barnett H.J.M., Jones M.W., Boughner Dr et al: Cerebral ischemic events associated with prolapsing mitral valve *Arch Neurol* 33:777–87, 1976.
17. McKay, Yacoub M.H. Clinical and pathological findings in patients with "floppy" valves treated surgically. *Circulation* 48 (suppl 3):63–73, 1973.

CHAPTER 23

The Elderly Patient with a Hip Fracture*

Jonathan Halevy

Case History. *A 83-year-old white female was brought to the hospital complaining of left hip pain after falling at home. She had been living alone, ambulating well prior to her admission, and was receiving daily assistance via the Meals on Wheels program in her neighborhood. Past history was significant for hypertension, which was controlled with a "water pill," and diabetes for which she took chlorpropamide every morning. Previous anesthetic experience included two D&Cs, and a right breast biopsy approximately 50 years ago. All procedures were without anesthetic sequelae. She smoked approximately half a pack of cigarettes per day for many years but had stopped 10 years before. Alcohol use was denied. Review of systems was negative for complaints of chest pain, shortness of breath, or syncope; however, she did report feeling weaker recently.*

Physical examination revealed a thin woman in moderate distress. Vital signs included: blood pressure 150/90mmHg, pulse 82/min, respiratory rate 18/min, temperature 37°C. Her neck had some restriction in movement but was supple and without carotid bruits or venous distention. Lung fields were clear to auscultation and percussion. Heart examination was normal.

Chest x-ray showed no acute infiltrates, but spondylitic changes were appreciated. Left hip films revealed a femoral neck fracture. Electrocardiogram showed occasional premature ventricular beats (2–3/min), rate 85/min, left axis deviation, and nonspecific ST-segment and T-wave changes.

Laboratory data base was: Hct 30%, Hb 10.2gm/dl, K+ 3.0mEq/L, glucose 294mg/dl. Urinalysis was unremarkable.

Introduction

The elderly comprise the most rapidly expanding segment of society. Perhaps because of this phenomenon, the age after which "elderly" is defined is increasing. The United States Census Bureau refers to those

---

*Reviewed by Dr. Patricia Underwood, Associate Professor of Anesthesiology, Albert Einstein College of Medicine of Yeshiva University, Bronx, New York.

persons over the age of 65 years as elderly. However, most data available delineate age groups that include a group greater than 65 years. In 1900, only 4% of the U.S. population was older than 65 years. In 1984 (the last year for which official statistics are available), 11.8% of the general population was over age 65. Improvements in health care and nutrition will support this trend; estimates for the year 2000 indicate that those older than 65 years will make up approximately 12.5% of the population.

In 1979, 18% of all operations in the U.S. were performed on patients over age 65, according to the Division of Health Care Statistics. Only four years later, those over age 65 underwent 25% of all surgical procedures.

Several institutions focus on an even more specialized group of elderly—those older than age 80. The statistics for this group are equally impressive. From 1970 to 1984, the number of persons in this group rose from 3.7 to 5.0% of the U.S. population. Approximately 20% of all operative cases performed in the Montefiore Medical Center operating rooms are in this "extra-elderly" subgroup. Fifty-eight percent of the total operating room caseload involves patients age 65 and older.

This elderly age group is not only expanding in itself, but new surgical technology, better diagnostic techniques, and anesthetic advances have made surgical procedures once considered too risky in this population routine.

Studies have indicated that perioperative morbidity and mortality are increased in the elderly.[1] One analysis of perioperative mortality showed that death within 7 days of anesthesia occurred in 1.5% of all surgical patients between 21 and 50 years of age, in 4.4% of those patients 61–70 years of age, in 6.8% of those 71–80 years of age, and in 8.2% of those patients over age 80.[2] The higher mortality seen in emergency cases compared to elective procedures was not related to age.

Both age and concomitant disease are important in predicting perioperative morbidity and mortality, and the two risk factors may be related. Systemic diseases are more common in the elderly. In one review of patients admitted to a special geriatric unit, the average number of diseases per patient was six.[3] Systemic hypertension was found in 40% of the patients. Mortality rose from 9.2% to 17–45% among patients over age 70 who also had cardiac or mental diseases.

The increased morbidity and mortality among the elderly are related to decreased organ function that can be appreciated as a two-stage process: First, a decrease in reserve ability occurs that manifests most frequently during times of stress. Ultimately, function at basal states is diminished to a critical level. See Figure 1.

Physiology of Aging

Metabolic and Endocrine Systems

The process of aging is a dynamic one. Physiologic systems progressively deteriorate. Between ages 30 and 40, the decline in organ function begins

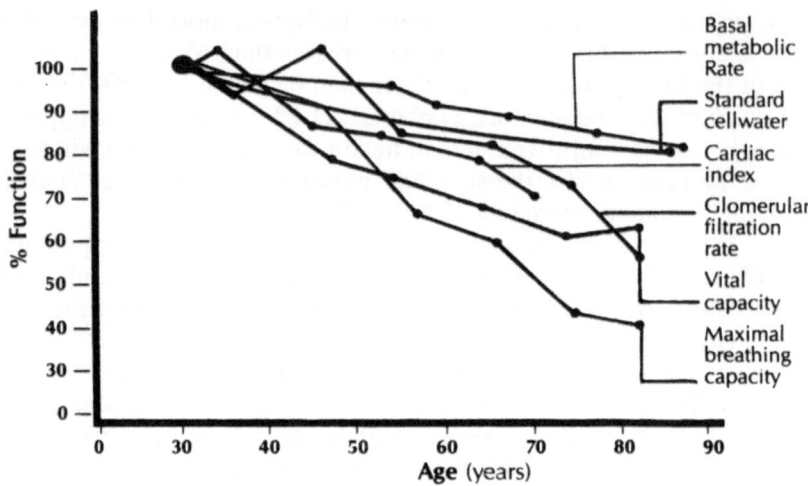

FIGURE 1. Decline of physiologic functions with age[4].

as the general basal metabolic rate decreases about 1% per year.[4] Decreased metabolic rate is an important factor to consider when estimating anesthetic drug metabolism and excretion curves. In addition, thermoregulatory ability is compromised. The temperature in most operating rooms is low, and elderly patient, in particular, are often hypothermic postoperatively. Compensatory shivering may double oxygen consumption.[5]

Changes in body composition are age dependent. Elderly individuals have a higher percentage of fat, where lipid-soluble anesthetic agents may be sequestered. See Figure 2.

Endocrinopathies occur frequently in the elderly. Diabetes mellitus is the most commonly found disorder and is most likely due to impaired peripheral tissue uptake of insulin and/or impaired insulin activity. Blood glucose levels should be adjusted individually. Some patients will require tight control, while in others more flexibility may be afforded. A previous history of clinically significant hypo- or hyperglycemic episodes will indicate to which group the patient belongs.

The presence of thyroid or adrenal dysfunction must be anticipated and defined in terms of excess or deficiency. Management is directed toward normalizing electrolyte and intravascular fluid status to avoid cardiac sequelae (arrhythmias, hypertension, hypotension). Stress doses of steroids may be needed in patients with adrenal cortical insufficiency to avoid acute adrenal crisis. Glucocorticoids, however, are lympholytic and immunosuppressive, and elevated levels may increase the patient's susceptibility to infection. The two most common complications of short-term

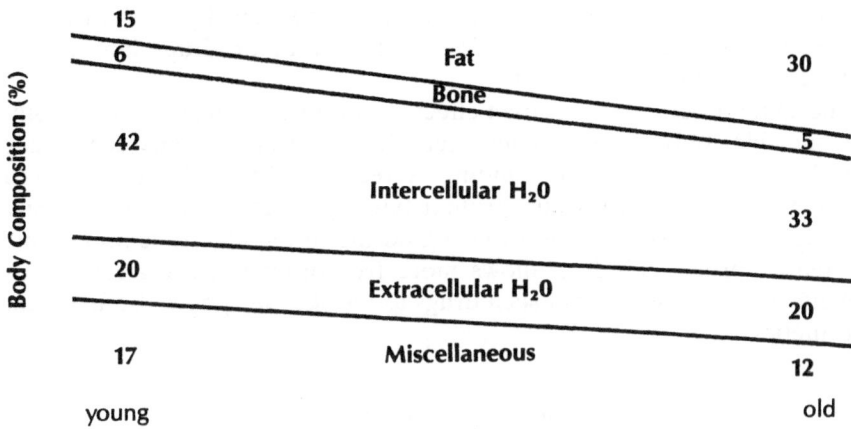

FIGURE 2. Changes in composition of body mass with aging (adapted from McLeskey C.H.: Anesthesia for the geriatric patient. *Adv Anesthesia* 1984; 2:31–68).

perioperative glucocorticoid supplementation are slower wound healing and increased incidence of infection.[6]

Renal and Hepatic Systems

Renal blood flow and glomerular filtration rate (GFR) decrease approximately 1.5% per year after age 30.[7] These changes are due to a decline in cardiac output and as a consequence of intrarenal aging, which is also manifested by glomerular fibrosis, capillary degeneration, and changes in cortical and medullary perfusion. The ability to excrete metabolized drugs and normal body-waste products is decreased.

Absolute creatinine level is often a misleading laboratory value in the elderly patient. The decline in renal function is offset by loss of lean body mass and decreased creatinine production. Thus, creatinine levels may be reported within the normal range. Renal compromise has been estimated by creatinine clearance values to be 33% of normal by age 70.[7]

Renal tubular function (and thus concentrating capacity) is also impaired as a consequence of aging. Therefore, the doses not only of anesthetics, but muscle relaxants and other drugs that depend on renal excretion, must be carefully titrated.[8] A peripheral nerve stimulator is essential for rational dose titration of muscle relaxants.

As with renal blood flow, hepatic blood flow decreases with age; this is evidenced by diminished bromsulphthalein clearance.[9] Although liver function parameters may appear within normal ranges (eg, coagulation studies, clotting factor levels, SGOT, SGPT, alkaline phosphatase) because of the liver's large reserve ability, hepatic function in the elderly is critically overestimated. As hepatic metabolism decreases, the capacity of the liver to conjugate (and thus convert) lipid-soluble anesthetic drugs into water-soluble metabolites is impaired.

The aging process has a distinct effect on serum protein levels, especially albumin. Not only is the absolute quantity of serum proteins decreased, but the affinity for protein binding is reduced. Since the relationship between anesthetic drugs and protein binding is significant with respect to drug action, close attention to drug dosing in the elderly is important. Decreased protein binding allows more free drug; thus, a greater clinical effect may be seen from such drugs as barbiturates, opioids, and local anesthetics.

Central Nervous System

As with other systems, the physiologic function of the central nervous system (CNS) declines with age. Smaller brain mass with age is documented (especially in cerebral and cerebellar cortices),[10] although correlations with brain function are not as well appreciated. But, aging causes changes in cognitive, sensory, motor, and autonomic functions.

Cerebral perfusion pressure is decreased in the elderly along with cerebral oxygen consumption. A laboratory study showed impaired autoregulation in aged rats during hypotension.[11] In the clinical setting, chronic hypertension can shift the autoregulatory curve to the right, exposing the patient to a greater risk of cerebral ischemia during periods of hypotension (eg, following barbiturate administration during induction).

Neurotransmitter effects decline with age due to either loss of the actual neurotransmitter or to receptor changes. The significance of this decline is not well defined.

Varying degrees of dementia due to localized areas of microemboli or perhaps decreases in cerebral blood flow and CNS activity are common. Organic mental syndromes may exist, resulting in emotional lability and unreliability as a historian both for recent and past events. As further sensory deprivation is imposed (eg, removal of familiar surroundings or extinguishing a light), the patient may become quite confused and obstreperous, putting himself at risk of injury and tempting the medical staff to apply excessive physical or pharmacologic restraints.

There is a decrease in anesthetic drug requirements applicable to local anesthetics, opioids, barbiturates, and inhalation agents. This may be due to a lower density of neuronal cells within the CNS and/or because of a lowered sensitivity of the pain receptors in the substantia gelatinosa.

Respiratory System

Deterioration in both parenchymal tissue and supportive lung structures has been described in elderly patients. Both pharyngeal and laryngeal, as well as general airway reflexes are less effective with increasing age.[12]

Thus, the possibility of pulmonary aspiration exists. Several important physiologic changes occur in the respiratory system with aging. Assessment of mechanical ventilatory function, alveolar gas exchange, and control of breathing are essential to properly manage the elderly patient.[13]

Concern must also be directed to general airway assessment when intubation is a consideration. The effects of any spinal deformities, arthritic changes of the spine and temporomandibular joint, and loss of dentition must be assessed. During the preanesthetic visit, the patient should be asked to perform a full range of motion of the neck, including lateral rotation. Should paresthesias or any feelings of light-headedness develop, plans should be made for fiberoptic or awake intubation.

Four primary changes in mechanical ventilation take place with aging that contribute to loss of function: 1) decreased size of intervertebral spaces; 2) decrease in elastic recoil; 3) stiffening of the chest wall; and 4) loss of motor power. With age, intervertebral disks shrink and become less flexible thus leading to kyphosis. Total lung capacity (TLC) is decreased by at least 10% in the elderly. Loss of compliance of the thoracic cage (due to costal and intercostal and intervertebral cartilage stiffening) changes the shape of the aging chest into a barrel contour.

There are also changes within the distribution of the lung volumes. Absolute functional residual capacity (FRC) decreases minimally with aging, but the FRC/TLC ratio *increases* with age. Vital capacity (VC) decreases by about 20–30cc/year after age 20. Dynamic lung volumes also decrease with age due to loss of motor power and increased chestwall stiffness. Forced expiratory volume in the first one second of expiration (FEV_1) decreases by 27cc/year and 22cc/year for men and women, respectively. Age-induced parenchymal changes of the lung closely resemble those of emphysema: dilation of alveolar ducts, loss of intraalveolar septa, and a decreased number of alveoli. Thus, total lung surface area is reduced. All the above changes lead to compromise in the framework of the terminal bronchiolar units. This in turn allows for terminal airway collapse during early expiration, so the closing volume of the lung is increased.[13] See Figure 3.

Increased closing capacity is associated with obesity and the supine position (eg, intraoperatively). As closing capacity increases, greater portions of tidal ventilation occur at lung volumes below closing volume and, thus, air trapping and pulmonary shunting ($\dot{V}/\dot{Q}$ mismatch) is exacerbated, leading to hypoxemia.

Several changes in alveolar gas exchange occur. There is a decrease in PaO_2 of about 0.5mmHg/year after age 20. Several causes for this phenomenon have been identified. Total lung surface area decreases to about $60m^2$ by age 70, and pulmonary shunting increases.[13] Aging also leads to impairment of membrane permeability. In addition, the elderly are less able to compensate for increased shunting during anesthesia due to a less efficient hypoxic pulmonary vasoconstrictor reflex pathway. Many of these problems become exaggerated in the perioperative period.[13] Baseline arte-

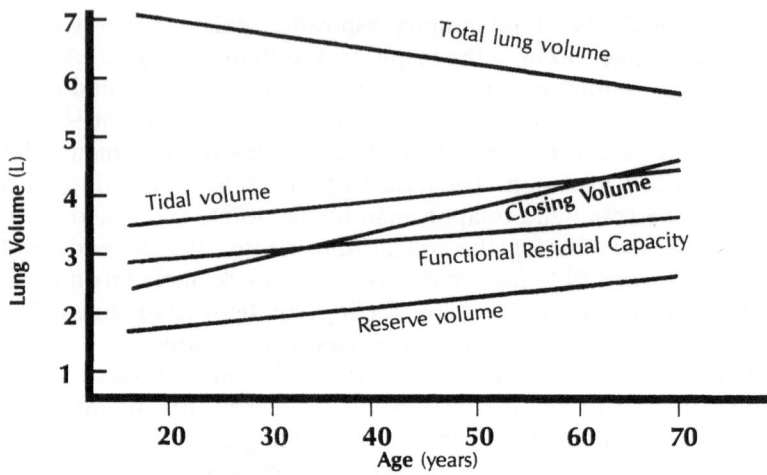

FIGURE 3. Changes in pulmonary volumes with aging (adapted from Pontoppidan H., Geffins B., Lowenstein A.: Acute respiratory failure in the adult. *N Engl J Med* 1972; 287:690–698).

rial blood gas values should be obtained and any hypoxemia during spontaneous ventilation detected. Then, supplemental oxygen may be given as necessary or respiratory therapy exercises commenced.

Aging alters the control of breathing. Kronenberg and Drage[14] have demonstrated a marked reduction in the ability to respond to induced hypercarbia and hypoxia in elderly males. Despite a $PaCO_2$ level of 55mmHg, the ventilatory response was negligible. In addition, the ability of the heart to increase its rate in response to hypoxia and hypercarbia was significantly decreased. Ventilatory drive in the elderly is further blunted by the use of opioids and/or inhalation agents intra- and postoperatively. Loss of respiratory tract cilia prevents effective clearing of foreign matter from the respiratory tract. With the concomitant decrease in laryngeal and tracheal reflexes, coughing is less efficient because of reduced volume, force, and flow rates.

Cardiovascular System

Accurate assessment and optimal manipulation of the cardiovascular system are the most important factors in assuring a successful outcome to surgery for the elderly patient. Issues in the elderly to be considered in the preoperative assessment include cardiac rhythms, myocardial function, and the presence of ischemia, valvular heart disease, or hypertension.[15]

The incidence of cardiac arrhythmias (whether at rest or exercise) increases with age. Common arrhythmias include sinus bradycardia, sinoatrial block, sinus arrest, sick sinus syndrome, and atrial fibrillation or flutter. Occasional premature ventricular contractions have been found in

70% of elderly patients and frequent PVCs in 12%.[15] Atrial fibrillation is commonly found in 3–8% of the elderly. Ventricular ectopy is seen in 50%, and couplets, or bigeminy, occur in about 25%. Left bundle branch block, intraventricular conduction defect, and ST-segment and T-wave changes are commonly observed on ECG tracings.[15]

Port et al,[16] among others, have shown that there were no changes in resting left ventricular ejection fraction (LVEF), left ventricular end diastolic volume (LVEDV), or regional wall motion with aging; however, early diastolic filling may decline with age, perhaps due to decreased left ventricular (LV) wall compliance. This correlates to about a 30% increase in LV wall thickness. However, during exercise, LVEF did decrease although LVEDV and heart rate did not change. Thus, the changes in heart function with respect to aging are selective decrements in the inotropic response to stimuli, including drugs and catecholamines. There are many diffuse multistep abnormalities of excitation–contraction coupling and diminished energy production and delivery, including decreased blood flow in small coronary vessels.[17]

The incidence of coronary artery disease increases with age, with estimates ranging from 13 to 65%.[18] Both occult and nonoccult coronary artery disease exist, and although the elderly patient may be marginally stable at rest, myocardial decompensation can occur rapidly during stress.

Valvular heart disease is also common. Pomerance[19] found aortic calcification in 26% of postmortem studies among 240 elderly patients. Aortic stenosis was found in only 9%. The hemodynamic compromise that valvular disease can impose may be clinically significant. Vigilance for infective endocarditis and its sequelae should be kept in mind with regard to the need for preoperative antibiotics.

Hypertension and its sequelae are perhaps the most common cardiovascular changes in the elderly. Systolic hypertension occurs more frequently than diastolic hypertension. The etiology of the hypertension is varied, although it is most frequently classified as essential hypertension. Intravascular volume is decreased, which exaggerates the hypotensive response to many anesthetic agents. Peripheral vascular resistance is elevated due to thickened elastic fibers and increased collagen and calcium in the arterial walls. Overall cardiac output is reduced by 3 to 3.5% per decade.

Preanesthetic Assessment

An individualized anesthetic plan can be formulated by a comprehensive preanesthetic visit. Provided the patient has intact communicative and intellectual ability, much information regarding functional capacity can be gathered. In patients who have diminished mental function, family members or friends should be interviewed, past medical records reviewed, and current examinations analysed to ascertain reserve capacity.

As mentioned earlier, occult disease is common in the elderly and must be presumed until proven otherwise. After studying 148 consecutive patients over the age of 65, Del Guercio et al[20] reported that only 13.5% had normal measured hemodynamic, respiratory, and oxygen transport function after being "cleared" for general surgery by standard assessment methods. For example, when arterial oxygen tension while breathing room air was plotted against age, 44% of the patients were found to have abnormally low PaO_2 levels, and 12 of 148 (8.1%) were below 50mmHg. Assessment of LV function (shown by plotting left ventricular stroke work index versus pulmonary capillary wedge pressure) showed that only 24% of the patients had normal myocardial contractility, while 22.3% had poor LV function that was undetected by the routine preoperative evaluation. Appropriate therapy improved the preoperative status and decreased the anesthetic risk.

Documentation of the number and types of medications the patient may be taking is very important. Adverse drug interactions are common. In one study, only 6.3% of hospital patients less than age 60 versus 15.4% of those greater than 60 years experienced drug interactions.[21] Several other studies have shown that the elderly as a group ingest many and multicomponent medications, both over-the-counter (60%) and prescription (40%) preparations. The mean number of drugs taken was found to be 3.8 per person[22]. Only 8% of the elderly population used *no* drugs at all. The risk of drug interaction rises sharply after the ingestion of more than 10 drugs—a situation that may be quickly realized during anesthesia. Important effects include an increased duration of nondepolarizing neuromuscular blockade by propranolol and calcium channel blockers, a synergistic action between opioids and many tranquilizers, a decreased effect of digitalis in the presence of halogenated anesthetics (resulting in a relative overdose postoperatively), among many others.[23] In addition, alcohol and sedative drugs are commonly taken in excess by the elderly.[24]

Monitors are employed to enable early detection of abnormalities and prompt application of appropriate therapy. The risk/benefit ratio of the proposed monitoring system must be considered, however. Noninvasive monitors have low risks and can give pertinent medical data. Invasive monitors offer more information but increased risk of complications. Clinical expertise may be the determining factor in their use.

The anesthesiologist should pay close attention to positioning of the patient because of fragile bones and a paucity of subcutaneous tissue for protection about bony prominences.

Anesthetic Plan

Three main concepts apply to administration of general anesthesia in the elderly: Longer elimination half-lives, a lower volume of distribution, and decreased clearance all increase the intensity and duration of the effects of

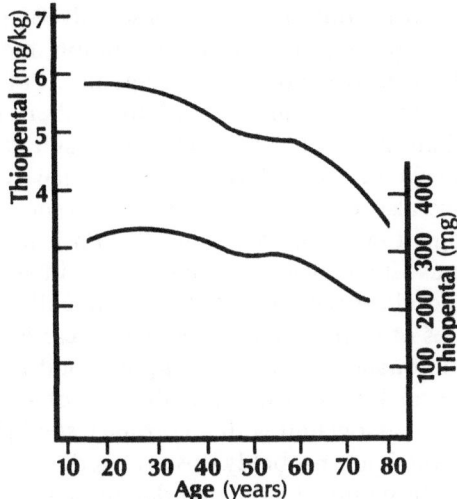

FIGURE 4. Dose of thiopental required to induce anesthesia as a function of age (adapted from Christensen J.H., Andreasen F.: Individual variation in response to thiopental. *Acta Anaesthesiol Scand* 1978; 22:303–313).

anesthetic agents. Smaller doses of thiopental are needed for the induction of anesthesia (ie, 1.8–2.5mg/kg). See Figure 4. Etomidate, which causes less cardiovascular depression, may be a suitable agent for induction, although some studies have shown that elderly patients may have a threefold decrease in the affinity constant for the binding of etomidate to plasma proteins.[25,26] Diazepam in the elderly has a greatly prolonged action and except in rare instances it is probably best avoided. There is insufficient experience yet with the new water-soluble agent, midazolam, to determine if it offers a significant advantage to the elderly patient.

Neuromuscular agents should be carefully titrated using nerve-stimulating devices. Reversal of neuromuscular blockade may be accomplished readily using a cholinesterase inhibitor combined with glycopyrrolate, an antimuscarinic agent which is associated with a low incidence of tachycardia. The recommended dose of glycopyrrolate is 0.2mg per 1.0mg neostigmine or 5.0mg pyridostigmine. The highly polar quaternary ammonium group of glycopyrrolate limits its passage across lipid membranes such as the blood brain barrier. When given intravenously the onset of action is generally evident within one minute. The vagal blocking effects last for 2–3 hours. Opioids, again in reduced dosage, are well tolerated primarily because of minimal cardiovascular depression. However, the elimination half-life of fentanyl is increased in the elderly by approximately 350%.[26] Thus, the dose interval should be increased. As always, respiratory support should be available until the ventilatory depressant effect has dissipated.

Because of lower cardiac output and increased alveolar ventilation, the rate of rise in alveolar partial pressure of inhalation anesthetic agents is very rapid (especially with the more-soluble agents). Pulmonary shunting counteracts this effect to some degree. In addition, there is a lower blood/ gas partition coefficient in the elderly.[27] The net result is rapid inhalation induction of anesthesia in the elderly. Maintenance requirements and MAC equivalents are also reduced. Because isoflurane is the least metabolized inhalation agent currently available (0.17%), it is well suited for elderly patients because it enables rapid emergence. In addition, isoflurane also has the lowest blood/gas partition coefficient and allows easy control of depth. Other qualities of isoflurane include lack of cardiac sensitization to catecholamines, maintenance of cardiac output, good muscle relaxation, little effect on cerebral blood flow, and absence of cortical excitation. Adverse effects may be associated with a coronary steal phenomenon and cardiac depression, which are probably dose related.

The choice of anesthesia may be difficult depending on the ability of the surgeon to accomplish an operation quickly and with minimal blood loss. There is debate over what constitutes the best anesthetic technique for patients with hip fractures.[28, 29] Probably lower mortality, less postoperative hypoxemia, and less-frequent mental status changes are associated with regional as opposed to general anesthesia.[28]

In the case study presented, a regional anesthetic technique is a reasonable choice. A contraindication might be pain in the hip, making it difficult or impossible for the patient to lie on the fracture site. Under these circumstances, the spinal anesthetic may be placed with the injured side uppermost. The patient must then be returned quickly to the supine position to minimize the possibility of unilateral anesthesia developing. An alternative technique is to administer the anesthetic with the patient in a sitting position which is usually not tolerated because of pain. A hyperbaric spinal technique may be useful in experienced hands. An added advantage in this situation is that the patient is already in an ideal position . . . ie injured side uppermost. Thus surgical preparation may be continued while the anesthetic is becoming effective. Spinal and epidural techniques are both acceptable. The incidence of postspinal headaches in the elderly is lower than in younger patients. Anesthetic dose to achieve adequate spinal block is not significantly different from that required in the general population; however, dosages are reduced for epidural anesthesia.

Premedication must be individualized. Altered pharmacokinetics and pharmacodynamics must be recognized and dosages reduced accordingly. Frequently, there is no need for sedative or opioid agents and an adequate preanesthetic state can be obtained by reassurance. Belladonna alkaloids are best avoided as the drying effect is most uncomfortable, and elderly patients who may not understand or simply forget, are likely to quickly quench their thirst.

Aging is a dynamic process that affects all systems. There is no single best anesthetic drug or technique. The physiologic changes that accompany aging and their impact on anesthetic application must be understood. Above all, care and understanding are needed for this very important but fragile group of our society.

References

1. Hospital Mortality, PAS Hospital U.S. 1974–1975. Ann Arbor, Mich., Commission on Professional & Hospital Activities, 1977.
2. Marx G.F., Mateo C.V., Orkin L.: Computer analysis of postanesthetic deaths. *Anesthesiology* 59:54–8, 1973.
3. Wilson L.A., Lawson I.R., Porass W.: Multiple disorders in the elderly. A clinical and statistical study. *Lancet* 2:841–3, 1962.
4. Evans T.I.: The physiological basis of geriatric general anesthesia. *Anesth Intensive Care* 1:319–22, 1973.
5. Bay J., Nunn J.F., Prys-Roberts C.: Factors influencing arterial PO_2 during recovery from general anesthesia. *Br J Anaesth* 40:398–407, 1968.
6. Engquist A., Backer O.G., Jarnum S.: Incidence of postoperative complications in patient subjected to surgery under steroid cover. *Acta Chir Scand* 140:343, 1974.
7. Rowe J.W., Andres R., Tobin J.D., et al: The effect of age on creatinine clearances in man—a cross sectional and longitudinal study. *J Gerontol* 31:155–63, 1976.
8. D'Hollander A., Massaux F., Nevelsteen M., et al: Age-dependent dose-response relationship of ORG-NC45 in anesthetized patients. *Br J Anaesth* 54:653–7, 1982.
9. Thompson E.N., William R.: Effect of age on liver function with particular reference to bromsulphtalein excretion. *Gut* 6:266–9, 1965.
10. Lytle L.D., Altar A.: Diet, central nervous system, and aging. *Fed Proc* 38:2017–22, 1979.
11. Fujishima M., Sadoshima S., Ogatha J., et al: Autoregulation of CBF in young and aged spontaneously hypertensive rats (SHR). *Gerontology* 30:30–6, 1984.
12. Pontoppidan H., Beecher H.K.: Progressive loss of protective reflexes in the airway with advance of age. *JAMA* 174:2209–13, 1960.
13. Wahba W.M.: Influence of aging on lung function—clinical significance of changes from age 20. *Anesth Analg* 62:764–76, 1983.
14. Kronenberg R.S., Drage G.W.: Attenuation of the ventilatory and heart rate responses to hypoxia and hypercapnia with aging in normal men. *J Clin Invest* 52:1812–9, 1973.
15. Martin A.: Cardiac rhythms in healthy elderly patients, in Coodley E.L. (ed), *Geriatric Heart Disease*. Littleton, Mass., PGS Publishing, 1985, pp 20–30.
16. Port S., Cobb F.R., Coleman R.E., et al: Effect of age on the response of the ventricular ejection to exercise. *N Engl J Med* 303:1133–7, 1980.
17. Lakatta E.G., Yin F.C.P.: Myocardial aging: Function alterations and related cellular mechanisms. *Am J Physiol* 242:H927–41, 1982.
18. Fisch C.: Electrocardiogram in the aged: An independent marker of heart disease. *AM J Med* 70:4–6, 1981.

19. Pomerance A.: Cardiac pathology in the elderly. *Cardiovasc Clin* 12(1): 5–9, 1981.
20. Del Guercio R.M., Cohn J.D.: Monitoring operative risk in the elderly. *JAMA* 243:1350–5, 1980.
21. Hurwitz N.: Predisposing factors in adverse reactions to drugs. *Br Med J* 1:536–9, 1969.
22. Chein C.P., Towsend E.J., Ross-Towsend A.: Substance use and abuse among the community elderly: The medical aspect. *Addict Dis* 3:337–56, 1978.
23. Nagashima H.: Drug interaction in the recovery room, in Frost E., Andrews I.C. (eds): *Recovery Room Care.* International *Anesthesia.* Clinics, Boston, Little Brown, 1983, pp 93–106.
24. Thompson T.L. II, Moran M.G., Nies A.S.: Psychotropic drug use in the elderly (Part 1). *N Engl J Med* 308:134–8, 1983.
25. Dagnino J., Prys-Roberts C.: Anesthesia in the aged hypertensive patient, in Stephen C.R., Assaf R.A.E. (eds): *Geriatric Anesthesia.* Boston, Butterworth Publishing Co, 1986, p 264.
26. Schmucher D.L.: Alterations in drug disposition, in Stephen C.R., Assaf R.A.E. (eds): *Geriatric Anesthesia.* Boston, Butterworth Publishing Co, 1986, pp 155–188.
27. Lerman J., Gregory G.A., Willis M.M., et al: Age and solubility of volatile anesthetics in blood. *Anesthesiology* 61:139–43, 1984.
28. McLaren A.D., Stockwell M.C., Reid V.T.: Anaesthetic techniques for surgical correction of fractured neck of femur. A comparative study of spinal and general anesthesia in the elderly. *Anaesthesia* 33:10–4, 1978.
29. McKenzie P.J., Wishart H.Y., Smith G.: Longterm outcome after repair of fractured neck of femur. Comparison of subarachnoid and general anesthesia. *Br J Anaesth* 56:581–5, 1984.

CHAPTER 24

The Patient with a Bleeding Disorder*

Gerald M. Scheinman

Case History. *A 63-year-old man was admitted for elective repair of a large recurrent inguinal hernia. The patient had a long history of alcohol abuse. For the past year, he had been taking approximately 8 aspirin tablets daily, for treatment of arthritic pain. He had not had surgery previously.*

When questioned, his wife reported that, after a recent bout of drinking, he had fallen, hit his face, and sustained a severe nose bleed. He had been taken to the local emergency room, where he was observed overnight. His wife seemed to recall that he had required blood transfusion. Although he had been told to return to the "blood clinic," he had not done so, for fear of contracting AIDS.

Physical examination revealed an obese (255lb), white male. Multiple small purpuric lesions were seen on his hands and legs. Several larger bruises were also apparent. Other vital signs were within normal limits.

Laboratory data included the following: Hct 29%, Hb 9.1g, PT 45 sec (normal 12), PTT 60 sec (normal 30), platelet count 52,000mm³, bleeding time 15 min. The patient was scheduled for hernia repair.

Introduction

Hemostasis requires the coordinated interaction of the following three elements: vasculature, platelets, and coagulation factors. The process is delayed by abnormalities in any of these components. Trauma to the vasculature causes a reflex vasoconstriction in an attempt to divert blood from areas of damage. This response does not result in hemostasis but does aid the hemostatic process in small vessels. Damage to the endothelial lining of a blood vessel exposes subendothelial structures to blood. In the presence of von Willebrand's factor, platelets adhere to these structures. This results

---

*Reviewed by Dr. Paul Goldiner, Department of Anesthesiology, Albert Einstein College of Medicine of Yeshiva University, Bronx, New York.

in platelet activation and a release reaction that causes further platelet adherence and the formation of a hemostatic plug.[1] Interactions of the coagulation proteins form fibrin strands that reinforce the platelet plug.[2] Formation of a plug stops the bleeding if (1) damage to the vessel wall is small, (2) vascular constriction has occurred, and (3) intravascular pressure does not dislodge the friable plug.

These three components of the coagulation process occur simultaneously in response to vascular damage. The failure of one of these components is apparent in the different forms of coagulation defects that can occur. In elderly people who have lost the connective tissue supporting cutaneous blood vessels, or in patients receiving corticosteroids, the vascular response to vessel injury becomes deficient. Purpuric skin lesions may appear even without abnormalities in platelet function or the coagulation pathways. Defects in platelet function cause ecchymoses at the sites of minor trauma or petechiae in areas of increased intravascular pressure. Abnormalities in the coagulation pathways cause rebleeding after initial hemostasis, because of lack of reinforcement of the hemostatic platelet plug.

Mechanisms of Blood Coagulation

Coagulation involves formation of an insoluble fibrin clot through interaction of a series of blood and tissue components. See Figure 1. Thrombin production is the critical step in clot formation.

Thrombin: Production and Activity

Complex mechanisms ensure that thrombogenesis remains localized, since leakage of active enzyme into the general circulation would have serious consequences. The enzyme thrombin catalyzes the conversion of soluble fibrinogen to fibrin monomers; these coalesce to form the insoluble fibrin clot. Thrombin also activates Factor XIII, which catalyzes the formation of irreversible covalent bonds between adjacent fibrin monomers. This changes the clot from an easily dissociated structure to a highly cross-linked, soluble network firmly holding the platelet plug in place.

Thrombin exists in the circulation as an inactive zymogen, prothrombin. Prothrombin is cleaved to thrombin by another enzyme, Factor Xa. This reaction requires calcium and a lipid surface to form the enzyme complex necessary for the conversion of prothrombin to thrombin. The lipid surface is provided by the membranes of platelets (platelet factor 3) which adhere to the sites of vascular damage and limit the activation of thrombin to these areas. The enzyme Factor V accelerates conversion of prothrombin to thrombin 100,000-fold in the presence of platelets. Activated Factor V apparently comes from platelet secretory granules. The final thrombin-generating complex consists of platelet membrane phospholipid, calcium, Factor Va, and Factor Xa.[1,2,3]

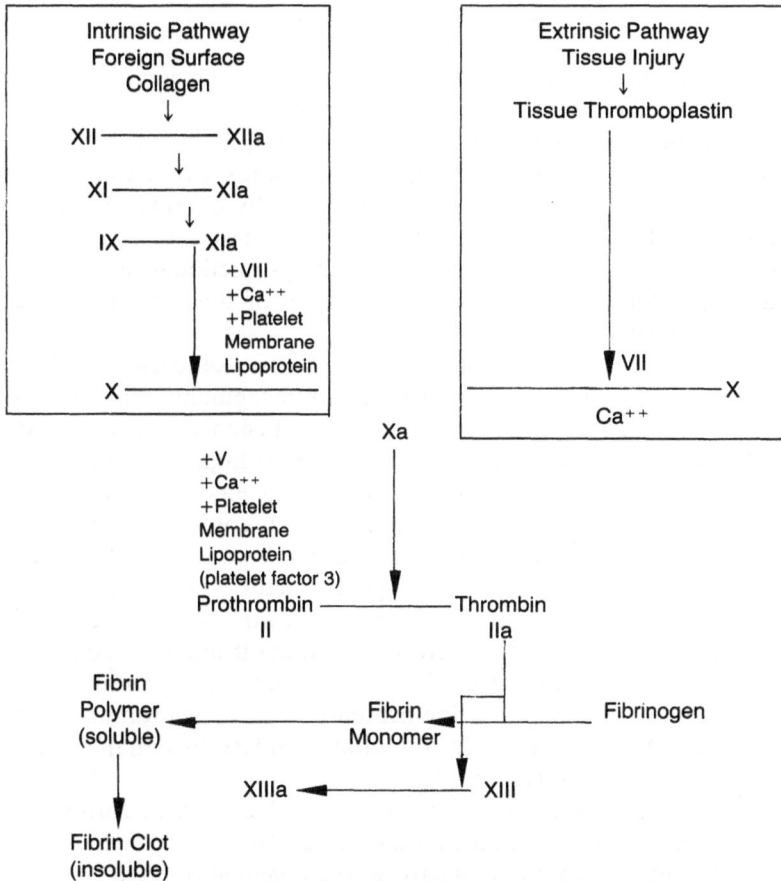

FIGURE 1. Several blood and tissue components interact to cause coagulation.

Intrinsic and Extrinsic Pathways

Formation of activated Factor X occurs by two different pathways, classically described as intrinsic and extrinsic. The intrinsic pathway uses factors present only in plasma. The extrinsic pathway requires both tissue and plasma factors. The extrinsic pathway is activated when damaged tissue releases, into the bloodstream, tissue factor—a lipoprotein found in many tissues such as placenta, lung, brain, and blood vessels. The intrinsic mechanism operates when coagulation components within the blood are exposed to collagen in a damaged vascular surface. This activates the first enzyme in the pathway, Factor XII, which in turn activates the next step. Factor VIII (deficient in hemophilia A) is important in the intrinsic pathway and serves to accelerate the activation of Factor X to physiologic rates.[1,2,3]

Regulatory Processes

Mechanical and biochemical factors exist to keep the coagulation cascade under control. The efficiency of these regulatory processes is apparent through the blood's ability to remain fluid despite intense stimuli for coagulation, such as massive trauma. Continuous circulation of blood through an area of trauma prevents coagulation by diluting the local concentration of activated factors and transporting these factors to the liver, where they are degraded. When the liver is dysfunctional or when shock prevents rapid blood flow, inadequate control of the enzymatic cascade may cause abnormalities in clotting.[1,2]

Inhibition of coagulation occurs through two different biochemical mechanisms. The first involves preformed anticoagulants that circulate in the bloodstream. These anticoagulants limit diffusion of the activated factors from the site of clot formation. The two most important inhibitors are antithrombin III (AT III) and protein C. AT III mediates the anticoagulant activity of heparin, inactivates enzymes that contain a serine at their active site, and inhibits the activity of thrombin, Factors Xa, IXa, XIa, and XIIa, plasmin, trypsin, and chymotrypsin; Factor VIIa seems to be relatively resistant to inhibition by AT III. Heparin catalyzes the reaction between AT III and the serine esterase, making it almost instantaneous. The synthesis of protein C occurs in the liver and is dependent upon vitamin K. Protein C becomes a serine protease upon activation and destroys Factors Va and VIIIa; it also helps to initiate clot lysis by enhancing release of tissue plasminogen activator.[1,4]

Alpha 2-macroglobulin is another plasma inhibitor that forms irreversible complexes with thrombin, although at a slower rate than AT III. Additional inhibitors that can inactivate the coagulation factors are alpha 1-antitrypsin and C1-esterase inhibitor.[1,4]

The second type of biochemical, regulation of the coagulation cascade consists of feedback inhibition. Thrombin production is important to this inhibition. Thrombogenesis not only leads to the formation of the fibrin clot but also has a biphasic effect on the activity of Factors V and VIII. Initially, thrombin acts to increase this activity, but as more thrombin is produced, the activity ceases.

During formation of the fibrin clot, simultaneous initiation of an enzymatic system that can remodel or remove the clot assures prompt reestablishment of flow through the damaged vessel. The principal enzyme of this system exists in the plasma in its inactive form, plasminogen. Its active form, plasmin, is a non-specific endopeptidase that is capable of cleaving a variety of proteins, such as fibrinogen, fibrin, Factors V and VIII, complement, ACTH, and growth hormone.[1] Plasminogen has a high binding affinity for fibrin as it polymerizes to form a clot. Fibrin-bound plasminogen is converted to plasmin by tissue plasminogen activators present in endothelial cells and other tissues. The general circulation is protected from the effects of plasmin by this local activation as well as by alpha 2-antiplasmin, which rapidly inactivates any plasmin released from the dissolving clot. Plasmin, by degrading fibrinogen and fibrin to fibrin degradation products (FDP), smooths out the rough surface of the forming clot to prevent uncontrolled platelet aggregation and fibrin deposition. Later, it also dissolves the established clot to restore vessel patency.[5]

Diagnosis of Bleeding Disorders

Once problems with surgical hemostasis have been ruled out as the cause of perioperative bleeding, the four major nonsurgical causes of coagulopathies are abnormalities in platelets or the coagulation factors, excessive fibrinolysis, or the presence of an anticoagulant. Several tests must be considered.

The basic laboratory tests necessary to establish the diagnosis of a bleeding disorder include the following:

- Hct, Hb, white blood cell and platelet count;
- prothrombin time (PT), partial thromboplastin time (PTT), thrombin time (TT);
- standardized template bleeding time.

The available laboratory tests of coagulation supplement information gathered in the history and physical examination. The initial evaluation consists of a complete blood count and a peripheral blood smear. If these are normal but a platelet-type bleeding abnormality seems possible, a standardized template bleeding time is an appropriate test. A prolonged bleeding time may signify either qualitative or quantitative platelet abnormalities.[6]

Coagulation abnormalities sometimes can be detected by the PT and PTT, which measure the extrinsic and intrinsic pathways, respectively. Unfortunately, neither test measures Factor XIII; further, both lack sensitivity. Therefore, laboratory values may be normal, despite significant depressions of various factors. In fact, activity loss of the various coagulation factors must approach 60–80% to prolong the PT or PTT. Patients with liver disease may have normal laboratory values, with moderate depletion of factors, but still be at increased risk of surgical bleeding. This emphasizes the importance of obtaining an adequate history.

The prothrombin time measures the extrinsic coagulation pathway and involves the addition of Ca^{++} and tissue factor to plasma that has been anticoagulated with a calcium chelator. Normal values for this test range from 12–16 seconds. A prolonged time may occur when Factors V, VII, X, or prothrombin are low, when the concentration of fibrinogen is less than 100mg%, or when heparin is present.[1]

The partial thromboplastin time measures the intrinsic pathway. It involves adding kaolin or celite for maximal surface activation, and a phospholipid emulsion to plasma that has been anticoagulated with citrate. Calcium is then added. The time required for clot formation is normally about 30–45 seconds. The PTT is prolonged when there are deficiences in Factors XII, XI, X, IX, VIII, II, or V, when the fibrinogen concentration is less than 100mg%, or in the presence of FDP or heparin. Only decreased Factor VII does not prolong PTT.

Thrombin time directly indicates the ability of thrombin to convert fibrinogen to fibrin by forming a gelatinous clot. The test is performed by adding a fixed concentration of thrombin to the patient's plasma. A thrombin time of 10–13 seconds is considered normal. Thrombin time can detect a deficiency or abnormality of fibrinogen or defects in the polymerization of fibrin. Heparin and FDP can both prolong thrombin time by affecting the polymerization of fibrin. The fibrinogen concentration can be calculated by mixing known concentrations of fibrinogen with samples of the patient's plasma and comparing the time required for clotting to the thrombin time.

The standardized template bleeding time assesses the overall hemostatic role of platelets in vivo by determining the duration of bleeding from a standardized skin incision during maintenance of increased venous pressure. It is typically done on the forearm with a blood presure cuff applied to the upper arm and maintained at 40mmHg. Two longitudinal incisions are made 1cm apart and 1mm deep with the template. The persistence of bleeding is monitored every 30 seconds, by seeing if filter paper can absorb any blood oozing from the cut. The normal range is 5–7 minutes. An abnormal result signifies either decreased platelet number, normal platelet number with abnormal function, or an intrinsic vascular defect.[6,7]

Role of Platelets

Platelets are critical to hemostasis by maintaining vascular integrity, forming platelet plugs, and stabilizing the hemostatic plug by contributing a phospholipid (PF 3) to the process of fibrin formation. The endothelium apparently is nourished by some platelet constituent or by incorporation of platelets into the vessel wall itself. Less than 10% of the normal platelet concentration is necessary to maintain normal vascular integrity. When platelets are absent from the circulation, red blood cells can migrate through the vessel wall in large numbers; they enter the lymphatic drainage or appear as petechiae or purpura in the skin or mucous membranes.

A break in the endothelium exposes the underlying collagen, microfibrils, and basement membrane to the flowing blood. When platelets contact the wound site, they change shape, become activated, and extrude their stored granules (release reaction). Located in these granules are various factors, such as serotonin, ADP, catecholamines, and other nucleotides.

These aggregating agents release arachidonic acid from the platelet membrane phospholipid, leading to irreversible platelet aggregation and the formation of a platelet plug. Cyclooxygenase converts arachidonic acid to labile prostaglandin intermediates (PGG2/PGH2) and thromboxanes (thromboxane A_2 produces vasoconstriction) to induce the platelet aggregation. A bleeding diasthesis may result from abnormalities in any biochemical event mediating platelet function despite normal platelet concentrations.[6]

Important factors regarding platelets include:

- normal range—150,000–400,000/mm³;
- 50,000/mm³—minimal level to prevent surgical bleeding;
- 100,000/mm³—minimal level to allow normal bleeding time (provided there are no other platelet abnormalities);
- qualitative and quantitative defects in platelet function occur in immune thrombocytopenia, leukemia, and in association with aspirin consumption.

Decreased Platelet Production

Platelets are produced in the bone marrow by megakaryocytes. A normally functioning marrow responds to thrombocytopenia by compensatory increases in megakaryocyte number, size, cytoplasmic maturation, and release. Platelet transfusions will be of no benefit if the bone marrow demonstrates normal reactive hyperplasia of the megakaryocytes. Inadequate platelet production may be due to the mechanical effects of marrow infiltration by tumor, granuloma, or fibrosis. Drugs may also cause decreased production by direct toxic effect. See Table 1. Implicated medications include thiazides, estrogens, ethanol, and chemotherapeutic agents.[1,6,7] In replenishing platelets the estimated duration of therapy should be con-

TABLE 1. Drugs associated with platelet abnormalities

Acetaminophen	Cephalosporins
Ampicillin	Ibuprofen
Aspirin	Indomethacin
Carbenicillin	Nitrofurantoin
Clofibrate	Papaverine
Diphenhydramine	Penicillin compounds
Dipyridamole	Phenothiazines
Furosemide	Propranolol
Gentamicin	Sulfinpyrazone
Glyceryl guaiacolate	Tricyclic amines
Chlorpropamide	Digitalis preparations
Meprobamate	Phenobarbital
Phenytoin	Quinidine
Streptomycin	Thiazide diuretics

TABLE 2. Causes of decreased platelet count

I. Decreased production
   A. aplastic anemia
   B. myelophthisic disorders (tumor, granuloma fibrosis)
   C. drugs (chemotherapeutic thiazides, estrogens, ethanol)
   D. ineffective thrombopoiesis (decreased folate or B_{12}, erythroleukemia, PNH, refractory anemia)
   E. X-ray therapy

II. Decreased survival
   A. immunologic
      1. autoantibodies (TTP, sepsis, SLE, drugs)
      2. isoantibodies (post-transfusion purpura, isoimmune neonatal purpura)
   B. nonimmunologic
      1. disseminated intravascular coagulopathies
      2. infection
      3. thrombotic thrombocytopenic purpura
      4. hemolytic-uremic syndrome
      5. artificial heart valves, extracorporeal circulation

III. Abnormal distribution
   hypersplenism (cirrhosis, Gaucher's disease, lymphoma, sarcoid, infections, myeloproliferative disorders)

IV. Platelet loss
   massive transfusions

sidered. Platelet concentrates are adequate for short-term support, but for the long term, single donor human leukocyte antigen (HLA) matched platelets are better.[6]

Other causes of decreased platelet numbers are listed in Table 2. The most common problems arise from decreased production and loss during massive transfusions. During acute blood loss, patients may receive many units of bank blood, which can cause dilutional thrombocytopenia. Deficiency also occurs following cardiopulmonary bypass; this is due to hemodilution from the pump prime and destruction by the pump rollers and oxygenator.[8] Platelets can survive only 72 hours at room temperature. Bank blood that has been stored for up to 21 days at temperatures of 0–4°C has almost no surviving platelets. It is recommended that after 8–10 units of blood have been transfused platelet concentrates be adminstered, if bleeding continues.[9]

Platelet count may be decreased by shortened platelet life span. Idiopathic thrombocytopenic purpura is the most common immune cause of thrombocytopenia. It most often is an acute childhood illness but can be a chronic disease in adults. Platelet counts increase in more than 70% of patients on corticosteroids (40–60mg/day of prednisone or 1mg/kg/day in children). However, more than 80% of these patients eventually require splenectomy for persistent or recurrent thrombocytopenia.

Platelet counts of less than 10,000 may be tolerated by these patients without serious bleeding, but platelets should be transfused as soon as the splenic vessels are clamped during splenectomy. Preoperative transfusion of platelets is not recommended unless the patient is actively bleeding since the platelets will be destroyed rapidly.

Other causes of immune thrombocytopenia include:

- lupus erythematosus;
- lymphoproliferative disorders;
- medications, via attachment of drug/antibody complex to "innocent bystander" platelets. Medications implicated include quinidine, sulfonamides, gold salts, phenytoin, alpha methyldopa, and digoxin. Discontinuation of treatment is mandatory. Once the drug is stopped and cleared from the circulation, the destruction ceases and the platelet count rises;[5, 7]
- isoimmune thrombocytopenia, usually associated with transfusion. Ninety-eight percent of the population is positive for platelet antigen 1 (PLA 1). When blood that is PLA 1-positive is transfused into a PLA 1-negative patient, post-transfusion purpura may occur. Thrombocytopenia occurs approximately one week after the transfusion. Newborns may suffer from a similar type of thrombocytopenia in a situation that resembles erythroblastosis fetalis. The bleeding may occur several hours after birth, but the greatest danger is at the time of delivery, because of trauma.

Several nonimmune causes of increased platelet destruction have been identified:

- Disseminated intravascular coagulation (DIC)—Increased platelet utilization occurs because of intense activation of the coagulation mechanism.
- Infection, which may cause marrow suppression or decreased platelet survival.
- Hemolytic-uremic syndrome (HUS)—usually a disease of childhood, associated with the acute onset of microangiopathic hemolytic anemia, renal failure, and thrombocytopenia.
- Renal disease, and fluctuating neurologic symptoms such as confusion, seizures, lethargy, or focal motor weakness. Patients with this syndrome should be treated with plasma replacement and plasmapheresis.
- Preeclampsia and eclampsia—coagulopathies may occur in up to 30% of patients.[6, 10]

Qualitative platelet abnormalities are fairly common and may be inherited or acquired. Acquired problems usually are due to an aspirin like effect. The increase in the bleeding time is due to an irreversible acetylation of the cyclooxygenase enzyme. This prevents production of prostaglandin products that initiate the second wave of aggregation. Since the inhibition is irreversible, aggregation is abnormal for the life of the platelets and thus lasts for 7–10 days after the last ingestion of aspirin-like products. Platelets inhibited by aspirin can aggregate when exposed to exogenous ADP released from transfused platelets, but do not undergo a release reaction. Treatment of bleeding problems involves transfusing normal platelets to increase the platelet count by 30,000/mm³. Platelet aggregation inhibition has also been described during the administration of the vasodilators sodium nitroprusside and nitroglycerine, although the mechanism is unclear.[11,12,13] Lesser platelet inhibition is seen with phenothiazines, phentolamine, ethanol, sulfinpyrazone, dipyridamole, dextran, propranolol, and carbenicillin.[6,14] In renal failure with uremia, qualitative platelet abnormalities may result from accumulation in the serum of certain dialyzable compounds. A bleeding time should be done on all uremic patients preoperatively. If the result is markedly prolonged, surgery should be carried out immediately after dialysis and the administration of cryoprecipitate. Platelet abnormalities may be present in other disorders, including dysproteinemias, liver disease, systemic lupus erythematosus (SLE), alcohol, myeloproliferative disorders, and leukemias.[9]

Increased Platelet Production

An increased platelet count may be due to either reactive or autonomous changes. Reactive thrombocytosis refers to a platelet increase that is part of a physiologic response to conditions such as inflammatory disease, nonhematologic malignancies, trauma, or iron deficiency. This is usually a benign condition and tests of platelet function, including the bleeding time, are generally normal. Autonomous thrombocytosis may be associated with production of abnormal platelets.[4,7] It can be due to myeloproliferative diseases such as polycythemia vera, chronic myeloid leukemia, acute leukemia, or essential thrombocythemia. Risk of bleeding may be increased when the platelet count exceeds 1,000,000/mm³. The platelets are unable to undergo the release reaction although they may be able to aggregate normally. Management of the patient who is bleeding consists of transfusing platelets (approximately 4 platelet packs) to bring the level of normal platelets to 30,000/mm³.

Specific Coagulopathies

Disseminated Intravascular Coagulation

DIC is a syndrome characterized by accelerated clotting in a vascular system that consumes factors faster than they can be replaced by the liver. Subsequent activation of the fibrinolytic system occurs with widespread destruction of the newly formed clots. Many causes have been identified, including Gram-negative sepsis, complications of pregnancy (amniotic fluid embolus, retained dead fetus, and abruptio placentae), liver disease, extracorporeal circulation, hemolytic transfusion reaction, shock, acidosis, cardiac arrest, snake bites, malignancy—including prostate, gastric pancreas, and promyelocytic leukemia—chemotherapy, and massive trauma.[14] The initiating event is probably activation of the coagulation cascade in the microvasculature, usually secondary to fibrin deposition. Activation of plasmin also occurs with lysis of fibrin and the formation of FDP, which leads to interference with clot formation.

Laboratory studies reveal prolonged PT, PTT and TT, decreased platelets and fibrinogen, and increased FDP. Anemia may also occur from fragmentation of red blood cells as they try to pass through the fibrin-laden capillaries. This can be demonstrated on a peripheral blood smear.

DIC is often associated with bleeding, but occasionally only thrombotic phenomena are seen. Bleeding may occur in the mucous membranes, at any wound or operative site, or manifest as hematuria or gastrointestinal bleeding. The severity of bleeding appears to correlate inversely with the levels of fibrinogen and circulating platelets. Since DIC is always secondary to some initiating cause, therapy is directed at that cause and only later at the coagulation disturbance itself. Replacement with platelet concentrates and fresh frozen plasma (FFP) temporarily replaces the deficient factors. Heparin is used in select patients to neutralize thrombin and other factors and prevent further factor utilization. However, since the hazard of potentiating bleeding exists, heparin should be given along with FFP and platelets. Therapy must be guided by a hematologist. Epsilon aminocaproic acid should not be used since it retards fibrinolysis and may initiate widespread intravascular clotting with severe thrombotic complications. The only indication for its use is prostate surgery complicated by massive local bleeding. Urine has high concentrations of urokinase that act like plasmin to cause fibrinolysis. Aminocaproic acid should be given only after heparin has been administered. Mortality in this syndrome is due ultimately to organ system dysfunction as a result of microcirculatory occlusion. Survival depends on correction of the underlying cause.[2, 6, 15]

Hepatic disease

Hepatic disease causes coagulopathies because the liver is responsible for producing all the coagulation proteins except Factor VIII, as well as inhibitors of coagulation. Parenchymal liver disease may lead to a deficiency of any or all of the proteins involved in hemostasis. Advanced liver disease may also be associated with portal hypertension with thrombocytopenia secondary to hypersplenism. Patients with advanced liver diseases are prone to DIC, because the liver is not able to clear the activated clotting factors from the plasma. Since no specific therapy exists for bleeding due to liver disease, treatment is basically supportive. Parenteral administration of vitamin K may be tried for 3 days, but will be beneficial only if the liver disease is so severe that little, if any, synthetic function remains. If bleeding develops acutely, administration of platelets, fresh frozen plasma, and cryoprecipitate are the best therapy.[15]

Shock

Shock may produce a bleeding diasthesis for many reasons. Poor tissue perfusion and stagnant blood flow, damage to the endothelial surface of the vasculature, and decreased liver perfusion with subsequent diminished production of coagulation proteins and decreased clearance of activated factors all contribute to the diffuse intravascular thrombosis and bleeding that may occur. Treatment involves correction of the syndrome's underlying cause. Fresh frozen plasma may help to reestablish the balance between clot formation and lysis, because it contains both clotting factors and inhibitors.[15]

Hemophilia

Hemophilia A is due to a deficiency in Factor VIII and is transmitted as a sex-linked recessive trait, occurring in approximately 1 of every 10,000 male births. Hemophilia B (Factor IX deficiency) resembles hemophilia A clinically but occurs far less frequently. Spontaneous bleeding is prevented by a 5% level of Factor VIII activity. Higher levels are needed for surgical hemostasis. Major surgery requires at least 30% activity, both preoperatively and for 2 to 3 weeks postoperatively. As close to surgery as possible, the hemophilic patient should be given an initial dose of Factor VIII to raise the activity level to 70–100%. An additional dose may be required during surgery if significant blood loss occurs. Factor VIII has a half life of approximately 8–12 hours; therefore, transfusion must take place every 8–12 hours during the first 2–3 weeks of the postoperative period. Factor VIII may be replaced as fresh frozen plasma, cryoprecipitate, or antihemophilic factor (AHF) concentrate. Although AHF concentrate has the highest concentration of Factor VIII, it also carries the highest risk of transmitting hepatitis and AIDS because it is pooled from many donors. The concentrate is best for those patients in whom volume administration is a problem.[1,2,9,15]

Vitamin K Deficiency

Although vitamin K is important in the synthesis of coagulation Factors II, VII, IX, and X, these factors are still produced in its absence, but without coagulant activity. Vitamin K deficiency can result from severe malnutrition, intestinal malabsorption, obstructive jaundice, or protracted antibiotic treatment. Patients with obstructive jaundice lasting more than 2 weeks should be given parenteral vitamin K to correct their PT. Vitamin K is poorly absorbed in biliary tract obstruction because bile salts do not enter the duodenum to facilitate uptake. Prolonged antibiotic therapy may eradicate the intestinal flora that produces vitamin K, leading to decreased production.[5]

Preanesthetic Assessment

Assessment of the severity of a bleeding disorder depends upon obtaining an accurate history. Areas to pursue include the following:

- difficulties with bleeding during prior surgical or dental procedures;
- history of transfusions;
- epistaxis, menorrhagia, easy bruising;
- bleeding abnormalities in other family members;
- all medications that the patient has been taking (both prescription and nonprescription)—gold, thiazide diuretics, quinidine, sulfonamides, aspirin, acetaminophen, phenytoin, digoxin, alpha methlydopa, sodium warfarin;
- history of biliary tract disease—this may lead to decreased absorption of the fat-soluble vitamins, eg, vitamin K;
- ethanol abuse or a history of hepatitis causing cirrhosis and portal hypertension;
- other associated disease, concurrent infections, or malignancy.

The physical examination should look for:

- enlarged spleen or unexplained lymphadenopathy, petechiae, ecchymoses, or joint deformities—all of which may point to bleeding disorders or platelet dysfunction;
- telangectasia—eg, in Osler Weber Rendu disease. Bleeding is due to the presence of multiple arteriovenous malformations. Brown skin pigmentation occurs in hemochromatosis. This disease can cause bleeding due to liver failure that occurs secondary to iron accumulation;
- stigmata of chronic liver failure, such as spider angiomata, palmar erythema, jaundice, ascites, Dupuytren's contracture, gynecomastia, or enlarged parotid or lacrimal glands.

Preanesthetic preparation includes transfusion or platelet packs of vitamin K as indicated, immediately before surgery. Blood products should be available for intraoperative administration.

Anesthetic Plan

In patients with coagulopathies, regional anesthetic techniques are not recommended unless unavoidable or unless the bleeding time can be returned close to normal. No specific general anesthetic technique is indicated; however, nitrous oxide administration has been associated with decreased white cell and bone marrow function.

References

1. Bennett J.S.: Blood coagulation and coagulation tests, in: Cassileth P.A. (ed): *Symposium on Hematology and Hematologic Malignancies, Medical Clinics of North America*. Philadelphia, W.B. Saunders, 1984, 68(3):557–76.
2. Rodman G.H., Jr: Bleeding and clotting problems in the critically ill patient, in: Divette J.M. (ed): *Intensive Care Therapeutics*. New York, Appleton Century Crofts, 1980, pp 135–96.
3. Kessler C.M., Bell W.R.: Coagulation factors, in: Spivak J.L. (ed): *Fundamentals of Clinical Hematology*. Hagerstown, Md, Harper & Row, 1980, pp 319–33.
4. Lammee B., Griffin J.M.: Formation of the fibrin clot: the balance of procoagulant and inhibitory factors, in: Ruggeri A.M. (ed): *Coagulant Disorders, Clinics in Hematology*. Philadelphia, W.B. Saunders, 1985, 14(2) 281–343.
5. Schrier S.L.: Disorders of hemostasis and coagulation, in: Rubenstein E., Federman D.D. (eds): *Scientific American Medicine* New York, Scientific American, Inc.; 1986, Sec. 5, subset 6, pp 1–46.
6. Cooper B.S., Churchill W.H., Jr: Hematology, in: Vandam L.D. (ed): *To Make the Patient Ready for Anesthesia, 2nd edition*. Menlo Park, CA, Addison–Wesley, 1984, pp 152–86.
7. Murphy S.: Platelets, in: Spivak J.L. (ed): *Fundamentals of Clinical Hematology*. Hagerstown Md, Harper & Row, 1980, pp 299–318.
8. Mammen E.F., et al: Hemostasis changes during cardiopulmonary bypass surgery. *Semin Thromb Hemost* 11(3):281–92, 1985.
9. Colvin B.T.: Problems of hemostasis, in: Stevens J. (ed): *Preparation for Anesthesia, Clinics in Anesthesiology*. Philadelphia, W.B. Saunders, 1986, 4(3):667–86.
10. Colvin B.T.: Thrombocytopenia, in: Letsky E.A. (ed)· *Hematological Disorders in Pregnancy, Clinics in Hematology*. Philadelphia, W.B. Saunders, 1985, 14(3):661–81.
11. Lichenthal P.R., Dose related prolongation of the bleeding time by intravenous nitroglycerine. *Anesth Analg* 64:30–33, 1985.
12. Fitzgerald D.J. The effect of organic nitrates on pro stacyclin biosynthesis and platelet function in humans. *Circulation* 70:2 297–302, 1984.
13. Saxon A. Platelet inhibition by sodium nitrprusside, a smooth muscle inhibitor. *Blood* 47:957–61, 1976.
14. Bick R.L.: Hemostasis defects associated with cardiac surgery, prosthetic devices, and other extracoporeal circuits. *Semin Thromb Hemost* 11(3):249–80, 1985.
15. Rodman G.H., Jr: Bleeding and clotting disorders, in: Shoemaker W.C., Thompson W.L., Holbrook P.R. (eds): *Textbook of Critical Care*. Philadelphia, W.B. Saunders, 1984, pp 722–32.

CHAPTER 25

The Patient with a Ruptured Intracranial Aneurysm*

Catherine Gulati

Case History. *A 33-year-old woman with a long history of migraine headaches was brought to the emergency room complaining of unduly severe pain in her head. Two days prior to admission she had developed a sudden intense headache, blurred vision, and a stiff neck. She took some phenytoin and codeine tablets and believes she slept for some hours. The next day the headache persisted and was not ameliorated by ingestion of several nonprescription analgesic compounds. The patient felt nauseated and sleepy.*

She was a heavy smoker (2 packs per day for 15 years). There was no history of cardiovascular disease. A routine physical examination a year ago was reported as normal. General anesthesia for a cesarean section (necessitated by prolonged labor) two years ago was uneventful.

A CT scan showed a right subarachnoid hemorrhage. An angiogram confirmed the presence of a right ophthalmic artery aneurysm.

The patient was sleepy but readily arousable and oriented, and the neurologic examination was otherwise unremarkable. Vital signs were: blood pressure 180/100mmHg; pulse 68/min, respiratory rate 12/min. Serum chemistry analyses were normal. ECG showed nonspecific ST-segment and T-wave changes. Arterial blood gas analyses on room air were PaO_2 68mmHg, $PaCO_2$ 47mmHg, pH 7.36. The patient was scheduled for semi-emergent clipping of the aneurysm.

Introduction

Morgagni of Padua is said to have first described cerebral dilatation at autopsy. The first clinical account of cerebral aneurysm rupture was given by Buimi of Milan about 1770.[1] The word "aneurysm" is derived from the Greek "aneurysma"—a widening, from "ana"—across, and "eurys"—

---

*Reviewed by Dr. James Goodrich, Assistant Professor of Neurosurgery, Albert Einstein College of Medicine of Yeshiva University, Bronx, New York.

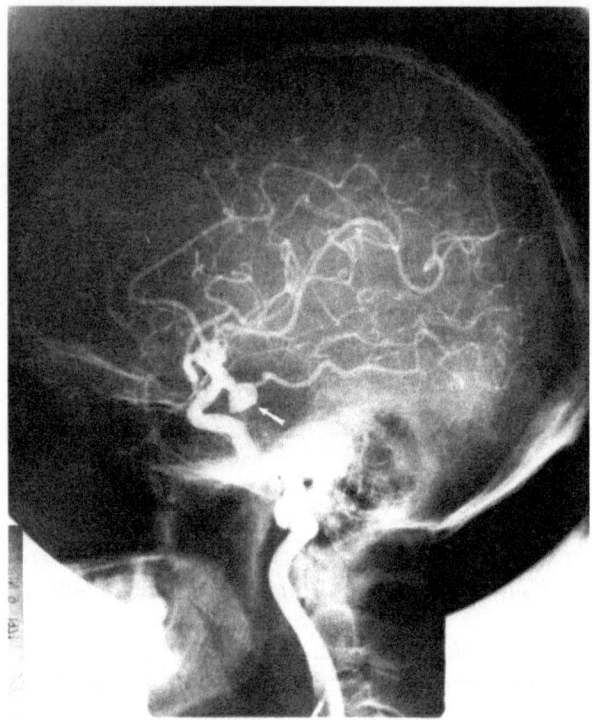

FIGURE 1. Posterior communicating artery aneurysm

broad. As intracranial aneurysms became recognized, the word "berry" was applied as an adjective referring to the shiny coats and rounded outlines. Also, aneurysms hang like berries on arterial stalks and are often multiple. (See Figure 1.)

Most reports calculating the incidence of intracranial aneurysm are derived from general autopsy series. Saccular aneurysms occur in all age groups past puberty, with an overall prevalence of 8%.[2] Twenty-five percent of cases present as multiple aneurysms. Approximately 25,000 patients suffer subarachnoid hemorrhages (SAH) annually. Cerebrovascular disease is the third highest cause of death in the United States; at least 5–10% of those cases are secondary to SAH.

There are about 6 cases of ruptured intracranial aneurysms per 100,000 population. The incidence of silent or undiagnosed SAH may be much higher. The immediate mortality after rupture of an aneurysm is 43%. With conservative management, 35% of survivors will die following

TABLE 1. Occurrence of single aneurysms according to artery of origin[4]

	Incidence %
Internal carotid artery	40%
Anterior circulation	30%
Middle cerebral artery	15%
Basilar artery	10%
Vertebral artery	5%

another bleed within one year and 51% will be dead from complications of the aneurysm within five years. The mortality rate is greater after recurrent hemorrhage—64% after the first rebleed and 96% after the second. Neurologic deficits occur in 30% of survivors.[3]

The occurrence of single aneurysms according to artery of origin is listed in Table 1.[4] The circle of Willis is commonly affected (Figure 2).

Pathophysiology

Aneurysms develop at arterial bifurcations, probably from medial defects in arteries. Women are affected more frequently than men; there is no racial predilection.

Although there apparently is an anatomic defect in the artery, intracranial aneurysm may be an acquired rather than a congenital disease since the abnormality has not been demonstrated at autopsy of infant brains; there is also a clinical association with smoking.

Bell's retrospective study of 208 patients with ruptured cerebral aneurysms revealed a significantly higher number of cigarette smokers among both men and women patients, compared with the expected incidence.[5] Continued cigarette smoking appeared to increase the risk of SAH from a cerebral aneurysm by a factor of 3.9 for men and 3.7 for women. Bell also showed angiographic evidence in smokers of atheroma on the internal elastic laminae—a factor associated with cerebral aneurysms.

Petitti and Wingerd followed 16,795 women for 6 years to determine the possible effects of contraceptive drugs and smoking. SAH occurred in 11 women, with a significant correlation in all of them between oral contraceptives and SAH, and between smoking and SAH, with a synergistic effect when both factors were combined.[6]

It is possible, however, that nonvisualized congenital weakness of vessel walls may predispose to subsequent changes.

Rupture of an aneurysm forces blood into the subarachnoid space at high pressure. As intracranial pressure (ICP) increases, cerebral perfusion pressure decreases. Blood in the subarachnoid space causes acute vasospasm of short duration (5–30 minutes) followed by a period of vascular

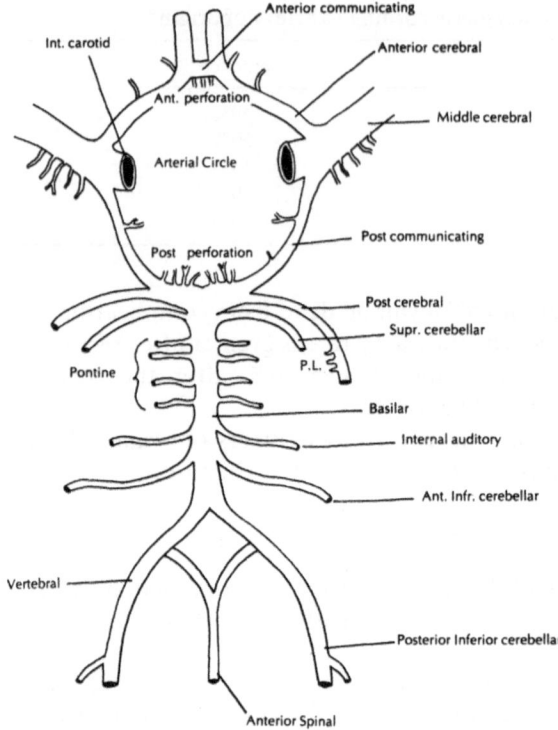

FIGURE 2. The circle of Willis.

relaxation. A second, longer-lasting arterial spasm can then develop later in the clinical course. In 45% of patients this second stage usually starts on the second or third day after rupture but may be delayed for 10–14 days. Spasm usually persists for 7–10 days but may last for 4 weeks. Patients are drowsy to comatose, and may exhibit focal neurologic deficits.

Although a decreased sensorium is usually associated with vasospasm, considerable arterial constriction may occur in intact individuals. This vasospasm is an exaggerated response to substances such as catecholamines, 5-hydroxytryptamine (serotonin), angiotensin, histamine, prostaglandins, calcium, and breakdown products of hemoglobin.

Signs and Symptoms of Rupture

The signs and symptoms of SAH are listed in Table 2. The commonest presenting symptom is headache, possible causes of which include: pain by traction or pressure of the aneurysm on the tentorial edge (first division of the trigeminal nerve supply); distention of the aneurysmal sac stimulating

TABLE 2. Signs and symptoms of ruptured intracranial aneurysms

Meningeal irritation	Headache
	Vomiting
	Stiff neck
Space-occupying effect	3rd nerve palsy
	Visual field defects
	Brain-stem compression
Cerebral edema	Headache
	Vomiting
	Papilledema
	Lethargy
	Coma
Hydrocephalus Vasospasm	Focal neurologic deficit
	Seizures
Antidiuretic hormone (ADH) secretion	Hyponatremia
Other	Hypertension
	ECG abnormalities
	Hyperglycemia

periarterial sensory fibers; giant aneurysms acting as tumors with increased ICP; hydrocephalus from blockage by the mass of the aneurysm or from adhesions secondary to previous bleeds. Outcome is related most closely to the initial condition of the patient.

Several grading systems (eg, Botterell, Hess, Hunt & Miller) have been used to categorize patients. The following is based on the Hunt and Hess system:

Grade   I: Asymptomatic; minimal headache.
Grade II: Moderate headache; nuchal rigidity; no neurologic deficit except in relation to a cranial nerve.
Grade III: Confusion; focal deficit.
Grade IV: Coma, hemiparesis.
Grade V: Moribund.

Preanesthetic Assessment

Perioperative care is aimed at prevention of further neurologic deficit from vasospasm or rebleeding, intracerebral hematoma, or seizures. Appropriate precautions also must be observed to prevent complications such as deep venous thrombosis, pulmonary embolism, sepsis, or the development of metabolic abnormalities such as hyperglycemia or hyponatremia. Preanesthetic assessment requires special attention to cardiorespiratory status and to evaluation of the patient's drug therapy.

Respiratory Assessment

As indicated earlier, smoking is a significant risk factor for subarachnoid hemorrhage. However, discontinuing smoking for a few weeks to reduce secretions is not usually feasible prior to surgery in the aneurysm patient. Cessation of smoking for as short a time as 48 hours, however, has been shown to decrease carboxyhemoglobin levels (thus increasing hemoglobin available for oxygen transport) and shift the oxyhemoglobin dissociation curve to the right (increasing available O_2).[7] In patients with reduced pulmonary reserve, this effect may confer a critical benefit as both general anesthesia and controlled hypotension increase pulmonary shunting.[8]

Baseline arterial blood gas values should be obtained. Vigorous respiratory therapy is clearly contraindicated as it may induce rupture of the aneurysm. However, simple bedside estimations of pulmonary function will be helpful as marginal values may indicate a need for higher inspiratory concentrations of oxygen or a decrease in the period or amount of induced hypotension intraoperatively.

Sudden pulmonary edema is rarely evident after rupture of an intracranial aneurysm, and no specific aneurysm site has been associated with this complication. However, autopsy studies of patients who died after aneurysm rupture showed up to 70% incidence of pulmonary edema.[9] The mechanism is unknown. Parasympathetic lesions may cause hyperactivity of an "edemogenic center," or direct stimulation of descending sympathetic pathways from the hypothalamus may cause cardiac failure.[4] However, since primary cardiac decompensation is rare, digitalis is seldom beneficial. Probably as ICP rises, increased sympathetic activity attempts to increase blood pressure and cerebral perfusion. Systemic vasoconstriction shifts blood to pulmonary compartments and causes pulmonary edema.

Treatment requires intubation and ventilation, head elevation, diuretic administration, and, if hypertension is severe, adrenergic receptor blockade with small doses of labetalol (5–10mg) or propranolol (1mg) repeated every 15–30 minutes until therapeutic effect is achieved.

Cardiac Assessment

Although most patients with SAH are hypertensive, this is probably a consequence rather than a cause of the disease. In patients with no evidence of elevated ICP, systemic arterial pressure should be brought under control to stabilize transmural pressure across the wall of the aneurysm. Appropriate drugs include propranolol or labetalol. If there is clinical evidence of ICP elevation, both ICP and systemic pressure should be measured directly and treated appropriately to ensure maintenance of adequate cerebral perfusion pressures.

Electrocardiographic changes are commonly associated with ruptured aneurysms. Prolonged QT-interval, T-wave inversion, and prominent U-waves are almost pathognomonic of SAH.[10] Although this is suggestive of myocardial ischemia, autopsy studies have not shown typical changes. Usually ECG changes occur early and are transient. Occasionally, abnormalities are associated with cerebral vasospasm. Pathogenesis is believed to be secondary to neural (autonomic), humoral (catecholamine), or metabolic (respiratory and hemodynamic) dysfunctions.

In a few cases, myocytolysis (loss of sarcoplasm from muscle), small areas of myocardial necrosis, and subendocardial hemorrhages have been demonstrated. In those cases, ECG abnormalities were preceded by severe hypertension and increase in ICP. Laboratory studies have correlated intracranial hypertension and myocardial lesions.[11] Also, stimulation of the brain stem and especially of the reticular formation can cause arrhythmias and zones of myocardial ischemia. The effects are blocked by propranolol.[12]

Therapy of cardiac arrhythmias requires documentation of the abnormality, serial enzyme analyses, bed rest, sedation, and propranolol.

Drug Evaluation

Pharmacologic management of the patient may include the administration of epsilon aminocaproic acid (EACA), 30–35gm/day I.V. EACA is an antifibrinolytic agent used to preserve clot formation, although use of this agent is rapidly losing favor. The drug is associated with nonspecific electrocardiographic ST-segment and T-wave abnormalities, changes that are not accompanied by other symptoms of myocardial ischemia and may be associated with blood in the subarachnoid space. Surgery should not be delayed pending resolution of these cardiographic abnormalities. A further complication of the use of EACA is hydrocephalus, which has been demonstrated radiographically in up to 43% of patients.[13]

Tranexamic acid, another antifibrinolytic agent, reduces the rate of rebleeding, but this is more than offset by a higher incidence of cerebral ischemic complications.[14]

Nimodipine, a calcium channel blocker with a greater specificity for cerebral vessels, has been used effectively intravenously in one study to prevent and reduce the severity of ischemic neurologic deficits by decreasing vasospasm.[15] It may also afford neuronal protection during ischemia. This drug, which crosses the blood-brain barrier easily, is not yet available in parenteral form in the United States (October 1987).

Steroids have been used, although there is little evidence of beneficial effect after SAH. Theoretically at least, steroids may decrease the incidence of aseptic meningitis and the formation of arachnoid adhesions, thus reducing the risk of hydrocephalus. On the other hand, steroids may mask fever from pneumonitis or pulmonary embolism, induce gastritis or peptic ulcers, suppress normal adrenal gland function, and inhibit scar formation around the wall of the aneurysm. Certainly, blood sugar levels are elevated by steroid use, and even slight degrees of hyperglycemia have been associated with increased size of infarcted areas.[16]

Timing of Surgery

Previously, the presence or absence of vasospasm on angiographic studies determined the timing of aneurysm surgery. Current neurosurgical practice suggests that a better outcome is achieved by early operation (within 24–48 hours) in patients who are neurologically intact (grade I and II) whether or not vasospasm has been demonstrated (91% of grade I and 73% of grade II patients do well). Such emergency intervention decreases the likelihood of rebleeding. There is no need for other potentially harmful therapy such as antifibrinolytics, sedatives, antihypertensives, bed rest, or fluid restriction that may cause further complications. However, only 53% of grade III patients do well, indicating that the gross neurologic condition preoperatively is the best prognostic indicator of good survival.

Anesthetic Plan

Adequate sedation is essential. Agitation raises blood pressure and increases transmural pressure. The organizing clot in the rent in the aneurysm must be protected. Premedication with a large dose of oral diazepam (10mg) is usually adequate. Atropine causes tachycardia and should be avoided.

Mild to moderate fluid restriction reduces cerebral edema and has been associated with a lower mortality rate; a high fluid intake, however, may combat vasospasm. Whole blood administration expands intravascular volume and increases cardiac output without improving cerebral blood flow. However, reducing blood viscosity by hemodilution with plasma expanders appears to increase cerebral blood flow but tends to raise ICP. Sugar-containing solutions should not be used.

The primary goal is to maintain a stable transmural pressure. Induction into anesthesia can be achieved with relatively large doses of sodium thiopental (4–5mg/kg), lidocaine (1–1.5mg/kg), fentanyl (2μg/kg), and adequate relaxation with atracurium (0.5mg/kg). Labetalol (5–10mg) is useful in attenuating the hypertensive response to intubation and liberal use of a laryngotracheal spray of lidocaine 4% is also helpful.

Maintenance of anesthesia is achieved with isoflurane (0.7–1%) in air and oxygen supplemented by a fentanyl infusion (2μg/kg/hr).

Lumbar cerebrospinal fluid drainage is established to better control the size of the contents of the intracranial space and to continuously record lumbar subarachnoid pressure.

Other monitors are listed in Table 3. Prior to insertion of the pin head-holder, local anesthesia should be injected into the scalp. Epinephrine

TABLE 3. Monitoring during intracranial aneurysm surgery (Monitors necessary and desirable for anesthetic management)

Necessary	Desirable
Electrocardiogram	Television monitor
Esophageal stethoscope	Video recorder
Pulse oximeter	Blood gas apparatus
Capnograph	3-channel trend recorder
Urine output	Swan-Ganz catheter
2 intravenous routes	Somatosensory evoked potential monitor
Continuous blood pressure display	Automated record-keeping
Ventilator	
Thermistor	
Drip counter	
Airway humidifier	

should be used with caution as subsequent absorption of the drug causes hypertension in about 30 minutes. Patients are usually operated on in the supine position. Common flaps are shown in Figure 3.

Prevention of premature rupture of the aneurysm during surgery most often is achieved with pharmacologically induced hypotension to decrease the pressure to which the aneurysmal wall is exposed. Several drugs have been recommended. Currently the most frequently used are isoflurane (which decreases metabolic rate of oxygen consumption) and sodium nitropursside (which has an evanescent action because of its rapid conversion to thiocyanate). Reduction in mean pressure to a level of 40 or 50mmHg has

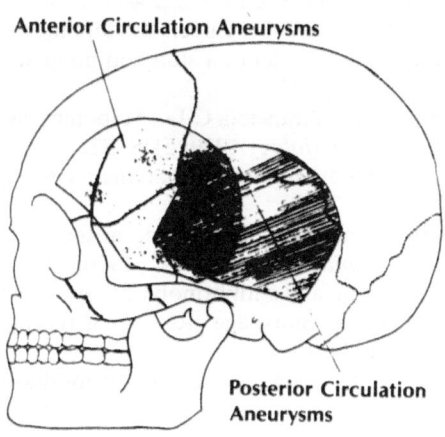

FIGURE 3. Sites for craniotomy flaps.

only negligible effect on cardiac output, but vascular resistance is significantly decreased. If sodium nitroprusside is started only when the surgeon begins to work in the immediate area of the aneurysm, the total dose rarely exceeds 10–15mg and duration of administration is generally less than 1 hour. At this dosage range, the adverse effects of tachyphylaxis, cyanide toxicity, rebound hypertension, and platelet abnormalities are rarely encountered. Should arterial pressure rise more than 20–30mmHg above baseline when sodium nitroprusside infusion is discontinued, hydralazine in increments of 10mg with small doses of propranolol (1mg) may be given.

If the patient was neurologically intact preoperatively, the same state should be realized postoperatively. Ideally, the patient should be awake and responsive in the operating room prior to transfer to the recovery room.

References

1. Johnson H.C.: Surgery of cerebral vascular anomalies, in: Walker A.E. (ed): *A History of Neurological Surgery*. New York: Hafner Publ. Co., 1967, p 250.
2. McCormick W.F.: The natural history of intracranial saccular aneurysms, in: *Weekly Update, Neurology and Neurosurgery*. Miami: Biomedica Inc., 1978; 1:3.
3. Winn H.R., Almaani W.S., Berga S.L., et al: The long-term outcome in patients with multiple aneurysms. *J Neurosurg* 59:642–51, 1983.
4. Fox J.L.: *Intracranial Aneurysms*. New York: Springer-Verlag, 1983; pp 19–26.
5. Bell B.A., Symon L.: Smoking and subarachnoid hemorrhage. *Br Med J* 1:577–8, 1979.
6. Petitti D.B., Wingerd J.: Use of oral contraceptives, cigarette smoking and risk of subarachnoid hemorrhage. *Lancet* 2:234–5, 1978.
7. Davies J.M., Latto I.O., Jones J.G.: Effects of stopping smoking for 48 hours on oxygen availability from the blood: a study on pregnant women. *Br Med J* 2:355, 1979.
8. Frost E.A.M., Tabaddor K., Arancibia C.U.: Hypotensive drugs and outcome in aneurysm surgery. *Anesthesiology* 1979; 51:S–82.
9. Weir B.K.: Pulmonary edema following fatal aneurysm rupture. *J Neurosurg* 49:507, 1978.
10. Keller A.Z.: Hypertension, age and residence in the survival with subarachnoid hemorrhage. *Am J Epidemiol* 91:139–47, 1970.
11. Corkill G.: Earlier operation and antifibrinolytic therapy in the management of aneurysmal subarachnoid haemorrhage. Review of recent experience in Tasmania. *Med J Aust* 1:468–70, 1974.
12. Hugosson R., Hogstrom S.: Factors disposing to morbidity in surgery of intracranial aneurysms with special regard to deep controlled hypertension. *J Neurosurg* 38:561–7, 1973.
13. Park B.E.: Spontaneous subarachnoid hemorrhage complicating hydrocephalus: epsilon aminocaproic acid: a possible predisposing factor. *Surg Neurol* 11:73–8, 1977.

14. Vermeulen M., Lindsay K.W., Murray G.D.: Antifibrinolytic treatment in subarachnoid hemorrhage. *N Engl J Med* 311:432–7, 1984.
15. Allen G., Sahn H.C., Preziosi T.J.: Cerebral arterial spasm—a controlled trial of nimodipine in patients with subarachnoid hemorrhage. *N Engl J Med* 308:619–24, 1983.
16. Siesjo B.K.: Cell damage in the brain: A speculative synthesis. *J Cereb Blood Flow Metab* 1:155–85, 1981.
17. Ropper A.H., Zervas N.T.: Outcome 1 year after SAH from cerebral aneurysm. *J Neurosurg* 60:909–15, 1984.

CHAPTER 26

The Patient with Scoliosis*

James B. Mueller

Case History. *A 23-year-old woman with idiopathic scoliosis was admitted for Harrington rod instrumentation. The diagnosis of scoliosis was made when she was 13 years old, at which time the curvature was between 20 and 30°. She was initially treated conservatively with application of a Milwaukee brace, which was used for 5 years. The curvature increased, and at time of admission measured 62°.*

The patient had no respiratory, cardiac, or neurologic symptomatology. She reported allergies to penicillin, erythromycin, and iodine. Physical examination was normal except for an obvious scoliosis with the hump convex to the right and a lumbar compensatory curve. Chest x-ray showed a normal heart and lungs, and a thoracic curve to the right, with a Cobb angle of 62°. The electrocardiogram indicated a normal sinus rhythm; normal axis; and borderline peaked P waves in leads II, III, aVF.

Pulmonary function tests: forced vital capacity (FVC) 2.2L (53% of normal); forced expiratory volume (FEV$_1$) 16.1L (50% of normal); vital capacity (VC) 2.3L (57% of normal); functional residual capacity (FRC) 1.7L (59% of normal).

Other laboratory values were: hemoglobin 14.4gm/dl, hematocrit 43.7%, white blood cell count 6.3/mm³, potassium 3.7mEq/L, glucose 120 mg/dl.

Introduction

Scoliosis is a lateral and rotational deformity of the spinal column that may be associated with many disease processes (see Table 1).

The patient with scoliosis presents the anesthesiologist with a unique set of problems:

- The patient, most often female, is usually a child or young adolescent.
- There is a high incidence of associated congenital anomalies.

---

*Reviewed by Dr. Stanley Hoppenfield, Associate Clinical Professor of Orthopedics, Albert Einstein College of Medicine of Yeshiva University, Bronx, New York.

TABLE 1. Classification of scoliosis

I. Idiopathic Scoliosis (65%)	II. Congenital Scoliosis (15%)
Age at onset	*Vertebral anomalies*
Infantile (first 3 years of life)	Vertebral column
Juvenile	Meningomyelocele
(skeletal ages 4–9 years)	Spina bifida occulta
Adolescent	
(skeletal ages 9 years to	
maturity)	

III. Neuromuscular Abnormalities (10%)
Neuropathic

Upper motor neuron lesion	Lower motor neuron lesion
Cerebral palsy	Poliomyelitis
Spinocerebellar degeneration	Meningomyelocele
Friedreich's ataxia	Dysautonomia
Syringomyelia	
Spinal cord tumor	*Myopathic*
Hemangioma	Muscular dystrophy
Astrocytoma	Myotonia
Teratoma	Hypotonia
Intramedullary cyst	
Spinal cord injury	

IV. Scoliosis Associated with Neurofibromatosis (5%)

V. Mesenchymal Disorders	VI. Trauma
Congenital	
Marfan's syndrome	
Acquired	
Rheumatoid arthritis	

VII. Bone Infections	VIII. Metabolic Disorders
	Osteomalacia
	Osteoporosis

- Varying degrees of cardiopulmonary embarrassment may coexist.
- Surgical correction requires continuous somatosensory evoked potential monitoring and/or an intraoperative wake-up test.
- Intraoperative blood replacement is often required.
- Respiratory support and pain control may present considerable postoperative problems.

Incidence

The incidence of scoliosis varies in several studies from 0.3–4.0/1000. Females outnumber males approximately 9:1. Idiopathic scoliosis appears to be transmitted as an autosomal dominant gene with incomplete penetrance.[1]

Onset is categorized into three peak periods: infancy—between birth and 3 years of age, more frequent in males (occurs very rarely in the United States); juvenile—between 4 and 10 years of age, with an equal ratio of male: female; adolescence—between 10 years of age and skeletal maturity, occurring in females in more than 80% of cases.

Etiology

The cause of scoliosis is unknown in approximately 65% of all cases. Most patients with idiopathic scoliosis present during periods of maximum growth. This growth is usually associated with menarche in girls and puberty in boys, periods of endocrine activity and increased protein synthesis and collagen production.[2] The remaining 35% of scoliosis cases are associated with congenital and acquired diseases. Since the development of the spinal cord, heart and great vessels, and the genitourinary systems are closely related, scoliosis is frequently associated with defects in these other systems. Patients with congenital heart disease, especially cyanotic disease, have an incidence of scoliosis increased by 2–12%.[3, 4]

Before the availability of the Salk and Sabin vaccines, polio was the leading cause of neuromuscular scoliosis. Paralysis related to meningomyelocele is now the leading cause of this type of abnormal curvature. Muscular dystrophy is an example of myopathic scoliosis that frequently progresses to severe spinal curvature. With myopathic disease, both the underlying disease and the scoliosis are progressive and increasing difficulty with breathing, swallowing, and decreased pulmonary function can lead to cor pulmonale and right-sided cardiac failure.

Forms of Scoliosis

Scoliosis can be classified as nonstructural and structural. Nonstructural scoliosis is a lateral curvature of the spine without structural defect of the vertebrae or disks. The curve is flexible and corrects by bending the convex side of the curve. This form is usually nonprogressive and can be found associated with several conditions (see Table 2). If the underlying conditions are not corrected during childhood, the abnormalities may progress to a structural scoliosis.

Structural scoliosis is characterized by four main features: (1) The curve does not straighten with bending. (2) The soft tissue contracts in the concavity of the curve. (3) Structural abnormalities occur, such as wedging of the vertebral bodies and variations in the sizes of the laminae, pedicles, and transverse processes of the individual vertebrae in the deformity.[4] A fixed rotary deformity develops in the vertebral bodies, usually in the direction of the curve.

The vast majority of scoliotic patients develop multiple curves, divided

TABLE 2. Nonstructural scoliosis

I. Postural
II. Hysterical
III. Compensatory
IV. Nerve root inflammation
    Herniated nucleus pulposus Tumors
V. Inflammatory sclerosis
VI. Anisomelia
VII. Spinal tumors

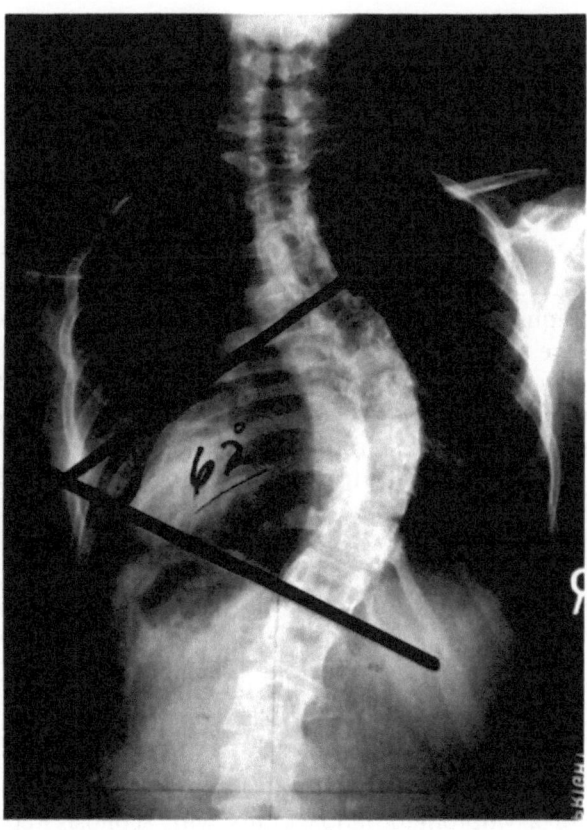

FIGURE 1. The Cobb angle assesses spinal deformity by measuring the angle subtended by the intersecting lines drawn perpendicular to the superior surface of the uppermost vertebra and the inferior surface of the lowest vertebra involved in the major curve.

into two types: (1) Structural curve (major angle), defined as the length of the spinal column over which the fixed deformity extends, is usually the most severe and largest curve, and most often is to the right. (2) Compensatory curves (minor angle), which the body forms in an attempt to maintain a balanced posture, are usually above and below the structural curve, are not as severe as the major angle curve, and are in the opposite direction.

Several methods have been derived to follow the progression or correction of scoliosis, measuring the curves by means of spinal roentgenograms. The most common method, first described by Cobb in 1948[5] gives an accurate assessment of the spinal deformity by measuring the angle subtended by the intersecting lines drawn perpendicular to the superior surface of the uppermost vertebra and the inferior surface of the lowermost vertebra involved in the major angle (see Figure 1).

Pathophysiology

The cardiopulmonary system is commonly affected (Figure 2). Most patients do not become symptomatic until the curves exceed 60° and/or the patients are older (30–40 years).

Respiratory Effects

Bjure et al studied 50 patients with untreated idiopathic scoliosis and found an increased frequency of respiratory impairment, especially in those patients with severe scoliosis. Seven of 50 patients were unable to walk (all had curves greater than 100°). None of the patients (ages 20–65 years) were able to engage in hard work and 22% of these patients were on disability pensions because of respiratory impairment.[6]

Restrictive lung volumes are usual. Total lung capacity (TLC), FRC, and residual volume (RV) are all decreased. Lung volumes as % of normal predictions correlate with degree of curvature:

	Degree of Curvature		
	<60	60–100	>100
TLC	85%	68%	52%
VC	83%	64%	46%
RV	95%	80%	62%

In a study of asymptomatic adolescents with scoliosis (curves <30°), 13.6% showed a restrictive defect with a vital capacity <80%. In 27.3% of these patients, maximum voluntary ventilation was reduced 80% of predicted normal values. FVC correlated with the maximum inspiratory and expiratory pressures and measures of respiratory muscle strength, but not

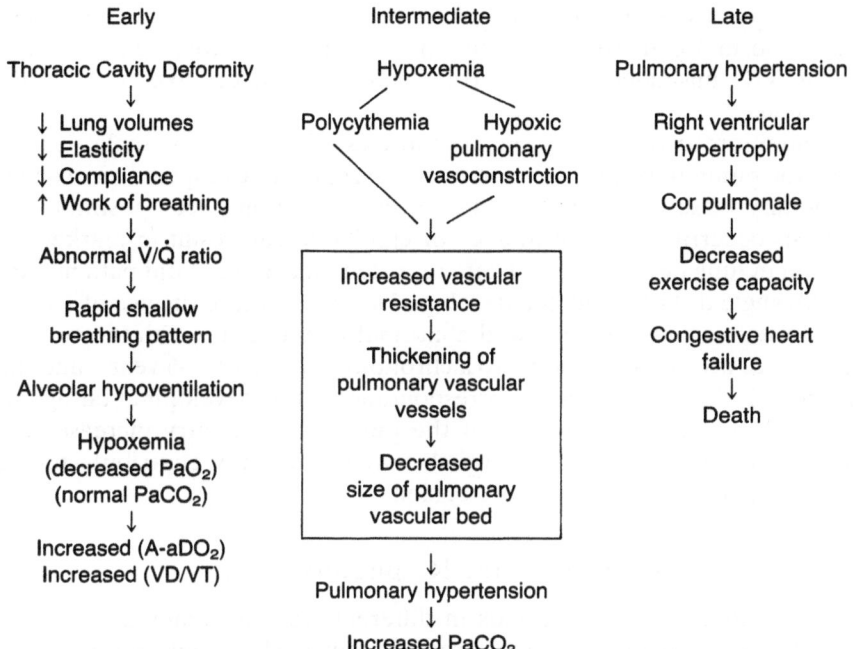

FIGURE 2. Progressive cardiopulmonary involvement in severe scoliosis.

to the degree of spinal curvature.[7] Thus ventilatory function may be impaired in mild scoliosis, and the force developed by the respiratory muscles is more important in determining respiratory impairment than the degree of curvature.

Respiratory function is impaired more with paralytic than with idiopathic scoliosis. In addition, the patient's overall prognosis is worse in poliomyelitis. This poorer prognosis may relate to paralysis of the respiratory muscles, which decreases the ability to cough, deep breathe, and clear secretions, resulting in atelectasis and secondary infection. Repeated infections are common, causing pulmonary fibrosis and continual worsening of pulmonary function.

The major abnormality in gas exchange associated with scoliosis is hypoventilation secondary to ventilation/perfusion defects. Because of the restrictive nature of scoliosis, the patient develops a rapid, shallow breathing pattern that helps to decrease the work of breathing. Increased dead space increases the volume of air in conducting airways and hypoventilates the alveoli. Arterial blood gas samples show reductions in arterial oxygen tension (PaO_2) with normal arterial carbon dioxide tension ($PaCO_2$). Also, the alveolar–arterial oxygen difference ($A–aDO_2$) and the dead space to tidal volume ratios (VD/VT) are increased. As the pulmonary disease worsens and the compensatory increase in ventilation subsides, hypercapnia is frequently seen. The slope of the ventilatory response to CO_2 is less than in normal patients, which may impair the ventilatory compensation for the $\dot{V}/\dot{Q}$ mismatching and further contribute to the hypercarbia and hypoxemia.[8]

In addition to the effects on the muscles of respiration, scoliosis also alters the pulmonary anatomy and microvasculature. Compression of small pulmonary vessels secondary to atelectasis is commonly seen postmortem. Scoliosis occurring early in infancy or childhood can result in marked alteration in lung development. Boffa reported on a 36-year-old patient with a Cobb angle of 140°, who had developed scoliosis before the age of 1 year. Postmortem examination showed abnormally small lungs with the volume and surface area corresponding to a chronological age of 5–6 years, and the number of alveoli per acinus corresponding to the developmental age of 1 year. The underdevelopment of the pulmonary circuitry increases the pulmonary vascular resistance, which may significantly contribute to the development of pulmonary hypertension.[9]

Response of the Respiratory System

The pulmonary system responds in different ways to maintain adequate systemic oxygen delivery during chronic hypoxia. The vasomotor mediated pulmonary vasoconstriction causes constriction of pulmonary precapillary arteries and arterioles. Shunting of blood balances the $\dot{V}/\dot{Q}$ ratio. Also, in response to chronic hypoxemia, polycythemia increases blood viscosity and pulmonary blood flow. Prolonged vasoconstriction and hyperviscosity cause changes in the caliber of the small blood vessels, leading to a permanent increase in pulmonary vascular resistance and promoting the development of pulmonary hypertension. Sustained pulmonary hypertension then results in cor pulmonale (see Figure 2). Shneerson et al performed cardiac catheterization on 40 patients with thoracic scoliosis and unexplained dyspnea or suspected pulmonary hypertension. The average patient age was 30 years, age of onset was 7 years, and the average angle was 75°. There was no correlation between the mean pulmonary artery pressure and etiology or severity of scoliosis. However, the mean pulmonary artery pressure rose as the PaO_2 fell, especially when the PaO_2 fell below 70mmHg. This rise in pulmonary pressure was secondary to hypoxic pulmonary vasoconstriction. The pulmonary pressure did not return to normal when the oxygen was raised above 70mmHg, indicating vascular hypertrophy and sustained increased vascular resistance.[10]

Cardiovascular Effects

Cardiac disease associated with scoliosis has long been recognized. Autopsies of scoliosis patients revealed right ventricular hypertrophy associated with moderately severe lung abnormalities. In 1899, Bachmann reported right ventricular hypertrophy in 82% of 197 autopsies in patients with kyphoscoliosis.[10]

Chronic respiratory insufficiency affects the cardiovascular system. Changes in the arterial oxygen and carbon dioxide levels as well as in the intrathoracic pressures alter both the cardiac filling pressures and cardiac output. In patients with pulmonary hypertension, the effects of hypoxia, hypercarbia, and acidosis increase right ventricular afterload. As the pulmonary hypertension becomes more pronounced and lung function deteriorates further, the decrease in pleural pressure associated with inspiration increases venous return to the right ventricle. Increased impedance obstructs right ventricular output.[11]

Because pulmonary hypertension develops slowly, right ventricular hypertrophy is usually not seen until late in the disease process. As the right ventricle decompensates, dyspnea with decreasing amounts of exertion occurs. Right ventricular afterload, and respiratory failure with associated hypoxia, are the major factors regulating the cardiac response to exercise.

Management of Scoliosis

The best treatment is early detection. The prognosis and specific form of therapy depend on the underlying causes, age of the patient, and the rate of progression of the scoliosis. Since the majority of cases are idiopathic and pain is not usual, the diagnosis is often delayed until the curvature is fairly well advanced. Also, the adolescent patient, because of modesty, is usually not seen fully undressed by his/her parents. Consequently, the scoliotic change is usually not noticed until the patient is observed during a routine physical exam or has trouble being fitted for clothes.

Currently, the two treatment alternatives commonly used are: (1) bracing (Milwaukee and Boston); and (2) surgery for spinal instrumentation and fusion. The Milwaukee brace, introduced in 1946, aims to prevent the deformity from increasing rather than to correct it,[12, 13] although some improvements have been described over 2–3 years of use. The brace is usually used when the curve is less than 30°.

Fusion of the spine can be performed anteriorly or posteriorly, although the posterior approach is usually used. The laminae of the vertebrae are exposed and fused with iliac crest bone graft. Harrington rods are inserted to produce spinal correction by longitudinal distraction. Postoperatively, the patients are immobilized in lightweight plaster casts for 6 months to provide time for additional spinal fusion to take place. This method was first described by Harrington in 1962.[14] In 1977, Luque offered a new technique involving the internal fixation by instrumenting each vertebra involved in the curve.[15] By sublamina wiring each vertebra, the force of the repair over the length of the fused spinal segments was evenly distributed.

The Luque method offers the patient early stability and does not require casting, allowing earlier ambulation.

Preanesthetic Plan

Routine requirements include full chart review, knowledge of the planned procedure, history and physical examination, chest x-ray (PA and lateral), review of spinal x-ray, ECG, and laboratory tests (CBC, SMA-6 and creatinine, urinalysis, clotting studies, and blood sample for type and screen).

Additional tests should include pulmonary function studies (PFTs), [pre- and postbronchodilator during erect and supine position], arterial blood gas analysis); cardiovascular studies (cardiology consult, echocardiogram); blood banking consult (if autologous blood transfusion is to be used or if there is a history of antigen–antibody reaction).

Informed consent should be based on an explanation of procedures (preoperative, monitoring, wake-up test, blood transfusion, postoperative care), and answers to questions from the patient and family.

Evaluation

Changes in the PFTs reflect the patient's tolerance to position changes as well as a response to bronchodilators, which may be required postoperatively. Immediately postoperative pulmonary function is significantly reduced. Thus any indication of borderline respiratory reserve requires great caution prior to early extubation. In one study after surgery, FRC, VC, and TLC were reduced $44 \pm 11\%$, $81 \pm 6\%$, and $61 \pm 10\%$ respectively, from preoperative values. Although FRC returned to within normal limits during the first several postoperative days, VC and TLC continued to be significantly reduced for at least 10 days.[16] Postoperative vital capacity is reduced below 50% of predicted values. Since these patients will remain supine and relatively inactive until plaster casting is completed, the reduced pulmonary function will place the patient at increased inability to cough and clear secretions.

If there is any indication of cardiac disease, a cardiology consult should be obtained. Studies have shown that peaked P-waves, enlarged pulmonary arterial diameters, and prolonged intervals between pulmonary valve closure and tricuspid valve opening are reliable indicators of increased pulmonary pressures.[10] Echocardiography is a reliable method for demonstrating right ventricular size and hemodynamic status. If a patient shows any signs of right ventricular hypertrophy, decompensation, and pulmonary hypertension, a pulmonary artery catheter should be inserted to assist in intraoperative monitoring and management.

Patients with other associated disease processes may be particularly sensitive to muscle relaxants or other anesthetic agents. Any questions about specific disease processes should be answered before entering the operating room and not after an accident has happened.

Intraoperative Monitoring

Spinal Cord Function

A catastrophic complication of spinal cord surgery for scoliosis is paraplegia. Currently, two methods are used to monitor spinal cord function during surgery.

Somatosensory evoked potentials (SSEPs) are electrical manifestations of the central nervous system's response to an electrical stimulus. The clinical usefulness of SSEPs is based on their ability to demonstrate abnormal sensory system function and integrity of pathways that cannot be clinically assessed under anesthesia. In spinal column surgery, loss of or changes in SSEPs are sensitive indicators of spinal cord damage or compromise.[17]

The blood supply to the normal spinal cord is extremely variable and there is limited collateral blood flow.[18] Moreover, the spinal cord and associated structures have little tolerance for hypoxia. Changes that occur because of scoliosis may cause further compromise of the blood supply and stretching of the nerve roots, increasing the sensitivity to hypotension and hypoxia. Grundy et al have shown that intraoperative SSEPs are very sensitive indicators of the hypoxia and ischemia associated with spinal column manipulation.[19] When changes are discovered, rapid reversal of spinal manipulation may prevent permanent spinal cord damage.[17]

Electrodes are applied to the patient preoperatively. After induction of anesthesia, baseline evoked potentials are obtained. Continuous SSEP monitoring is begun after positioning. The most common potentials monitored during Harrington rod surgery are generated from the posterior tibial nerves in both lower extremities and the scalp overlying the corresponding sensorimotor cortex (Cz'—Fz; C_5—Cz'). However, since intact SSEPs cannot always assure adequate motor function, intraoperative wake-up tests are often performed.

The wake-up test provides a reliable measure of gross motor function of the upper and lower extremities after spinal manipulation.[20] If compromise is noted, the surgeon can decrease the distraction and another wake-up test can be performed. Removal or modification of the Harrington rods within 3 hours after discovery of neurologic deficits decreases the risk of permanent neurologic sequelae.[21]

Preoperatively, the anesthesiologist should discuss the wake-up test with the patient. It is important to tell the patient that pain will not be felt and that recall will not be a problem. The patient should rehearse the wake-up drill several times with the anesthesiologist. Essentially, the test involves reversing the anesthetic effect and asking the patient to move his extremities. After satisfactory completion of the task, diazepam can be given to ensure amnesia.

Blood Loss and Replacement

Blood loss during scoliosis correction can range from 75–175ml per segment instrumented.[22] Losses as high as 50% of calculated blood volume have been reported. Blood loss is affected by surgical skill, proper patient positioning, use of subcutaneous epinephrine, and controlled hypotension.

The prone position on the Wilson frame or on chest rolls is designed to interfere minimally with venous return and ventilation. Improper patient positioning can obstruct venous return and lead to increased pressures in the epidural venous channels as well as requiring increased inspiratory pressures for ventilation. These higher pressures increase bleeding during surgical manipulation.

Subcutaneous infiltration of the surgical field with a large volume of diluted epinephrine (1:400,000) will promote vasoconstriction and help decrease blood loss during exposure of the spinal column. Controlled hypotension, with sodium nitroprusside as the drug of choice, has been shown to be safe and reliable in decreasing blood loss without endangering spinal cord blood flow and peripheral tissue perfusion.[23] Mean pressures of 60–80mmHg may be maintained for 30–60 minutes. Acid-base balance should be monitored to detect any signs of cyanide toxicity.

Today there is growing concern over the risk of infection from receiving blood products. Autologous blood transfusions offer a safe alternative, and may be achieved by intraoperative blood salvage (cell saver), hemodilution, and preoperative blood harvesting and intraoperative infusion.

The use of a cell saver to salvage and recirculate lost blood is common during cardiac surgery and should be considered for Harrington rod procedures if blood loss is expected to exceed 2 units of packed red blood cells. This volume of use justifies the cost of setting up the equipment. There is however, concern about increased soft tissue and bone damage when the cell saver is used, as well as decreased red blood cell survival time after reinfusion.[24]

Hemodilution is effective for blood replacement provided the patient is free of significant cardiopulmonary disease. Careful attention should be paid to fluid replacement during bloodletting to prevent hypotension or fluid overload. Cardiac output rises in response to a decrease in oxygen-carrying capacity and decreased peripheral vascular resistance. Hemodilution has been shown to increase tissue perfusion and oxygenation.[25]

Preoperative blood harvesting usually requires 3–4 weeks to obtain 4–5 units of whole blood for perioperative blood replacement. This is a safe and effective means of obtaining blood preoperatively without endangering the patient.

Postoperative blood losses can be as high as one half of the intraoperative blood loss due to sequestration and tissue infiltration of blood. Careful monitoring of drainage blood loss as well as serial hemoglobin levels will serve as an adequate guide to postoperative blood replacement.

Anesthetic Plan

Preanesthetic sedation is desirable. However, in rare instances as when scoliosis is due to a neurofibroma, muscle spasm may be integral to maintenance of spinal function. Reversal of this support mechanism by a drug such as diazepam may cause severe pain. If respiratory function is compromised, narcotics should be avoided or used only in low dosages.

An intravenous induction with pentothal (2–5mg/kg), fentanyl (2µg/kg) or sufentanil (0.2µg/kg) with adequate muscle relaxation (pancuronium 0.1mg/kg or atracurium 0.4mg/kg) is preferable. If airway management difficulties are anticipated, a short-acting muscle relaxant and/or an awake intubation should be considered.

Maintenance anesthesia can be achieved using several techniques. A balanced technique employs air/O_2, a continuous narcotic infusion (fentanyl 1–3 µg/kg/hr, or sufentanil 0.3 µg/kg/hr), and supplemental isoflurane for controlled hypotension. If evoked potentials are being used, isoflurane concentrations should be kept to under 1% to prevent excessive depression of the electrical potentials. If further hypotension is indicated, the narcotic infusion can be increased and/or sodium nitroprusside can be employed.

The use of a balanced technique offers a stable hemodynamic course throughout surgery including patient positioning. Narcotic infusion effectively attenuates catecholamine release in response to surgical stimuli, allows titration to a specific clinical endpoint (ie, BP control) and offers a smooth, pain-free wake-up at the end of surgery.

If an intraoperative wake-up test is planned, the narcotic infusion is discontinued. Muscle relaxant effect is reversed. Blood pressure and CO_2 levels are normalized. The patient is given 100% oxygen. If necessary, naloxone may be titrated 0.04mg/ml until the patient responds to commands. After voluntary movement has been satisfactorily demonstrated, anesthesia is reinstituted with pentothal, narcotic infusion, diazepam, and muscle relaxation.

Pain Control

Postoperative pain control is an important aspect of scoliosis surgery. Pain control can be achieved by administration of narcotics as necessary, continuous infusion of narcotics, or subarachnoid opiate instillation.

Intermittent narcotic administration is the least effective method for pain control. Medications are characteristically administered in doses too small to be therapeutic or after the pain is unmanageable. To be effective, narcotics should be administered in doses large enough to make the patient free of pain without significant respiratory depression. Subsequent narcotic administration should parallel the initial dose and should be given as the patient first starts to feel discomfort.

Continuous narcotic infusions allow a specific endpoint to be reached (ie, pain free) by achieving and maintaining a constant plasma level of narcotic. With the patient in the intensive care unit postoperatively, the anesthesiologist can continue the intraoperative narcotic infusion, but at a lower infusion rate. Since the ICU patient is closely monitored, a continuous narcotic infusion allows a smoother recovery period. The infusion can be titrated to the patient's needs (comparable to patient-controlled analgesia).

Subarachnoid opiates can be placed by the surgeon at the end of spinal manipulation, eg, 0.01mg/kg of morphine in the lumbar subarachnoid space with a small amount of barbotage before closing the surgical wound. Patients receiving subarachnoid morphine have been free of pain for more than 30 hours postoperatively. Patients must be monitored for signs of respiratory depression and, if needed, naloxoine can be titrated to reverse depressed respiration.

References

1. Gibbons P.A., Lee I.S.: Scoliosis and anesthesia. *Int Anesthesiol Clin*, Boston, Little Brown, 1985; 23(4):143–61.
2. Harrington P.R.: Aetiology of idiopathic scoliosis. *Clin Orthop* 126:17–25, 1977.
3. Roth A., Rosenthal A., Hall J.E., et al: Scoliosis and congenital heart disease. *Clin Orthop* 93:95–102, 1973.
4. Luke M.D., McDonnell E.J.: Congenital heart disease and scoliosis. *J Pediatr* 73:725–33, 1968.
5. Cobb J.R.: Outline for the study of scoliosis, in: J.W. Edwards, ed, *Institutional Course Lectures*. Ann Arbor, Michigan: American Academy of Orthopedic Surgeons, 1948; 5:261.
6. Bjure J., Grimby G., Kasalicky J., et al: Respiratory impairment and airway closure in patients with untreated idiopathic scoliosis. *Thorax* 25:451–6, 1970.
7. Smyth R.J., Chapman K.R., Wright T.A., et al: Pulmonary function in adolescents with mild idiopathic scoliosis. *Thorax* 39:901–4, 1984.
8. Kafer E.R.: Idiopathic scoliosis: gas exchange and the age dependence of arterial blood gases. *J Clin Invest* 58:825–33, 1976.
9. Boffa P., Stovin P., Shneerson J.: Lung developmental abnormalities in severe scoliosis. *Thorax* 39:681–2, 1984.
10. Shneerson J.M., Venco A., Prime F.J.: A study of pulmonary artery pressure, electrocardiography, and mechano-cardiography in thoracic scoliosis. *Thorax* 32:700–5, 1977.
11. Robotham J.L.: Cardiovascular disturbances in chronic respiratory insufficiency. *Am J Cardiol* 47:941–9, 1981.

12. Blount W.P., Schmidt A.C., Keeven E.D., et al: The Milwaukee brace in the operative treatment of scoliosis. *J Bone Joint Surg* 40(A):511–25, 1958.
13. Moe J.H., Kettleson D.M.: Idiopathic scoliosis: analysis of curve patterns and preliminary results of Milwaukee brace treatment—169 patients. *J Bone Joint Surg* 52(A):1509–33, 1970.
14. Harrington P.R.: Treatment of scoliosis corrections and internal fixation of the spine by instrumentation. *J Bone Joint Surg* 44:591–610, 1962.
15. Luque E.R.: Segmental spine instrumentation for correction of scoliosis. *Clin Orthop* 163:192, 1982.
16. Schur M.S., Brown J.J., Kafer E.R., et al: Postoperative pulmonary function in children: a comparison of scoliosis with peripheral surgery. *Am Rev Respir Dis* 130:46–51, 1984.
17. LaMont R.L., Wasson S.L., Green M.A.: Spinal cord monitoring during spinal surgery using somatosensory spinal evoked potentials. *J Pediatr Orthop* 3:31–6, 1983.
18. Gillian L.A.: Vascular supply of the spinal cord: clinical significance, in: S.N. Chou, El Seljeskoy, eds, Spinal Deformities and Neurological Dysfunction. New York: Raven Press, 1978, pp 11–24.
19. Grundy B.L., Heros R.C., Tung A.S., et al: Intraoperative hypoxia detected by evoked potential monitoring. *Anesth Analg* 60(6):437–9, 1981.
20. Vauzelle C., Stagnara P., Jouvinrouk P.: Functional monitoring of spinal cord activity during spinal surgery. *Clin Orthop* 93:173–8, 1973.
21. Chamberlain M.E., Bradshaw E.G.: The "wake-up test": a new approach using drug infusions. *Anesthesia* 40:780–2, 1985.
22. Gardner R.C.: Blood loss after spinal instrumentation and fusion in scoliosis (Harrington procedure). *Clin Orthop* 71:182–5, 1970.
23. Malcolm-Smith N.A., McMaster M.J.: The use of induced hypotension to control bleeding during posterior fusion for scoliosis. *J Bone Joint Surg* 65B:255–61, 1983.
24. Viviani G.R.: Autotransfusion in scoliosis surgery. *Clin Orthop* 135:74, 1978.
25. Barbier-Bohm G., Desmonts J.M., Couderc E., et al: Comparative effects of induced hypotension and normovolemic haemodilution on blood loss in total hip arthroplasty. *Br J Anaesth* 52:1039–43, 1980.

Self-Assessment Questions

Self-Assessment Questions

Select the single letter response that most correctly answers the question or completes the sentence.

Chapter 1

1. The effect of aspirin on coagulation is best evaluated by which of the following laboratory tests?
   a. PT
   b. PTT
   c. platelet count
   d. bleeding time
2. Aspirin adversely affects coagulation through which of the following mechanisms?
   a. stimulation of autoimmune-mediated platelet destruction
   b. inhibition of platelet prostaglandin endoperoxidase and thromboxane A formation
   c. suppression of Factors II, VII, IX and X synthesis
   d. combination with antithrombin III and subsequent inhibition of thrombin and other serine proteases
3. Abrupt discontinuation of propranolol is associated with intraoperative:
   a. supraventricular tachycardia with AV block
   b. hypotension unresponsive to vasopressors
   c. myocardial ischemia
   d. bronchospasm
4. Proper management of a patient treated with propranolol for angina pectoris includes:
   a. gradual discontinuation of the drug two weeks prior to surgery
   b. administration of the normal daily dose until the time of surgery
   c. discontinuation of propranolol 24–48 hours prior to surgery
   d. tapering the daily dose to 1/4–1/2 normal one week prior to surgery
5. Anesthetic induction and tracheal intubation in a patient with skeletal muscle weakness resulting from stroke is best accomplished by:
   a. tracheal intubation with a short-acting nondepolarizing relaxant such as atracurium or vecuronium

    b. inhalation induction followed by succinylcholine in a dose of 0.75–1.5mg/kg prior to intubation

    c. pretreatment with a nondepolarizing muscle relaxant prior to succinylcholine

    d. intubation after succinylcholine and monitoring of twitch response prior to subsequent doses of muscle relaxant

6. Which statement is most accurate regarding the patient with symptomatic coronary artery disease undergoing carotid endarterectomy?

    a. Operative mortality approaches 7%.

    b. Operative mortality is reduced significantly when coronary artery bypass grafting and carotid endarterectomy are performed simultaneously.

    c. Operative mortality of carotid endarterectomy is significantly reduced by the use of regional or local anesthesia.

    d. Operative mortality is almost equal to that in patients with no coexisting symptomatic coronary artery disease.

7. Which of the following statements concerning cerebrovascular disease is *not* true?

    a. The disease is bilateral in 50% of patients.

    b. The most common site of lesions is at vascular bifurcations.

    c. The disease process becomes symptomatic when the vascular lumen becomes 60% occluded.

    d. Intracranial lesions may be bypassed by means of anastomosis between an extracranial vessel and the affected vessel proximal to the lesion.

8. Which of the following statements is correct regarding the patient with uncontrolled hypertension?

    a. Diastolic blood pressure should be lowered to less than 90mmHg prior to induction in order to reduce the risk of myocardial ischemia resulting from intubation.

    b. Chronic hypertension causes a leftward shift of the cerebral autoregulatory curve.

    c. A balanced anesthesia technique using nitrous oxide/narcotic/relaxant affords better protection against intraoperative myocardial ischemia than inhalation agents.

    d. A preoperative diastolic pressure of 110mmHg or less poses no additional risk provided close intraoperative monitoring is combined with prompt therapy for control of systemic blood pressure fluctuations.

9. Which of the following statements accurately describes the pharmacology of clonidine?

    a. Its primary site of action is on peripheral arterioles.

    b. Intraoperative hypertensive episodes may be treated with intravenous clonidine in a dose of 0.1–0.2mg.

    c. Abrupt discontinuation may result in hypertension and myocardial ischemia.

    d. Its negative inotropic action may cause significant myocardial depression when inhalation agents are used.

10. Regarding the hyperkalemic response to succinylcholine administration in patients with denervated skeletal muscle, the following is true:

    a. The hyperkalemic response is maximum eight days following denervation.

b. The response may develop as early as four days following denervation.

c. The response may be reliably prevented by pretreatment with a non-depolarizing relaxant.

d. The magnitude of the hyperkalemic response may be reliably prevented by hyperventilation prior to succinylcholine administration.

Chapter 2

1. All of the following factors must be considered when choosing the technique for emergency intubation of the trauma patient *except*:
   a. NPO status of the patient
   b. arterial blood gas values
   c. extent of thoracic injuries
   d. the possibility of cervical spine injury

2. A left tension pneumothorax can be differentiated from cardiac tamponade by the presence of:
   a. hypotension
   b. venous distension
   c. hyperresonance over the left lung field
   d. evidence of thoracic trauma

3. An unconscious adult presents to ER with extensive facial injuries and evidence of cervical spine injury. The best way to secure the airway is:
   a. endotracheal intubation
   b. nasotracheal intubation
   c. tracheostomy
   d. cricothyroidotomy

4. A pneumatic antishock garment may be used to do all the following *except*:
   a. stabilize pelvic fractures
   b. increase total peripheral resistance
   c. apply pressure to an arterial bleeder in the leg
   d. reduce preload in a patient with congestive heart failure

5. Treatment of hypovolemic shock (>35% loss of circulating volume) may include any of the following *except*:
   a. crystalloid (balanced salt) solutions
   b. blood component therapy
   c. vasopressors
   d. polysaccharide-type plasma expanders

6. Peritoneal lavage is indicated in all of the following situations *except*:
   a. spinal cord trauma
   b. head injury
   c. drug or alcohol overdose
   d. a gravid uterus

7. Mechanical ventilation via an endotrachael tube is *not* indicated in cases of:
   a. raised intracranial pressure
   b. flail chest
   c. open pneumothorax
   d. severe facial fractures with laceration of the tongue

8. The *first* management priority of the trauma patient is:
    a. reduction of displaced fractures
    b. establishment of the airway
    c. obtaining a chest x-ray and cervical spine films
    d. eliciting a medical history
9. Which of the following signs is *not* associated with hypovolemic shock?
    a. tachycardia
    b. tachypnea
    c. widened pulse pressure
    d. orthostatic changes
10. A patient given uncrossmatched, type-specific blood may develop any of the following *except*:
    a. citrate toxicity
    b. hepatitis
    c. Rh incompatibility
    d. ABO incompatibility

Chapter 3

1. The mechanism of action of cocaine is:
    a. blockage of reuptake of catecholamines
    b. inhibition of dopamine release
    c. inhibition of acetylcholinesterase
    d. release of enkephalins locally
2. Use of metoclopramide and/or a phenothiazine in a cocaine-addicted patient can result in postoperative:
    a. delayed awakening
    b. hyperphagia
    c. depression
    d. all of the above
3. Acute injection of cocaine:
    a. raises MAC requirements
    b. causes no change in MAC requirement
    c. lowers MAC requirements
    d. has not been adequately studied
4. Present antimicrobial prophylaxis for the intravenous drug abuse patient includes:
    a. a penicillin and an aminoglycoside
    b. ampicillin
    c. gentamycin
    d. chloramphenicol
5. The decreased diastolic pressure often seen in heroin addicts is due to:
    a. hypovolemia
    b. hypoxia
    c. decreased sympathetic tone
    d. increased peripheral vascular resistance

6. Heroin addicts often have:
   a. pulmonary hypertension
   b. decreased peak expiratory flow rate
   c. granulomatous disease
   d. all of the above
7. The relative chance of a heroin addict being HBsAG positive relative to the general population is:
   a. four times
   b. two times
   c. five times
   d. no different
8. Which of the following drugs may safely be administered to a heroin addict?
   a. ketamine
   b. etomidate
   c. morphine
   d. all of the above
9. One mg heroin is equal in analgesic activity to:
   a. 1mg methadone
   b. 8mg morphine
   c. 60mg meperidine
   d. 100μg fentanyl
10. The preferred inhalation agent for use in intravenous drug abusers is:
   a. isoflurane
   b. enflurane
   c. halothane
   d. methoxyflurane

Chapter 4

1. The minimum systolic blood pressure (mmHg) considered normal in a healthy full-term infant is:
   a. 70.
   b. 60.
   c. 50.
   d. 40.
2. When using an inflatable cuff to measure blood pressure:
   a. The width of the cuff should equal two-thirds the length of the upper arm.
   b. Use of a narrower cuff leads to pressure measurements lower than actual pressures.
   c. The width of the cuff should equal one-half the length of the upper arm.
   d. Pressures measured in the leg are lower than those measured in the arm.
3. A child presents with a runny nose. Which of the following statements is *false*?
   a. It may be a prodrome of an asthmatic attack.
   b. The remainder of the physical examination may be normal even if the etiology is infectious.
   c. A chest x-ray should be routinely obtained.
   d. An elevated white cell count suggests a bacterial infection.

4. The routine preoperative laboratory work-up in a child scheduled for day surgery includes:
   a. chest x-ray
   b. hematocrit and urinalysis
   c. electrocardiogram
   d. sickle cell prep
5. The management of a child with a low preoperative hematocrit includes all of the following *except*:
   a. postponement of elective surgery
   b. appropriate laboratory work-up
   c. blood transfusion
   d. iron supplementation, if the cause of the anemia is dietary
6. The risks of anesthetizing a child with a low hematocrit include all of the following *except*:
   a. increased risk of intraoperative bradycardia
   b. an increased risk of cardiac arrest
   c. increased risk of hypoxemia
   d. the possibility of sickling in the perioperative period, if sickle cell disease is the cause
7. The most effective means of decreasing psychological trauma in a child presenting for surgery and anesthesia is:
   a. premedication
   b. use of audio-visual aids
   c. establishing rapport with the child
   d. use of transparent face masks
8. The criteria for the selection of children for day surgery include all of the following *except*:
   a. the need for endotracheal intubation
   b. the duration of the operation
   c. the physical status of the patient
   d. willing parents
9. The normal values for a healthy full-term newborn are all of the following *except*:
   a. a tidal volume of 6ml/kg
   b. a minimum systolic blood pressure of 60mmHg
   c. an average hematocrit of 55%
   d. a heart rate of 80 beats/minute
10. The advantages of outpatient surgery include all of the following *except*:
    a. economy
    b. less emotional disturbance to the child
    c. lower incidence of nosocomial infections
    d. fewer laboratory tests are necessary

Chapter 5

1. Which of the following statements about anemia in the patient presenting for renal transplantation is *true*?
   a. The anemia is primarily due to gastrointestinal bleeding.
   b. A hemoglobin level of at least 10g% is required prior to transplantation.

c. The physiologic effect of anemia in end-stage renal disease is overcome by production of 2,3-DPG.

d. Decreased erythropoiesis and increased RBC destruction are common.

2. Hyperkalemia in the patient with chronic renal failure:
   a. is definitively treated by dialysis or administration of ion exchange resins
   b. is always excessive following the administration of succinylcholine
   c. is best treated by the administration of calcium salts
   d. presents as a prolonged Q-T interval

3. Which of the following laboratory tests is *most* important prior to renal transplantation?
   a. chest x-ray
   b. serum potassium
   c. blood glucose
   d. white blood count

4. Which of the following chronic medications need *not* be continued preoperatively?
   a. propranolol
   b. steroids
   c. methyldopa
   d. diuretics

5. Which of the following statements about hypertension and renal transplantation is false?
   a. Blood pressure is directly related to time of last dialysis.
   b. A preoperative diastolic BP >110mmHg increases anesthetic risk.
   c. Intra- or postoperative hypertension may endanger the vascular anastomosis.
   d. Hypertension is common in patients with end-stage renal disease.

6. Renal transplantation became a routinely successful therapy for end stage renal disease in:
   a. 1930
   b. 1950
   c. 1960
   d. 1970

7. Factors influencing graft survival include all of the following *except*:
   a. immunosuppression
   b. etiology of renal disease
   c. histocompatibility
   d. duration of end-stage renal disease

8. Which of the following statements is *false*?
   a. Patients with diabetes mellitus are particularly at risk for hyperkalemia during renal transplantation.
   b. Dextrose and water is the fluid replacement of choice during renal transplantation.
   c. Metabolic acidosis is relatively benign at a bicarbonate level >15mEq/L in patients with end-stage renal disease.
   d. Patients with end-stage renal disease may have platelet dysfunction.

9. Which one of the following statements about dialysis as a modality for treating end-stage renal disease is *false*?
   a. Sepsis is the most common cause of death in dialysis patients.

    b. Hemodialysis should be performed at least 6–8 hours prior to surgery.

    c. Peritoneal dialysis should be continued up until the time for surgery.

    d. It is important to know the patient's pre- and postdialysis weight.

10. Which of the following statements is *true*?

    a. Diazepam must not be given to the transplant recipient.

    b. Renal transplantation must frequently be performed on an emergency basis.

    c. Perfusion of kidneys for transplantation is superior to preservation in cold electrolyte solution.

    d. All currently available anesthetic agents and techniques have been successfully used in the management of patients for renal transplantation.

Chapter 6

1. Regarding symptoms associated with pheochromocytoma, which of the following statements is *false*?

    a. The classic triad consisting of sweating, palpitations, and headache is highly suggestive of pheochromocytoma.

    b. Biochemical confirmation of excess catecholamine secretion should be obtained to make a definitive diagnosis.

    c. Pheochromocytoma may be mistakenly diagnosed as depression or a psychiatric disorder.

    d. There is usually no correlation between severity of symptoms and degree of hypertension.

2. The hypertension of pheochromocytoma:

    a. is a constant feature

    b. does not respond to antihypertensive medications

    c. may be episodic or sustained

    d. is best managed by β-blockade

3. Regarding the diagnosis of pheochromocytoma, which of the following statements is *true*?

    a. Since pheochromocytoma has familial tendencies, equivocal cases should by karyotyped to confirm the diagnosis.

    b. Assay of serum catecholamines is probably the most sensitive of available biochemical diagnostic tests.

    c. Results of serum catecholamine assays are most reliable if samples are obtained during a hypertensive episode.

    d. Localization should be confirmed by angiogram or selective venous sampling prior to surgery.

4. Which of the following statements is *false* as it applies to urinary diagnostic tests for pheochromocytoma?

    a. They are dependent on renal function.

    b. Under most circumstances, they will confirm or exclude a diagnosis.

    c. They are probably not as reliable as assays of serum catecholamines.

    d. Of the four substances that are routinely measured, elevated levels of vanillylmandelic acid correlate best with presence of pheochromocytoma.

5. Which of the following statements is *true* regarding phentolamine and phenoxybenzamine?

    a. A hazard of preoperative α-adrenergic blockade is worsening myocarditis with progressive ECG changes.

b. Decreased hematocrit is an indication of the effectiveness of α-blockade.
c. A side effect of α-blockade is worsening hyperglycemia.
d. Preoperative α-blockade is optimal when it is total.

6. Preoperative goals for the pheochromocytoma patient include all of the following, *except*:
   a. weight loss
   b. an increase in intravascular volume
   c. absent or infrequent PVCs
   d. resolution of ST-T-wave abnormalities

7. Which of the following is *not* essential for "state of the art" monitoring of the patient for excision of pheochromocytoma?
   a. 5-lead electrocardiogram
   b. precordial Doppler
   c. neuromuscular blockade monitor
   d. arterial catheter

8. All of the following should be prepared or be immediately accessible prior to the induction of anesthesia *except*:
   a. lidocaine, propanolol, and a defibrillator
   b. dantrolene
   c. a potent antihypertensive agent such as sodium nitroprusside
   d. a vasopressor

9. Which statement is *true* regarding drug administration to a patient with a pheochromocytoma?
   a. Succinylcholine is contraindicated because of documented episodes of lethal hyperkalemia which have occurred during the induction of patients with pheochromocytoma.
   b. The first line of treatment for hypotension following tumor isolation should be a norepinephrine, dopamine, or phenylephrine infusion.
   c. If a narcotic is to be used, morphine is the best choice.
   d. Pancuronium and gallamine should be avoided because they are vagolytic, and may give rise to sympathetic reactions.

10. Overall, it is important to:
    a. maintain a high index of suspicion of pheochromocytoma when hypertension occurs in an unusual setting or presentation
    b. confirm diagnosis with biochemical evidence of hypersecretion of catecholamines, and if possible, localize lesions with noninvasive testing
    c. obtain consultations from an endocrinologist, and, in most cases, administer α-blocking agents preoperatively
    d. all of the above

Chapter 7

1. Which of the following is the most common indication for diagnostic muscle biopsy for MH susceptibility?
   a. positive response to dantrolene
   b. history of masseter muscle rigidity after succinylcholine
   c. history of severe muscle cramps
   d. well-documented MH episode during anesthesia

2. MH is a genetic disorder of:
   a. neonates

   b. first two years of life
   c. children and young adults
   d. middle-aged adults

3. In investigation of MH susceptibility, the most important factor is a:
   a. history of MH in the family
   b. history of Duchenne's muscular dystrophy
   c. history of a well-documented MH crisis during anesthesia
   d. positive muscle biopsy (caffeine and halothane contracture tests)

4. What would you advise patients with known MH susceptibility 2 weeks prior to surgery?
   a. normal activity without restrictions
   b. restricted physical activity
   c. normal activity with oral dantrolene twice a day
   d. limited activity and bed rest two days prior to admission

5. The incidence of positive muscle biopsy in patients who develop masseter muscle rigidity is?
   a. 10%
   b. 30%
   c. 60%
   d. 80%

6. What is the association between stress, exercise and awake episodes of MH in susceptible swine and humans?
   a. high incidence in humans, low incidence in swine
   b. high incidence in both swine and humans
   c. high incidence in humans
   d. low incidence in humans, high incidence in swine

7. The most efficient drug in preoperative preparation of MH patients to prevent an MH episode is:
   a. alpha-blocking agent and oral dantrolene
   b. beta-blocking agent and oral dantrolene
   c. calcium blocking agent and oral dantrolene
   d. intravenous dantrolene

8. The best choice of preoperative medication for MH susceptible patients is:
   a. reassurance alone
   b. reassurance and narcotic-anticholinergic combination
   c. reassurance and antianxiety medication
   d. reassurance and narcotic-sedative combination

9. A 19-year-old patient scheduled for elective hernia repair gives you a history of jaw rigidity which occurred 10 years ago when he was exposed to anesthesia. The surgery was cancelled. What should you do?
   a. cancel the case until the diagnosis of MH is confirmed
   b. manage the patient as MH susceptible by avoiding triggering agents
   c. give spinal anesthesia because it is completely safe
   d. postpone the surgery, obtain previous anesthetic records and contact the anesthesiologist involved

10. A 24-year-old black male on a college football team is scheduled for emergency open reduction of a fracture of the left humerus. During the preanesthetic visit, you find out that the patient's younger brother had a bad reaction to anesthesia 5 years ago when he was scheduled for tonsillectomy. What is the appropriate action?

a. delay the case until the family history is available
b. proceed with the case using an anesthetic technique "safe" for MH susceptible patients and have I.V. dantrolene available
c. refer the patient to an MH center
d. order additional laboratory tests including CPK and proceed, or delay the case based on laboratory results

Chapter 8

1. Which of the following statements is correct regarding the epidemiology of SCI?
   a. It most often occurs in the elderly in whom osteoporosis predisposes the spine to more extensive damage from trauma.
   b. The most frequently injured area is the lumbosacral.
   c. Mortality from SCI is 47% compared with an overall mortality from trauma of 6.7%.
   d. It is a self-limiting process which requires only a short period of hospitalization in order to stabilize the injury.
2. Concerning hypercalcemia in the SCI patient:
   a. The most frequent EKG changes manifest as ventricular ectopic beats.
   b. Initial treatment is hydration with normal saline and diuresis using furosemide.
   c. Proper treatment includes use of chelating agents and mithramycin.
   d. The primary cause of elevated serum calcium is parathyroid hyperactivity.
3. The acute phase of SCI (first 24–48 hours) is characterized by:
   a. The potential for development of autonomic hyperreflexia and renal failure.
   b. Osteoporosis, limb contractures and diffuse muscle spasm.
   c. Electrolyte abnormalities and negative nitrogen balance.
   d. Spinal shock and pulmonary insufficiency.
4. Spinal shock is best described as:
   a. hypotension, absent deep tendon reflexes and flaccid paralysis
   b. hypertension, hyperreflexic deep tendon reflexes and flaccid paralysis
   c. hypertension, absent deep tendon reflexes and skeletal muscle spasm
   d. hypotension, hyperreflexic deep tendon reflexes and skeletal muscle spasm
5. Regarding autonomic hyperreflexia in SCI:
   a. It occurs in over 85% of spinal cord transsections below the T5 level.
   b. The potential for occurrence declines 4 weeks after initial injury.
   c. Vasodilation below the site of injury, vasoconstriction above the site of injury and tachycardia are the major manifestations.
   d. The potential for occurrence is greatest 4 weeks after injury, but it may manifest any time thereafter following a period of dormancy.
6. Regarding the relationship between cervical cord lesions and pulmonary dysfunction:
   a. Total loss of diaphragmatic function results from lesions at C6 or below.
   b. Intercostal paralysis accompanying a spinal cord lesion at C6 may result in a 60% reduction in tidal volume.
   c. A lesion at C4–C5 results in only a minor impairment of respiratory function.
   d. Sleep apnea occurs due to abolition of the Hering-Breuer reflex.

7. Which of the following statements is correct regarding succinylcholine use in SCI patients?
   a. The potential for the hyperkalemic response may persist as long as 6 months following the initial injury.
   b. The hyperkalemic response is not likely to occur in lesions located below T6.
   c. Prior treatment with a small dose of a nondepolarizing drug (3mg tubocurarine) reliably prevents the occurrence of the hyperkalemic response.
   d. Hyperventilation prior to succinylcholine administration has been demonstrated to reduce the magnitude of the hyperkalemic response.
8. Which one of the following statements most accurately describes the sequelae of a spinal cord injury at the T1–T4 level?
   a. The potential for occurrence of autonomic hyperreflexia is almost nonexistent with lesions below this level.
   b. Spinal cord injury at this level is incompatible with life because of denervation of the diaphragm.
   c. Injury at this level results in loss of sympathetic innervation of the sino-atrial node.
   d. Only minor reductions in tidal volume and vital capacity result.
9. Therapy directed at minimizing further spinal damage during the acute phase of SCI includes:
   a. use of controlled hypotension to obtain a mean arterial pressure of 50mmHg in order to minimize bleeding at the site of injury
   b. high doses of β-adrenergic blocking agents to reduce the vasoconstrictive effect of endogenous catecholamines on spinal cord microvasculature
   c. maintaining optimal arterial oxygenation and cord perfusion pressure
   d. small doses of nondepolarizing muscle relaxants to prevent skeletal muscle spasm at the site of injury
10. What is the most frequent cause of death following high SCI (C2–T1)?
    a. acute respiratory failure due to loss of intercostal and diaphragmatic innervation
    b. myocardial dysfunction secondary to sino-atrial node denervation
    c. renal failure and electrolyte imbalance
    d. pulmonary embolus

Chapter 9

1. Respiratory papillomas are:
   a. predominantly subglottic
   b. benign and undergo spontaneous regression
   c. caused by viruses and bacteria
   d. characterized by stridor without hoarseness
2. Surgical treatment of laryngeal papillomas:
   a. is usually curative after two endoscopies
   b. always requires prophylactic tracheotomy
   c. aims at reduction of tumor mass
   d. requires concomitant antiviral agents
3. Stridor in laryngeal papillomas is:
   a. always high pitched
   b. present during inspiration and expiration

   c. decreased by reducing airflow rate

   d. diagnostic

4. Which of the following statements about lasers is *false*?

   a. Biological tissue is vaporized.

   b. The high-energy beam increases bleeding.

   c. The beam can be precisely focused.

   d. The energy is a form of electromagnetic radiation.

5. Which of the following is *not* a characteristic of the laser beam?

   a. spatial coherence, ie, waves are in step in space

   b. temporal coherence, ie, waves are in step in time

   c. polychromaticity, ie, many wavelengths

   d. well-defined wave fronts

6. The *correct* statement about laser beams is:

   a. They are invisible.

   b. The invisible beam requires alignment with a visible trace light.

   c. Energy density of the laser beam is independent of the source.

   d. The depth of the beam must be adjusted prior to use.

7. Respiratory distress following laser surgery is *most likely* due to:

   a. edema of the epiglottis

   b. foreign body in the trachea

   c. recurrent laryngeal nerve injury

   d. edema of the uvula

8. Appropriate anesthetic steps to reduce laser fire hazard include the use of:

   a. low oxygen concentration (25%)

   b. red rubber endotracheal tube

   c. water-soluble instead of oil-based lubricants

   d. nitrogen/oxygen rather than nitrous oxide/oxygen

9. Anesthesia for laser surgery of laryngeal papillomas requires:

   a. no belladonna premedication

   b. ketamine induction

   c. immobility of the target area

   d. no suction in the surgical field

10. In the recovery room, appropriate therapy should include:

   a. antibiotic therapy

   b. steroid coverage

   c. mechanical ventilation

   d. routine laryngoscopy to exclude supraglottic edema

Chapter 10

1. Symptoms of AS include all of the following *except*:

   a. angina pectoris

   b. hypertension

   c. congestive heart failure

   d. syncope

2. AS may be caused by:

   a. bacterial endocarditis

   b. hypertension

   c. rheumatic disease

   d. trauma

3. Which of the following statements is *false*?
   a. The normal aortic valve area is about 3cm^2/m^2.
   b. Acute AI is poorly tolerated compared with chronic AI.
   c. Concentric hypertrophy occurs with chronic AI.
   d. Risk of sudden death occurs with AS.

4. Symptoms of chronic AI include all of the following *except*:
   a. narrow pulse pressure
   b. head bobbing
   c. diastolic thrill
   d. bounding pulse

5. Anesthetic management for patients with AI should include:
   a. maintenance of sinus rhythm
   b. afterload reduction to improve cardiac output
   c. normal to increased blood pressure
   d. maintenance of normal heart rate

6. The best indicator of the severity of AS is:
   a. systolic blood pressure
   b. heart rate
   c. calculated valve area
   d. cardiac index

7. Which of the following is *false*?
   a. AI may be either acute or chronic.
   b. AI may be produced by trauma.
   c. Chronic AI is characterized by a wide pulse pressure.
   d. Concentric hypertrophy of the left ventricle is seen with chronic AI.

8. Pathophysiology of AI results in:
   a. obstruction to left ventricular ejection
   b. left ventricular volume overload
   c. reduced ventricular compliance
   d. symptoms of angina pectoris

9. A patient with AS scheduled for repair develops chest pain and diaphoresis. Blood pressure falls to 90/50 and heart rate increases to 140/min. The best treatment at this time should be:
   a. a sedative to calm the patient
   b. an inotropic drug to increase blood pressure and contractility
   c. a beta blocker to slow the heart rate
   d. nitrates to relieve chest pain

10. Pre-operative evaluation of a patient with valvular disease should include all the following *except*:
    a. history of symptoms and their progression
    b. evaluation for signs of congestive failure
    c. angiographic studies to determine ventricular function
    d. a graded stress test

Chapter 11

1. Factors predisposing to the development of diabetic ketoacidosis include all of the following *except*:
   a. pregnancy

   b. sepsis

   c. trauma

   d. obesity

2. The stress of surgery, trauma, and anesthesia is associated with elevated levels of all the following hormones *except*:

   a. insulin

   b. glucocorticoids

   c. aldosterone

   d. ADH

3. Diabetic ketoacidosis is associated with all of the following *except*:

   a. extracellular hyperglycemia

   b. intracellular glucopenia

   c. insulin deficiency

   d. deficiency of growth hormone

4. Each of the following processes *except one* contribute to the pathophysiology of diabetic ketoacidosis:

   a. osmotic diuresis

   b. hyperosmolality

   c. electrolyte depletion

   d. fluid overload

5. Important historical data that support the diagnosis of diabetic ketoacidosis may include all of the following *except*:

   a. prior history of diabetes mellitus

   b. nausea and vomiting

   c. sudden onset of illness, without prodrome

   d. confusion

6. Physical examination of the patient in diabetic ketoacidosis may reveal all of the following *except*:

   a. signs consistent with dehydration

   b. Cheyne-Stokes respiration

   c. alterations in vital signs

   d. acetone-tainted breath

7. In the patient suspected to be in diabetic ketoacidosis, the most practical and informative initial laboratory examination is:

   a. SMA-6

   b. arterial blood gases

   c. reagent testing of urine for glucose and ketones

   d. calculation of serum osmolality

8. Guidelines for preoperative management of diabetic ketoacidosis include all of the following *except*:

   a. observation of urine output, cardiac filling pressures, and changes in vital signs as guides to volume resuscitation

   b. aggressive administration of alkalinizing solutions to maintain pH 7.30–7.40

   c. serial serum potassium levels

   d. frequent arterial blood gases to assess degree of ketosis

9. Which statement is *false* about crystalline insulin and the treatment of diabetic ketoacidosis?

   a. in vivo half life is about 5 minutes

b. traditionally administered in large boluses
c. because it sticks to the walls of standard containers, it is ineffective if administered by infusion
d. intravenous administration is preferable to subcutaneous injection
10. Important principles in the preoperative management of diabetic ketoacidosis include:
a. correction of fluid, electrolyte, and acid-base abnormalities
b. modification of therapy to account for coexisting systemic illness
c. return to glucose metabolism by judicious use of insulin
d. all of the above

Chapter 12

1. An 18-year-old male who is 25% above ideal weight is considered:
a. overweight
b. obese
c. normal
d. morbidly obese
2. Body mass index is calculated as:
a. weight in pounds divided by height in inches
b. weight in kilograms divided by height by inches
c. weight in kilograms divided by height in meters
d. weight in kilograms divided by height in meters squared
3. The most useful index of morbid obesity is:
a. body mass index
b. Broca index
c. insurance company data
d. body densitometry
4. Height in centimeters minus 100 is equal to:
a. ideal body weight
b. Broca index
c. a measurement of adiposity
d. body mass index
5. Which of the following characterizes complex morbid obesity?
a. hyperventilation syndromes
b. pulmonary hypotension
c. systemic hypertension
d. predisposition to cor pulmonale
6. A frequent feature of the Pickwickian syndrome is:
a. left ventricular failure
b. systemic hypertension
c. cyanosis related to left ventricular hypertrophy
d. periodic respiration
7. Total metabolism in the morbidly obese is:
a. in linear relation to increased body weight and surface area
b. frequently associated with an abnormal respiratory quotient
c. a minor factor controlling cardiac output and minute ventilation
d. up to 4 times normal
8. Pulmonary dysfunction in the morbidly obese is usually associated with:
a. markedly increased chest wall compliance

b. decreased ERV, FRC, and vital capacity
c. decreased lung compliance
d. abnormal closing volume and inspiratory reserve volume

9. Associated cardiovascular changes in the morbidly obese include:
   a. decreased cardiac output and polycythemia
   b. increased systolic and diastolic pressures with elevated SVR
   c. decreased fibrinolytic activity but elevated fibrinogen levels
   d. systemic hypotension

10. Which of the following is the least crucial factor during the preanesthetic visit?
    a. assessment of psychologic status
    b. pulmonary function testing
    c. SGOT of 56
    d. PaO_2 of 74 on room air

Chapter 13

1. The anticholinesterase drug of choice for the treatment of myasthenia gravis is:
   a. edrophonium
   b. neostigmine
   c. ambenonium
   d. pyridostigmine

2. The most common respiratory abnormality in myasthenia gravis is a decrease in:
   a. forced maximum inspiratory force
   b. vital capacity
   c. tidal volume
   d. peak flow

3. The dose of pancuronium to produce 95% twich depression in patients with myasthenia gravis compared with normal patients is less by a factor of:
   a. 2
   b. 4
   c. 10
   d. 16

4. MG is most commonly diagnosed by:
   a. curare testing
   b. edrophonium challenge
   c. assay for ACh antibody
   d. electrophysiologic testing

5. The defect in myasthenia gravis at the neuromuscular junction is:
   a. decreased release of ACh from the presynaptic membrane
   b. decreased density of postsynaptic ACh receptors
   c. increased metabolism of ACh
   d. decreased affinity of ACh for the postsynaptic receptor

6. Patients with myasthenia gravis who are given succinylcholine initially demonstrate:
   a. resistance
   b. increased sensitivity
   c. increased metabolism
   d. normal response

7. Duration of action of oral pyridostigmine is:
   a. 1–2 hours
   b. 2–3 hours
   c. 3–4 hours
   d. 4–5 hours
8. All of the following are characteristic signs of a myasthenia crisis *except*:
   a. sweating
   b. mydriasis
   c. salivation
   d. miosis
9. The most frequent initial complaint of myasthenic patients involves which of the following muscle groups?
   a. respiratory
   b. extremity
   c. bulbar
   d. ocular
10. MG patients on chronic anticholinesterase therapy should be managed preoperatively by:
   a. increased dose the morning of surgery
   b. medication discontinued 24 hours prior to surgery
   c. no medication change
   d. medication administered I.M. while in hospital

Chapter 14

1. Missile injuries are associated with epidural, subdural, or intracerebral hematomas in what percentage of cases?
   a. 10%
   b. 20%
   c. 50%
   d. 90%
2. In general, which of the following injuries (size and severity being equal) should be considered the most urgent of intracranial emergencies requiring immediate surgical intervention?
   a. compressed skull fracture
   b. arterial epidural hematoma
   c. subdural hematoma
   d. intraparenchymal bleed
3. The first priority in the anesthesiologist's care of the head injured patient is always:
   a. obtaining a complete history
   b. sedation in the combative patient
   c. establishment of the airway
   d. reduction of intracranial pressure
4. Regarding the practice of controlled hyperventilation in head injured patients:
   a. All patients with major head injury should be hyperventilated.
   b. Hyperventilation to $PaCO_2$ 23mmHg has no known deleterious effects.
   c. Hyperventilation is not beneficial if cerebral hyperemia exists.
   d. Hyperventilation shifts the CO_2 dissociation curve to the right.

5. Common electrocardiographic abnormalities in the head injured patient include all of the following *except*:
   a. ST and T-wave changes
   b. prolonged QT-interval
   c. prominent U-waves
   d. extreme bradycardia
6. Intracranial hypertension in the head injured patient is *least well* controlled by:
   a. hyperventilation
   b. barbiturate infusion
   c. craniotomy
   d. steroid administration
7. The Glasgow Coma Scale:
   a. is a prognostic indicator of outcome after head injury
   b. must be performed every hour
   c. depends on patient cooperation for accurate measurement
   d. indicates good outcome at values of 8 or less
8. The primary preventable cause of death after head injury is:
   a. intracranial hypertension
   b. bradycardia
   c. respiratory obstruction
   d. blood loss
9. Epidural hematoma:
   a. is a frequent complication of head injury
   b. is rarely emergent
   c. is more common in older age groups
   d. usually results from laceration of middle meningeal vessels
10. The most common cause of hypoxia following head injury is:
    a. mechanical obstruction
    b. aspiration
    c. neurogenic causes
    d. drug overdose

Chapter 15

1. The incidence of pregnancy induced hypertension (PIH) is approximately:
   a. 0.1–0.2%
   b. 1–2%
   c. 5–7%
   d. 12–15%
2. The clinical feature that is least useful to establish a diagnosis of PIH is:
   a. blood pressure exceeding 140/90
   b. systolic blood pressure increase of 30mmHg or diastolic blood pressure increase of 15mmHg from prepregnancy values
   c. proteinuria exceeding 2 grams in 24 hours
   d. edema
3. The most common cause of maternal mortality in PIH is:
   a. abruptio placentae
   b. cerebral hemorrhage and pulmonary edema

    c. renal failure

    d. bleeding diathesis

4. Definitive therapy for PIH is:

    a. strict bed rest with left uterine displacement

    b. antihypertensive and anticonvulsant therapy

    c. cautious hydration

    d. delivery of the placenta

5. There is convincing evidence for elevations in cardiac output and renal and placental perfusion with:

    a. continuous infusion of magnesium sulfate

    b. lumbar epidural analgesia (LEA)

    c. hydralazine

    d. left uterine displacement

6. The first priority in managing a patient who has had an eclamptic seizure is:

    a. administration of phenytoin

    b. steroid administration

    c. seizure control and airway management

    d. treatment of malignant hypertension with sodium nitroprusside

7. The main objection to the administration of LEA to patients with PIH is:

    a. high incidence of dural puncture

    b. the majority of patients have platelet counts of less than $50,000/mm^3$

    c. blood levels of local anesthetic could exacerbate seizures

    d. the fetus is particularly vulnerable to hypotension

8. Suggested guidelines for the administration of LEA in patients with severe PIH include:

    a. prevention of hypotension by the prior administration of ephedrine 25mg intramuscularly

    b. a double catheter technique

    c. the inclusion of 1:200,000 epinephrine to detect intravascular injection

    d. cautious volume infusion using central venous pressure as a guide

9. If magnesium sulfate has been administered

    a. required doses of muscle relaxants are higher

    b. precurarization is mandatory

    c. LEA is contraindicated

    d. potentiation of neuromuscular blocking agents can be expected

10. Uterine atony can be managed by:

    a. methylergonovine administered intramuscularly

    b. small intravenous boluses of oxytocin

    c. 2–3% halothane

    d. uterine massage and a dilute oxytocin infusion

Chapter 16

1. Classical neurofibromatosis is transmitted as an:

    a. autosomal recessive trait

    b. autosomal dominant trait

    c. sex-linked trait

    d. none of the above

2. Embryonic neural crest cells migrate to:
   a. pigmentary tissues
   b. endocrine tissues
   c. neural supportive tissues
   d. all of the above
3. The three defining features of neurofibromatosis are:
   a. neurofibromas, café-au-lait spots, kyphoscoliosis
   b. intersitital alveolitis, café-au-lait spots, neurofibromas
   c. café-au-lait spots, Lisch nodules, neurofibromas
   d. café-au-lait spots, Weber nodules, neurofibromas
4. Plexiform neurofibromas are associated with:
   a. pituitary tumor
   b. pheochromocytoma
   c. spinal cord tumor
   d. none of the above
5. What percentage of neurofibromatosis patients have intellectual impairment?
   a. 15
   b. 40
   c. 60
   d. 94
6. Difficulty in securing an airway in neurofibromatosis patients is due to involvement of:
   a. larynx
   b. pharynx
   c. cervical spine
   d. all of the above
7. Induction of anesthesia in the neurofibromatosis patient with elevated ICP requires all of the following *except*:
   a. hyperventilation
   b. barbiturates
   c. lidocaine
   d. ketamine
8. Prolonged neuromuscular block has been reported in patients with neurofibromatosis with *all* of the following agents *except*:
   a. pancuronium
   b. atracurium
   c. d-tubocurarine
   d. succinylcholine
9. Which statement regarding autonomic hyperreflexia is true?
   a. Succinylcholine produces hyperkalemia.
   b. Bladder stimulation may trigger such a response.
   c. Patients with a spinal cord lesion below T7 are at special risk.
   d. Vasodilatation below the level of the lesion is characteristic.
10. Which of the following is most specific in the diagnosis of pheochromocytoma?
   a. 24-hour collection of urinary vanillylmandelic acid
   b. 24-hour collection of urinary catecholamines
   c. 24-hour collection of urinary metanephrine
   d. 24-hour collection of urinary tyrosine

Chapter 17

1. The drug of choice for the management of trigeminal neuralgia is:
   a. phenytoin
   b. carbamazepine
   c. baclofen
   d. valproic acid
2. Trigeminal neuralgia is most commonly diagnosed by:
   a. CAT scan with contrast
   b. neurologic examination
   c. history
   d. all of the above
3. Trigeminal neuralgia is caused by:
   a. viral infection
   b. trauma
   c. degenerative demyelination
   d. all of the above
4. Tic douloureux is characterized by the following, *except*:
   a. Tic pain is so severe it keeps the patient awake at night.
   b. It afflicts women more often than men.
   c. It can coexist with multiple sclerosis.
   d. Typical onset is after age 40 years.
5. Surgical management of trigeminal neuralgia is:
   a. the primary modality in the treatment of tic pain
   b. palliative but not curative
   c. not recommended for the elderly or debilitated
   d. by chemical or thermal destruction of the trigeminal nerve
6. Among the pharmacologic agents used in the management of tic pain, which is a gamma aminobutyric acid (GABA) analog?
   a. phenytoin (Dilantin)
   b. carbamazepine (Tegretol)
   c. baclofen (Lioresal)
   d. chlorphenesin carbamate (Maolate)
7. Anesthetic considerations for percutaneous trigeminal neurolysis include:
   a. It can be performed under local anesthesia because it is not too painful a procedure.
   b. Tracheal intubation is needed for positioning the needle electrode through the foramen ovale.
   c. Monitoring of blood pressure, electrocardiogram, heart, and breath sounds are essential.
   d. Patients are preferably heavily premedicated.
8. The most sensitive readily available method for the detection of venous air embolism is:
   a. right atrial catheter
   b. precordial Doppler ultrasound unit
   c. end-tidal carbon dioxide monitor
   d. electrocardiogram
9. Posterior fossa craniectomy for microvascular decompression of the trigeminal nerve:

    a. is reserved for those patients in whom medical treatment has failed
    b. can be done only in the sitting position
    c. spares the nerve and treats the apparent cause of the pain
    d. requires right atrial catheterization at all times for aspiration of air in case of air embolism
10. The best choice of preoperative medication for posterior fossa craniectomy for microvascular decompression of the trigeminal nerve is:
    a. reassurance alone
    b. reassurance and opioid-antihistaminic combination
    c. reassurance and opioid-anxiolytic combination
    d. reassurance and antianxiety medication

Chapter 18

1. The HIV is:
    a. subject to antigenic variation
    b. resistant to heat
    c. readily destroyed in banked blood
    d. most easily transmitted by heterosexual activity
2. AIDS cases associated with transfusion in the U.S. are:
    a. due to administration of pooled plasma
    b. less than 3% of the total number of cases
    c. the leading cause of death in hemophiliacs
    d. rarely reported
3. HIV seropositivity means that:
    a. The AIDS virus is definitely present.
    b. The patient has been exposed to the AIDS virus in the past 24 hours.
    c. The AIDS syndrome will develop in 1–2 years.
    d. Observation and follow-up testing are indicated.
4. The major characteristics of AIDS infection in the U.S. include:
    a. It is a disease of homosexuals.
    b. It is transmitted most commonly by heterosexual contact.
    c. Kaposi's sarcoma is only a late complication.
    d. The primary manifestations are neurologic.
5. The estimated number of persons infected with the AIDS virus in 1987 is:
    a. 2000
    b. 18,000
    c. 50,000
    d. 1,000,000
6. The pathology of AIDS infection includes:
    a. infection of the lymphocytes of the human T-cell subset
    b. conversion of DNA to RNA by transcriptase
    c. mutation of cells to a leukemic-type state
    d. immediate seropositivity
7. Which of the following is *false* regarding the HIV:
    a. It can persist in asymptomatic individuals for at least 2 years.
    b. It is a poor pathogen.
    c. Virus has been cultured from more than 85% of seropositive individuals.
    d. It can be isolated form 68% of homosexual men.

8. The main therapy of AIDS is:
    a. vaccination
    b. radiation
    c. interferon
    d. treatment of associated infections
9. In children, AIDS:
    a. develops usually within the second year of life
    b. may be associated with craniofacial dysmorphism
    c. is rarely fatal
    d. is seldom complicated by pneumonia
10. In observing precautions that should be adopted in caring for AIDS victims, the *most important* statement is:
    a. Used needles should always be recapped immediately, since accidental sticks can transmit HIV.
    b. Separate instruments should be identified and used only for AIDS cases.
    c. The patient is at greater risk from the physician than vice versa.
    d. Glasses must be worn as AIDS can be transmitted by droplets.

Chapter 19

1. The inducible porphyrias are inherited as:
    a. autosomal recessive diseases
    b. sex-linked diseases
    c. autosomal dominant diseases with variable expression
    d. autosomal dominant diseases
2. Acute crises of all the inducible porphyrias are associated with:
    a. blistering skin lesions
    b. urine that turns black on standing
    c. elevated levels of fecal ALA and PBG
    d. elevated levels of urinary ALA and PBG
3. A basic screening test for the inducible porphyrias is:
    a. the Watson–Schwartz test
    b. the Weil–Felix test
    c. the Shick test
    d. the Remington–Steele test
4. The hyponatremia noted during crises of the inducible porphyrias is caused by:
    a. a salt-losing nephropathy
    b. inappropriate antidiuretic hormone secretion
    c. inadequate dietary intake due to vomiting
    d. secondary hypoaldosteronism
5. Heme has all the following biochemical functions *except*:
    a. feedback inhibition of ALA-S activity
    b. induction of ALA-S synthesis
    c. electron transport
    d. drug metabolism
6. The definitive diagnosis of an inducible porphyria requires:
    a. documentation of an acute attack
    b. positive family history
    c. measurement of urinary and fecal heme precursors
    d. biopsy of a skin lesion

7. Pregnancy is associated with increased disease activity because:
   a. the gravid uterus exerts aortocaval compression
   b. it induces vomiting
   c. there are increased levels of peptide hormones
   d. there are increased levels of steroid hormones
8. The unique clinical features of an acute porphyric crisis allow one to distinguish AIP from:
   a. hereditary coproporphyria
   b. variegate porphyria
   c. porphyria cutanea tarda
   d. variegate coprotoporphyria
9. Large amounts of glucose exert a therapeutic effect in acute porphyric crisis via:
   a. massive caloric intake
   b. establishment of osmotic diuresis
   c. inhibiting synthesis of ALA-S
   d. storage of hepatic glycogen
10. The usual cause of death from porphyric crisis is:
   a. respiratory failure
   b. massive hemolysis
   c. renal failure
   d. dementia

Chapter 20

1. The annual incidence of venomous snakebites in the U.S. is:
   a. 300,000
   b. 30,000
   c. 8000
   d. 15
2. The snake responsible for 95% of snakebites in the U.S. is:
   a. elapid
   b. Old World viper
   c. boomslang
   d. crotalid
3. The most typical anatomic site for a snake bite is the:
   a. eyes
   b. extremities
   c. head
   d. chest
4. The venom component responsible for spontaneous oozing of blood from capillaries is:
   a. fibrinogenase
   b. prothrombinase
   c. hemorrhagin
   d. hyaluronidase
5. The cause of hypoxia in systemic crotalid envenomation is:
   a. histotoxic, analogous at the cellular level to cyanide toxicity
   b. pulmonary edema from loss of pulmonary capillary integrity

   c. respiratory arrest
   d. anemia

6. A first-aid measure in crotalid envenomation is:
   a. incision and suction
   b. lightly constricting band
   c. immersion in ice water bath for six hours
   d. a shot of brandy

7. The purpose of fasciotomy in crotalid limb envenomation is:
   a. to remove the venom
   b. to inspect the tissues
   c. to decrease the compartment pressure
   d. all of the above

8. The intracompartmental pressure above which a compartment syndrome becomes likely is:
   a. 3mmHg
   b. 30mmHg
   c. 60mmHg
   d. 90mmHg

9. Placebo-controlled double-blind studies have demonstrated the efficacy of which of the following for systemic envenomation?
   a. crotalid antivenom
   b. elapid antivenom
   c. anticholinesterases
   d. none of the above

10. Intracompartmental pressures are measured using:
   a. an epidural catheter
   b. an intraarterial catheter
   c. a wick catheter
   d. a blood flow technique

Chapter 21

1. Apnea during sleep occurs:
   a. during non-REM sleep
   b. during REM sleep
   c. during the first half of night sleep
   d. most often in young women

2. Obstructive sleep apnea is characterized by:
   a. obstruction of the pharynx
   b. obstruction at the larynx
   c. cessation of diaphragmatic activity
   d. the presence of nasal polyps from an early age

3. Patients with sleep apnea have:
   a. normal control of ventilation
   b. reduced sensitivity to $PaCO_2$
   c. increased sensitivity to $PaCO_2$
   d. respiratory alkalosis

4. Obstructive sleep apnea may be associated with:
   a. craniofacial abnormalities
   b. neuromuscular disorders

   c. Down's syndrome

   d. all of the above

5. The most serious cardiovascular abnormality associated with sleep apnea is the development of:

   a. hypertension

   b. malignant ventricular arrhythmias

   c. sinus bradycardia

   d. all of the above

6. A patient scheduled for uvulopalatopharyngoplasty should:

   a. be sedated to relieve anxiety

   b. pose no problems to establishment of the airway

   c. require only routine postoperative care

   d. have adequacy of ventilation assessed intra- and postoperatively by measurement of arterial blood gases

7. Opioids and sedatives:

   a. are well tolerated by patients with sleep apnea once airway obstruction has been corrected

   b. may cause prolonged apnea in patients with sleep apnea irrespective of the etiology

   c. should be used as the primary agent to maintain anesthesia

   d. are not associated with airway obstruction in a semi-awake patient

8. Patients with craniofacial anomalies and obstructive sleep apnea:

   a. may be extremely difficult to intubate

   b. should have intravenous induction followed by a short-acting muscle relaxant whenever possible

   c. rarely require the use of a fiberoptic bronchoscope to facilitate intubation

   d. can easily be managed with ketamine

9. Patients with mixed sleep apnea are characterized by:

   a. marked obesity

   b. somnolence during the day

   c. hypoventilation and hypoxia

   d. all of the above

10. Tracheoplasty:

   a. may be required in patients whose obstructive episodes are not resolved by uvulopalatopharyngoplasty

   b. may be required in patients with central sleep apnea to allow for ventilation during sleep

   c. may be closed permanently after reestablishment of normal ventilatory control following relief of the obstruction

   d. all the above

Chapter 22

1. Mitral valve prolapse occurs:

   a. predominately in young women

   b. predominately in young men

   c. more frequently in older women than older men

   d. equally in women of all ages

2. The structural abnormalities associated ith MVP include:

   a. redundant mitral valve

    b. elongated chordae tendinae
    c. both
    d. neither

3. Conditions associated with MVP are:
    a. idiopathic hypertrophic subaortic stenosis
    b. Marfan's syndrome
    c. cardiomyopathy
    d. all of the above

4. Prolapse of the redundant mitral valve leaflet occurs during:
    a. early systole
    b. mid- to late systole
    c. early diastole
    d. mid- to late diastole

5. Factors that accentuate the degree of prolapse include:
    a. increased contractility
    b. decreased preload and afterload
    c. increased heart rate
    d. all of the above

6. Symptoms of MVP include:
    a. chest pain and palpitations
    b. increased exercise tolerance
    c. ventricular arrhythmias
    d. pansystolic click

7. The most beneficial effect of propranolol for symptomatic MVP is:
    a. the antiarrhythmic effect
    b. the hypotensive effect
    c. the increase in end-diastolic and systolic volumes
    d. all of the above

8. The anesthetic technique for MVP patients should not include drugs that:
    a. decrease myocardial contractility
    b. increase heart rate
    c. cause volume loading and decreased SVR
    d. have a negative chronotropic effect

9. Because of its myocardial depressant effect, the anesthetic agent of choice in patients with MVP is:
    a. isoflurane
    b. halothane
    c. morphine
    d. ketamine

10. The ventilatory pattern under anesthesia for patients with MVP should be one of:
    a. slow expiratory flow
    b. decreased I:E ratio
    c. slow inspiratory flow
    d. none of the above

Chapter 23

1. According to the U.S. Census Bureau, by the year 2000 persons over the age of 65 will comprise what percent of the general population?

a. 2%
b. 5%
c. 12.5%
d. 21.4%
2. Postoperative mortality in the elderly when compared to younger patients is:
   a. decreased
   b. increased
   c. about the same
   d. dependent on the surgery
3. The elderly patient is at greater risk for pulmonary aspiration because:
   a. laryngeal reflexes are impaired
   b. pharyngeal reflexes are impaired
   c. gastric emptying is delayed
   d. all of the above
4. Effects of the aging process on serum proteins are:
   a. increase in quantity
   b. decreased binding ability
   c. limited to albumin
   d. all of the above
5. Pulmonary changes with respect to aging include all of the following *except*:
   a. decreased closing capacity
   b. increased FRC/TLC
   c. decreased FEV_1 of 20–30cc/year
   d. decreased VC of 5–10cc/year
6. The most commonly observed cardiac arrhythmias in the elderly are:
   a. supraventricular arrhythmias
   b. ventricular arrhythmias
   c. sick sinus syndrome
   d. atrial fibrillation
7. Drug interactions in the elderly are:
   a. less commonly seen because the older person is used to more drugs
   b. equal in incidence to those seen in younger persons
   c. more commonly observed
   d. the most common cause of perioperative mortality
8. The antimuscarinic agent of choice for use with a neuromuscular reversal agent in the elderly patient is:
   a. atropine
   b. glycopyrrolate
   c. scopolamine
   d. edrophonium
9. The ventilatory response in persons over age 70 years to hypoxia and hypercapnia is:
   a. increased
   b. decreased
   c. the same as in younger persons
   d. has no bearing on anesthetic management
10. Preoperative assessment of the elderly patient must include:
   a. thorough history and physical exam
   b. investigation of past medical records when available

  c. knowledge of physiologic changes in the elderly
  d. all of the above

Chapter 24

1. Choose the correct statement:
   a. Hemophilia A is an autosomal recessive trait that leads to excessive bleeding.
   b. Hemophilia B is due to Factor VIII deficiency.
   c. The liver manufactures all coagulation factors except Factor VII.
   d. Hemophiliacs may require Factor VIII transfusions every 8–12 hours postoperatively, for several weeks.
2. The following statement is true regarding platelets:
   a. Estrogens can cause decreased platelet production.
   b. Spontaneous bleeding is likely with platelet counts below $50,000/mm^3$.
   c. The prothrombin time is prolonged if the platelet count is below $30,000/mm^3$.
   d. Rebleeding after initial hemostasis is suggestive of severe thrombocytopenia.
3. Parenteral Vitamin K would *not* be expected to correct coagulation factor deficiencies secondary to:
   a. antibiotic use
   b. obstructive jaundice
   c. cirrhosis
   d. intestinal malabsorption
4. Vitamin K-dependent factors include all of the following, *except*:
   a. Factor II
   b. Factor V
   c. Factor VII
   d. Factor X
5. The prothrombin time does not depend on:
   a. Factor V
   b. Factor VII
   c. Factor VIII
   d. Factor X
6. Neither the prothrombin time nor the partial thromboplastin time evaluates:
   a. Factor II
   b. Factor VII
   c. Factor X
   d. Factor XIII
7. A prolonged bleeding time can be caused by:
   a. decreased platelets
   b. abnormal platelet function
   c. intrinsic vascular defect
   d. all of the above
8. The anticoagulant activity of heparin depends on interaction with:
   a. Factor V
   b. antithrombin III

   c. fibrin
   d. complement
9. Decreased platelet count is commonly seen in:
   a. Hodgkin's lymphoma
   b. moderate hemorrhage
   c. iron deficiency
   d. hypersplenism
10. Laboratory abnormalities in DIC include all of the following, *except*:
   a. elevated PT
   b. decreased platelet count
   c. decreased fibrin split products
   d. elevated thrombin time

Chapter 25

1. The main goal in the anesthetic management of the patient with a cerebral aneurysm is:
   a. avoidance of mean arterial pressure below 50mmHg
   b. stabilization of cerebral perfusion pressure
   c. maintenance of systolic pressure to preanesthetic levels
   d. avoidance of decreases in intracranial pressure
2. An increased incidence of ruptured aneurysms has been associated with:
   a. smoking
   b. black race
   c. hypertension
   d. all of the above
3. Symptoms and signs of ruptured aneurysms include all of the following *except*:
   a. headache
   b. nausea and vomiting
   c. stiff neck
   d. decreased blood sugar
4. Epsilon aminocaproic acid administration is associated with all of the following *except*:
   a. hydrocephalus
   b. bradycardia
   c. ST-segment and T-wave abnormalities
   d. hyperglycemia
5. Nimodipine:
   a. does not easily cross the blood-brain barrier
   b. has a dilatory effect on pial arterial vessels
   c. affects cerebral and systemic vessels equally
   d. does not produce vasodilatation when topically applied
6. The mortality after rupture of an aneurysm is:
   a. 85% after the first rebleed
   b. 43% immediately following rupture
   c. 96% following the first rebleed within one year, with conservative management
   d. none of the above

7. Complications of ruptured aneurysms include:
   a. hydrocephalus
   b. hyponatremia
   c. seizures
   d. all of the above
8. ECG changes most often associated with ruptured aneurysms are:
   a. shortened QT-interval and peaked T-waves
   b. prolonged QT-interval, T-wave inversion and prominent U-waves
   c. atrial fibrillation
   d. bradycardia
9. The best prognostic indicator of good outcome after ruptured aneurysm is:
   a. normal or decreased intracranial pressure
   b. no demonstrable vasospasm on x-ray
   c. lack of neurologic deficits preoperatively
   d. no evidence of amnesia
10. Complications of sodium nitroprusside-induced hypotension include:
   a. rebound hypertension
   b. platelet abnormalities
   c. tachyphylaxis
   d. all of the above

Chapter 26

1. Scoliosis is transmitted to offspring as:
   a. an autosomal recessive trait
   b. a sex-linked trait
   c. an autosomal dominant gene with incomplete penetrance
   d. an unknown pattern of inheritance
2. The incidence of scoliosis is:
   a. more common in males than females
   b. averages 50 cases/1000 population
   c. very difficult to assess
   d. more common in females than males in a ratio of 5:1
3. The most common form of scoliosis is:
   a. congenital
   b. idiopathic
   c. acquired
   d. traumatic
4. All of the following statements concerning scoliosis are true *except*:
   a. structural curves are usually the largest and most severe curves
   b. patients with congenital heart disease have an increased incidence of scoliosis
   c. structural scoliosis is characterized by correction of the curve with bending
   d. the Cobb method is a common method for measuring the curve
5. In the treatment of scoliosis:
   a. Harrington rod manipulation is usually the first-line treatment
   b. idiopathic scoliosis is usually diagnosed before the curve is very noticeable
   c. the Milwaukee brace is used primarily to prevent the curve from increasing
   d. the Luque method requires postoperative plaster casting

6. Common pulmonary problems associated with scoliosis include:
   a. obstructive respiratory pattern
   b. restrictive respiratory pattern
   c. increased TLC, FRC, and VC
   d. hyperventilation of alveoli
7. All of the following statements are true *except*:
   a. prolonged hypoxemia and increased pulmonary vascular resistance lead to cor pulmonale
   b. in patients with pulmonary hypertension, $PaO_2 > 70$mmHg returns pulmonary artery pressure to within normal levels
   c. hypoxia, hypercarbia, and acidosis tend to increase right ventricular afterload
   d. right ventricular afterload and respiratory failure with hypoxia are the major factors regulating cardiac response to exercise
8. All of the following statements about spinal cord monitoring are true *except*:
   a. SSEPs are sensitive indicators of hypoxia and hypotension
   b. the most common lead monitored during Harrington rod manipulation is the median nerve
   c. the wake-up test monitors general motor function to extremities
   d. if changes in SSEPs are discovered, rapid reversal of spinal manipulation may prevent permanent spinal cord damage
9. Blood replacement by autologous blood transfusion includes all of the following methods *except*:
   a. hemodilution
   b. preoperative red blood cell harvesting
   c. specific type and cross-match transfusion
   d. cell saver transfusion
10. Pulmonary hypertension and right ventricular function can be assessed using:
   a. echocardiography
   b. ECG
   c. chest x-ray and pulmonary artery size
   d. all of the above

Answers to Self-Assessment Questions

Chapter 1	Chapter 2	Chapter 3	Chapter 4
1. d	1. b	1. a	1. b
2. b	2. c	2. d	2. a
3. c	3. d	3. a	3. c
4. b	4. d	4. a	4. b
5. a	5. c	5. c	5. c
6. b	6. d	6. d	6. a
7. c	7. d	7. a	7. c
8. d	8. b	8. c	8. a
9. c	9. c	9. d	9. d
10. b	10. d	10. a	10. d

Chapter 5	Chapter 6	Chapter 7	Chapter 8
1. d	1. d	1. a	1. c
2. a	2. c	2. c	2. b
3. b	3. b	3. c	3. d
4. d	4. d	4. a	4. a
5. a	5. b	5. c	5. d
6. d	6. a	6. d	6. b
7. d	7. b	7. d	7. a
8. b	8. b	8. c	8. c
9. a	9. d	9. d	9. c
10. d	10. d	10. b	10. a

Chapter 9	Chapter 10	Chapter 11	Chapter 12
1. b	1. b	1. d	1. b
2. c	2. c	2. a	2. d
3. c	3. c	3. d	3. b
4. b	4. a	4. d	4. a
5. c	5. b	5. c	5. d
6. b	6. c	6. b	6. d
7. b	7. d	7. c	7. a
8. c	8. b	8. b	8. b
9. c	9. c	9. c	9. c
10. b	10. d	10. d	10. c

Chapter 13	Chapter 14	Chapter 15	Chapter 16
1. d	1. c	1. c	1. b
2. b	2. b	2. d	2. d
3. b	3. c	3. b	3. c
4. d	4. a	4. d	4. c
5. b	5. d	5. d	5. b
6. a	6. d	6. c	6. d
7. c	7. a	7. d	7. d
8. d	8. c	8. d	8. b
9. d	9. d	9. d	9. b
10. c	10. c	10. d	10. b

Chapter 17	Chapter 18	Chapter 19	Chapter 20
1. b	1. a	1. c	1. c
2. c	2. b	2. d	2. d
3. d	3. d	3. a	3. b
4. a	4. a	4. b	4. c
5. c	5. d	5. b	5. b
6. c	6. a	6. c	6. b
7. c	7. d	7. d	7. c
8. b	8. d	8. d	8. b
9. c	9. b	9. c	9. d
10. d	10. c	10. a	10. c

Chapter 21	Chapter 22	Chapter 23	Chapter 24
1. b	1. a	1. c	1. d
2. a	2. c	2. b	2. a
3. b	3. d	3. d	3. c
4. d	4. b	4. b	4. b
5. b	5. d	5. d	5. c
6. d	6. a	6. b	6. d
7. b	7. c	7. c	7. d
8. a	8. b	8. b	8. b
9. d	9. b	9. b	9. d
10. d	10. c	10. d	10. c

Chapter 25	Chapter 26
1. b	1. c
2. a	2. d
3. d	3. b
4. d	4. c
5. b	5. c
6. b	6. b
7. d	7. b
8. b	8. b
9. c	9. c
10. d	10. d

Index